# CO-TRANSMISSION

# CO-TRANSMISSION

## Proceedings of a Symposium held at Oxford during the 50th Anniversary Meeting of the British Pharmacological Society

*Edited by*

## A. C. CUELLO
*University Department of Pharmacology,*
*Oxford*

*First published 1982 by*
**THE MACMILLAN PRESS LTD**
*London and Basingstoke*
*Associated companies in Delhi Dublin*
*Hong Kong Johannesburg Lagos Melbourne*
*New York Singapore and Tokyo*

*Typeset by Reproduction Drawings Ltd., Sutton, Surrey.*

Printed in Great Britain by

Unwin Brothers Limited
The Gresham Press, Old Woking, Surrey

ISBN 0 333 32592 3

# Contents

# Foreword

It is a pleasure to be asked to write a foreword to this volume, based on the symposium at the 50th Anniversary meeting of the British Pharmacological Society at Oxford, that was brought into being by the imagination and energy of my colleague, Claudio Cuello. It is particularly stimulating for one brought up scientifically in Dale's old laboratory, who remembers the period when neuro-transmission by one transmitter, let alone several, was not accepted and who was present when J. C. Eccles, at a Royal Society meeting, announced his conversion. Almost immediately, in the context of the intense interest in central transmission that Eccles had aroused, the idea that one neurone could release both an inhibitory and an excitatory transmitter was canvassed, but found to be unnecessary with the recognition of interpolated inhibitory interneurones. From then on the issue was not of multiple transmitters, but of being able to identify *any* transmitter as a valid candidate for each of the various distinguishable central synaptic mechanisms – a battle that is still not finished. There have been many subsequent additions to our knowledge: the recognition of presynaptic inhibitory processes, allowing a modulation of postsynaptic effect through the control by the transmitter from one nerve terminal of the transmitter output from a second – a biochemically more economical process than the two transmitters fighting it out postsynaptically; the extension of this to negative feedback by a transmitter onto its own terminals; the possibilities of control of receptor function ('up' and 'down' regulation) according to exposure to transmitter. Together with the delicate central control of response through the frequency of discharge down the nerve fibres, mediated by reflexes drawing on all the subtle connectivity of the central nervous system, the available mechanisms seemed to offer ample scope to allow physiological function to be accurately adjusted to any physiological need. A general conceptual requirement for the additional control mechanisms offered by co-transmission could hardly be said to have existed; and if there has been resistance to the idea, perhaps it was more on grounds of economy of hypothesis than anything else.

Thus it seems to me not only wrong when 'Dale's principle' is cited in the terms of 'one neurone-one transmitter', as though an established functional co-transmission would falsify some rule enunciated by him, but also to miss one of his creative insights. If one goes back to what he wrote in the Nothnagel lecture, or to his talks at the Royal Society and later to the students of St. Andrews in 1952, the issue is a different one. He brought the new knowledge about cholinergic and

vii

adrenergic transmission into relation with old work on cross-innervation, pointing out how the latter could now be 'summarized by stating that any cholinergic fibre will functionally replace any other cholinergic fibre, and that any adrenergic fibre will replace any adrenergic fibre, but that neither can assume the function of the other'. These phenomena appeared 'to indicate that the nature of the chemical function, whether cholinergic or adrenergic, is characteristic for each particular neurone and unchangeable'. To this he added the past work on antidromic vasodilatation, brought again into prominence by Sir Thomas Lewis's demonstration that the 'flare' evoked by histamine in skin was due to an axone reflex in sensory nerves. Was it possible that discovery and identification of a chemical transmitter of axon-reflex vasodilatation would provide a clue to the central transmission process? He was suggesting not a particular number of transmitters, but what might be called a 'principle of biochemical consistency' within a neurone, that might bring with it the great prize of a way to identify the transmitter at the first sensory synapse. Dr W. Feldberg has reminded me of Dale's letter to him (recently published in Notes and Records of the Royal Society **30** 231, 1976) written during the preparation of the Nothnagel lecture, which is worth transcribing.

4th September, 1934

My dear Feldberg,

I was very glad to hear from you, and to hear that you and
your family are enjoying Cornwall. Reading between the lines,
I am sorry to get the impression that you are not having the
best of weather. As a matter of fact, however, the English
coast and country look at their best and most characteristic
when the fine weather is broken by rainstorms.

I am very grateful to you for your trouble, and the progress
which you are making with my Nothnagel Lecture. If you
would like to send me what you have already done, by post, I
should get it just in time to take with me to America; and I
might use the return journey to familiarise myself with it a
little, and mark any points for discussion. However, that is a
matter which I would gladly leave entirely to your judgment.
If you would prefer to retain the whole of the MS until your
translation is completed, by all means do so. You might then,
when you return, consult Mrs. Cutts about the possibility of
getting some of it, at least, into typescript before I return.

There is one point which I propose to add at the end, even
if it involves sacrificing some earlier passages. All the evidence
seems to point to chemical function being a characteristic of
nerve fibre, or, perhaps, of the cell from which it originates. A

fibre arising from a sympathetic ganglion cell appears to be adrenergic, and to be incapable of changing its function. Thinking on those lines, it seems to me that there is a good deal of probability that chemical transmission of antidromic vasodilatation at the *peripheral* end of a sensory neurone might be expected to use the same susbtance as transmission of a sensory impulse to a motor cell at a central synapse. It is, of course, merely a guess, but it is a point of some interest, I think and one worth mentioning in a lecture. It would be extremely interesting if identification of the chemical transmitter for antidromic vasodilatation should lead directly to the problem of chemical transmission in the central nervous system. However, I can think what is appropriate to say on that point, if anything, when I return from America. I am glad you are taking a full holiday, and getting fit for a good winter's work.

Yours very sincerely,
H. H. Dale


Today, Sir Henry might well demand evidence as cogent as that which he and his colleagues put forward for cholinergic transmission, before accepting cotransmission; yet one cannot believe he would object in principle. Indeed, if one reads another letter to Feldberg in 1962 in the same collection, where he puzzles over the functional vasodilatation of the salivary gland, it seems more likely that he would have been delighted at the new evidence about VIP and at the combination of histochemical and physiological experiment behind it.

Yet perhaps he would also come back to the question, with all the new evidence this volume presents, of the 'characteristic chemical function' of a neurone. Is it possible that it is less unchangeable than he suggested and that the selective repression of the genetic capacity to synthesize all known and unknown transmitters in each cell is not always complete, or immutable? Considering the present knowledge of the ultrastructure of the neurone, is it possible that differential release might indeed take place, between (say) release from the dendrites, with short supply lines, compared with release at nerve terminals at the end of a long axone? Could re-innervation experiments help to disentangle the biochemically consistent from the biochemically mutable functions of the neurone? How does it come about that the most commonly chosen partners in the neurochemical dance seem to be adrenaline and the enkephalins?

Perhaps it is not unfitting to think of him reading and discussing this volume, unruffled by some mentions of his name, as searching as ever in his questioning of the experimenters, but as eager as they to see where the new work would lead.

W. D. M. Paton

ix

# Preface

The committee organising the celebratory meeting of the 50th Anniversary of the foundation of the British Pharmacological Society considered it appropriate to include a main symposium on an emerging subject in pharmacology. **Cotransmission** could not be a more appropriate problem, as the possible existence of multiple transmitters in single neurones can profoundly change our understanding of the pharmacology of central and peripheral nervous systems. This book represents a collection of papers from distinguished colleagues who have made great contributions to the development of this idea, many of whom have strong links with the Society. Some of the contributions were presented within the frame of the meeting, while others were invited papers.

I am most grateful to the authors for their co-operation towards the speedy publication of this volume and for accepting minor editorial changes. I would also like to acknowledge the enthusiastic co-operation received from Macmillan Press for both the meeting and the publication of this book. In this connection, I would particularly like to acknowledge the personal interest of Mr Alexander Macmillan on the success of the meeting and to thank Dr Sharrock and Mr Harry Holt for their enthusiastic contribution to the efficient production of the book. The secretarial assistance of Ella Iles was invaluable, dealing with correspondence, editing references and indexing.

From Oxford I would like to express my gratitude to Professor Sir William D. M. Paton and Dr Richard Green for their direct involvement in the materialisation of the Symposium, and The Rector and Bursar of Lincoln College for their help in lodging our guests and for offering a home for social events. The celebration of the 50th Anniversary of the Society and the Co-transmission symposium at Lincoln College were particularly pleasant events, as we were distinguished by the presence of honorary members of the Society such as Professors Blaschko, Bülbring, Feldberg, Kosterlitz, Paton and Vogt, together with many eminent colleagues.

Finally, I would also like to thank my wife, Martha, for her support in this endeavour.

A.C.C.

# 1

# Coexistence of traditional neurotransmitters with peptides in the mammalian brain: 5-hydroxytryptamine and substance P in the raphe and γ-aminobutyric acid and motilin in the cerebellum

Victoria Chan-Palay (Department of Neurobiology, The Harvard Medical School, Boston, Massachusetts 02115, USA)

## INTRODUCTION

This chapter will deal with two examples of the coexistence of neuroactive substances in single neurones of the mammalian central nervous system: first, the 5-hydroxytryptamine (5-HT; serotonin)-containing neurone in the raphe and other brain stem nuclei that have coexistent substance P; second, the γ-aminobutyric acid (GABA)-containing Purkinje neurones of the cerebellum which have coexistent motilin.

In the context to be discussed here, coexistence denotes a situation in which more than one neuroactive substance can be localised by cytochemical means in an individual neurone. Usually this has meant the combination of a traditional neurotransmitter, such as acetylcholine (ACh) or noradrenaline (NA) or an amino acid, together with a peptide, such as substance P or enkephalin. This definition, however, does not exclude the presence of more than one traditional neurotransmitter in the same cell or more than one neuroactive substance, such as peptides. The issue of the presence of multiple neuroactive substances in neurones is not

1

limited to the mammalian central nervous system (CNS); the peripheral nervous system of vertebrates and identified neurones in a number of invertebrates also have examples of this phenomenon (Pearse, 1969; Burnstock, 1976; Osborne, 1979; see also Osborne, chapter 9), but for the sake of brevity they will not be reviewed here.

True "coexistence" of neuroactive substances in single neurones as defined here must be distinguished from the looser definitions used by many investigators to denote the simultaneous existence of mutliple neuroactive substances in different nerve cells in a particular geographical area of the brain. This can be illustrated by specific examples. Single 5-HT neurones in the medulla and raphe nuclei have also been shown to contain substance P (Chan-Palay *et al.*, 1978; Chan-Palay, 1979; Hökfelt *et al.*, 1978). Purkinje cells in the cerebellum have been found to contain motilin and glutamic acid decarboxylase (Chan-Palay *et al.*, 1981). However, enkephalin, substance P and glutamic acid decarboxylase immunoreactivity have been demonstrated in separate cell types in the neostriatum (Panula *et al.*, 1980); somatostatin and substance P have been distinguished in separate cell groups in primary afferent neurones (Hökfelt *et al.*, 1976); and 5-HT, tyrosine hydroxylase, and enkephalin exist simultaneously in separate cells elsewhere in the rat CNS (Beaudet *et al.*, 1980). As it is clear that one geographical area of nucleus in the brain consists of many nerve cells which may be heterogeneous, it would be expected that these neurones could utilise a number of different chemicals in neural communication. Thus, the simultaneous existence of a number of neuroactive compounds in a nerve cell group is not surprising. The phenomenon of true coexistence, of multiple neuroactive substances in a single cell is, however, more interesting and calls for careful investigation of the parameters of such coexistence, its function, the cytological substrates that allow for orderly synthesis, transport and release of the compounds, and, of course, its significance in the complexity of nerve circuits.

## 5-HT/SUBSTANCE P NEURONES

Since the first biochemical demonstration of 5-HT in the CNS (Twarog and Page, 1953) and the subsequent fluorimetric confirmation of its existence (Bogdansky *et al.*, 1956), the major thrust of investigations concerning this important neurotransmitter has depended upon the development of methods for localising it in nerve cells. The formaldehyde-induced fluorescence method has permitted the initial mapping of some 5-HT cells and their terminals by means of the evanescent fluorescence of their endogenous 5-HT in fragile preparations (Dahlström and Fuxe, 1964). Procedures to improve this basic fluorescence approach have been attempted (Bjorkund *et al.*, 1972), along with selective destruction of indole-amine neurones by 5,6-dihydroxytryptamine (5,6-DHT) (Fuxe and Jonsson, 1967), 5,7-dihydroxytryptamine (5,7-DHT) (Baumgarten and Lachenmeyer, 1972) and other pharmacological manipulations to locate 5-HT cells, such as the use of *p*-chloroamphetamine (Massari *et al.*, 1978).

The 1970s witnessed the development of a host of more specific, direct and permanent methods for the localisation of 5-HT, based upon the biochemistry of 5-HT synthesis and the selective uptake of exogenous 5-HT by these neurones combined with sophisticated morphological tools for the localisation of these processes. First, the enzyme tryptophan hydroxylase, which is responsible for conversion of tryptophan to 5-hydroxytryptophan (5-HTP) before the synthesis of 5-HT, was isolated and characterised. Polyclonal antibodies raised against this enzyme were used for immunocytochemical localisation of some 5-HT cells and their processes (Joh *et al.*, 1975; Pickel *et al.*, 1976). Unfortunately, subsequent deterioration of the antibody has caused this important 5-HT marking method to fall into disuse. Concurrently, however, autoradiography was initiated to detect 5-HT processes after local injection of [$^3$H]-5-HT (Bloom *et al.*, 1972*b*). This approach was perfected by the introduction of intraventricular infusions of [$^3$H]-5-HT of low molarity, which permitted mapping of the entire brain in permanent autoradiograms for study at light and electron microscope levels (Chan-Palay, 1975; 1976; 1977*a,b*; 1978*a*) or allowed the analysis of single discrete areas of the brain (Beaudet and Descaries, 1979; Gershon, 1981) (see figure 1.1*a*). Subsequent developments in immunocytochemistry have resulted in the mapping of 5-HT-like immunoreactivity in the brain, in cells and terminals, with antibodies directed against 5-HT itself (Steinbush, 1981; Consolazione *et al.*, 1981) (see figure 1.1*b*).

The possibility that 5-HT and a peptide, substance P, might coexist began to be suspected in the mid-1970s. In the course of our studies with the development and application of intraventricular infusion methods for [$^3$H]-5-HT and autoradiography for mapping 5-HT cells and fibre systems in the brain (Chan-Palay, 1975; 1976; 1977*a,b*; 1978), we were also involved with immunocytochemical demonstrations of substance P-containing cells. Using the polyclonal antibodies against substance P conjugated to thyroglobulin (produced by Dr S. Leeman at Harvard Medical School), we applied (Chan-Palay and Palay, 1977*a,b*) the existing methods of immunocytochemistry at the light and electron microscope levels. With autoradiography for 5-HT cells and immunocytochemistry for substance P, we observed that 5-HT and substance P (a) exist separately in discrete cell and fibre types in some areas of the brain, for example, the paratrigeminal nuclei (Chan-Palay, 1978*b,c*) and the raphe nuclei; and (b) coexist in individual 5-HT/substance P neurones and processes, for example, in the neurones surrounding the exit of the hypoglossal nerves (Chan-Palay *et al.*, 1978). To prove conclusively that 5-HT and substance P coexist in single neurones, we have used the formaldehyde-induced fluorescence method on selected 5-HT cells, documented the 5-HT nature of each neurone by microspectrofluorimetry, and then processed the same cells with the peroxidase-antiperoxidase immunocytochemical method to show that these cells contained substance P-like immunoreactivity (Chan-Palay *et al.*, 1978). These studies showed that a traditional transmitter could coexist with a peptide in the CNS. Confirmation of these results appeared later in the same year (Hökfelt *et al.*, 1978), when positive reactions for substance

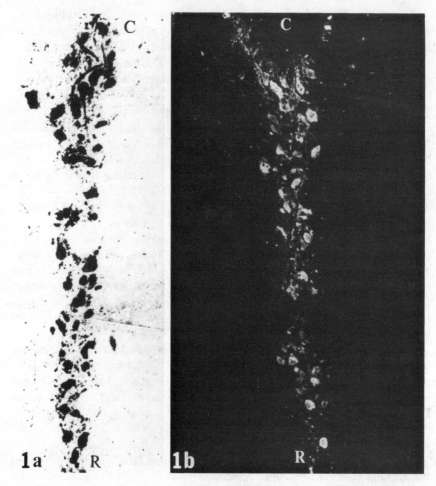

Figure 1.1  5-HT neurones and their axonal and dendritic processes in the rat raphe pallidus demonstrated (*a*) by autoradiography after intraventricular infusions of [³H]-5-HT and (*b*) by immunofluorescence using anti-5-HT antibody and a fluorescein isothiocyanate conjugate. The rostral (R) and caudal (C) aspects of the brain are indicated.

P and for 5-HT immunoreactivities were demonstrated using the indirect fluorescence method (Coons, 1958) on separate or alternative sections through cells in the raphe. Both approaches, however, were not suitable for further analysis by electron microscopy.

The next task was obvious. We needed to develop methods to demonstrate 5-HT and substance P in permanent single preparations suitable for ultrastructural analysis. Efforts in this direction advanced after two major developments: first, use of monoclonal antibodies against substance P (Köhler and Milstein, 1975; Cuello *et al.*, 1979; 1981), which are single molecular species with well defined specificity; and second, the direct labeling of substance P neurones by microinjection of monoclonal anti-substance P antibodies *in vivo*, combined with the infusion of [³H]-5-HT and subsequent autoradiography (Chan-Palay, 1979*b*). This method provided reliable labeling of single neurones and their processes in the raphe pallidus nucleus with demonstrable 5-HT and substance P in permanent preparations on single sections of the same cells or processes (Chan-Palay, 1979*b*) (see figure 1.2*a,b* and *c*).

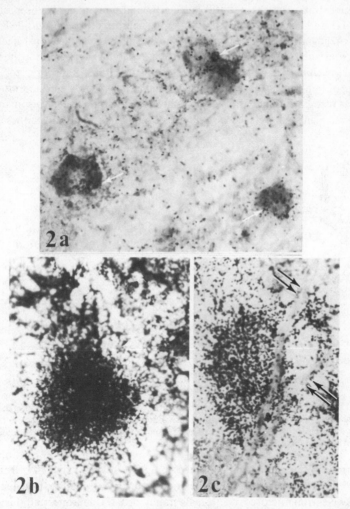

Figure 1.2 Double label preparations using immunocytochemistry with monoclonal anti-substance P antibody and [³H]-5-HT uptake autoradiography to demonstrate (*a*) three small neurones containing only immunoreactivity to antisubstance P, (*b*) a larger neurone with both substance P immunoreactivity and silver grains from [³H]-5-HT uptake, and (*c*) a neurone with only silver grains from [³H]-5-HT uptake innervated by two substance P immunoreactive axons (arrows). Rat raphe pallidus nucleus after *in vivo* injections of [³H]-5-HT and monoclonal anti-substance P antibodies, followed by peroxidase immunocytochemistry and autoradiography.

Two other examples of the possible coexistence of 5-HT with a peptide have
been suggested in the literature. The nucleus raphe dorsalis has been demonstrated
to have 5-HT neurones (Dahlström and Fuxe, 1964; Chan Palay, 1977*a*; Steinbusch,
1981; Consolazione and Cuello, 1982) as well as separate GABA-containing cells
(Gamrani *et al.*, 1979). More recently it has been suggested (Nanopoulos *et al.*,
1981) that both substances may coexist in some cells, but a rigorous experimental demonstration of these is still lacking. In addition, it has also been suggested
that 5-HT and enkephalin may exist in raphe neurones (Glazer *et al.*, 1981).

The recognition that a single neurone can contain a traditional neurotransmitter and another neuroactive substance necessitates the search for the internal
cellular machinery that can facilitate the manufacture, transport, storage, and
release of multiple substances and the membrane-related mechanisms for the
specific recognition and the differentiation of multiple mediators at receptors
on the recipient cell surface (see figure 1.3). Especially significant in these studies

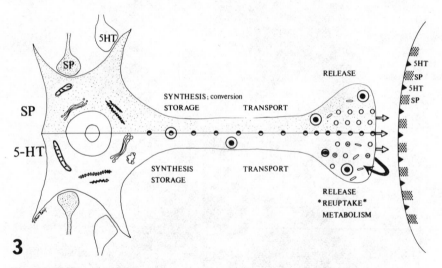

**3**

Figure 1.3  Schematic diagram of a neurone with 5-HT and substance P (SP) coexisting in
its soma and processes. Internal cellular machinery to facilitate the synthesis, transport,
storage and release of peptide and amine transmitter, as well as the separate mechanisms
required for re-uptake and metabolism of the amine, are depicted.

is the recognition that a potent, specific uptake system exists for serotonin in
these cells and that none has yet been defined for the peptide. Detailed studies
exist by electron microscope autoradiography of 5-HT neurones and their axonal
projections in the mammalian brain, in locations as different as the cerebellum
(Chan-Palay, 1975; 1977*a,b*) (figure 1.4), the supraependymal plexus (Chan-
Palay, 1976) (figure 1.5), the locus coeruleus (Mouren-Mathieu *et al.*, 1976;
Pickel *et al.*, 1976), the cerebral cortex (Descarries *et al.*, 1975), the reticular
paragigantocellularis lateralis nucleus (Chan-Palay, 1978*b*; Andrezik and Chan-
Palay, 1977), and the paratrigeminal nucleus (Chan-Palay, 1978*b,c*). These

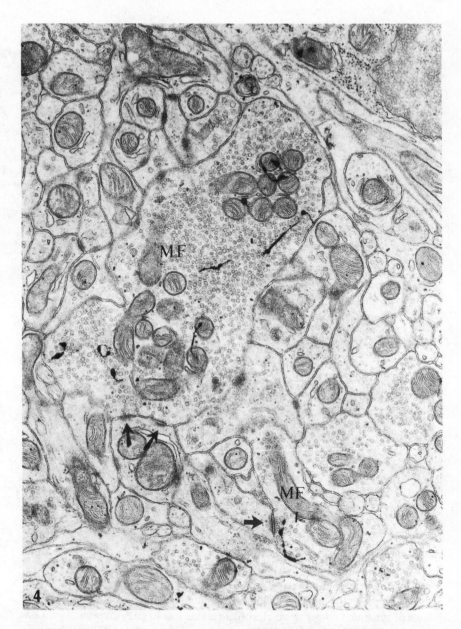

Figure 1.4 Cerebellar mossy fibre rosette specifically labelled by silver grains from [³H]-5-HT uptake and electron microscope autoradiography. Portions of the labelled rosette (MF) with obvious synaptic junctions (arrows) made upon unlabelled granule cell dendrites. Rat cerebellar cortex, paraflocculus (×30,000).

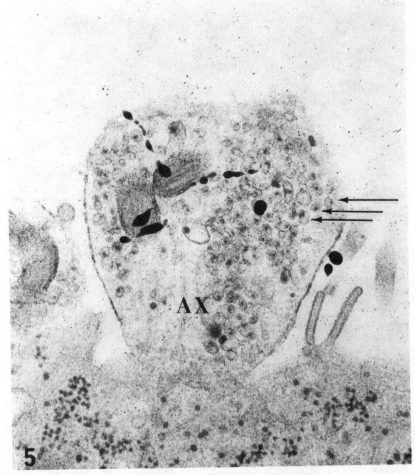

Figure 1.5 Supraependymal axon from the fourth ventricle labelled by silver grains from [³H]-5-HT uptake and electron microscope autoradiography (×68,000).

studies show that there is no consensus on a single constellation of ultrastructural features of the axoplasm that differentiate 5-HT axons from those of other neurones. In fact, identified 5-HT axons are different from one another in one specific region of the brain and they may contain a number of different populations of synaptic vesicles when classified carefully as to size, shape, and content (Chan-Palay, 1977*b*) (figure 1.6). There is a remarkable variety of vesicle populations: small pleomorphic, clear or granular, large granular, large granular alveolate, and small tubular profiles. The non-synaptic boutons are generally associated with the unusual small tubular profiles. The synaptic boutons have a large number of different synaptic vesicle morphologies (see figure 1.6). Regardless of the

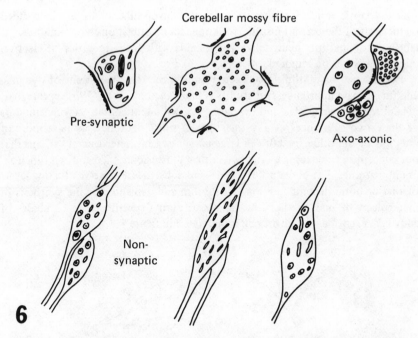

Figure 1.6  Six types of axon terminals labelled by autoradiography after intraventricular infusions of [$^3$H]-5-HT. Sizes and shapes of axonal varicosities and their synaptic vesicles are diagrammed. Each axonal variety has a different internal synaptic vesicle content, style of synaptic junctional complex, and incidence of a morphologically identifiable synaptic junction. There are synaptic 5-HT axons (upper three examples) and non-synaptic 5-HT axons (lower three examples).

presence or absence of the small vesicles or their form, all these axons contain large granular vesicles (LGVs). There can be exclusively LGVs or there may be a small number of smaller vesicles scattered in the axoplasm. Seemingly, LGVs may be the only consistent feature in all 5-HT axons; however, even they vary in morphology, size and content from one 5-HT axon to another. Can it be presumed that all these vesicular forms have something to do with 5-HT storage, transport, release and uptake? Or conversely, is this heterogeneity in synaptic vesicle morphology an expression of the multiplicity of their neurotransmitter content?

A review of the studies of substance P-containing axons identified by positive immunoreactivity indicates that there too, there is no consensus on whether a single constellation of ultrastructural features and of synaptic vesicle population identifies substance P content in an axon (Chan-Palay and Palay, 1977*b*; Pickel *et al.*, 1977; Hökfelt *et al.*, 1977; Cuello *et al.*, 1977; Barber *et al.*, 1979). In the light of the present evidence for coexistence of multiple putative transmitters in 5-HT/substance P neurones and their terminals, it would be unwise to assume that there are vesicular populations primarily identifiable with substance P content alone or with 5-HT alone. The question of which chemical mediator for which synaptic vesicle, or whether vesicles are involved at all, cannot be decided on the basis of the present insufficient evidence. Investigations with simultaneous labelling for multiple neuroactive compounds with high resolution at electron microscope level are required.

Coexistence of mutliple neuroactive substances raises questions of dynamic and functional importance. Our studies (Chan-Palay, 1978*a*; 1979*b*) suggest that, in addition to having 5-HT and substance P, a cell might contain varying amounts of these two substances at any one time. A single neurone may have more of one, less of the other, or both in large amounts. This heterogeneity means that our concept must encompass the two critical dimensions: time and cell function. Could neurones that contain both 5-HT and substance P have fluctuating levels of one or both, depending upon cell rhythm and demands for the synthesis of metabolism of one or the other mediator during specific types or phases of activity? A scheme of such a cycle is illustrated in figure 1.7.

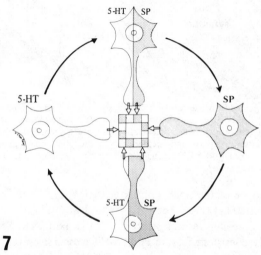

Figure 1.7  Schematic diagram to illustrated the concept of dynamic relationships between 5-HT and substance P (SP) in a single neurone. A neurone with both substances in coexistence may have fluctuating levels of one or both substances depending upon parameters of rhythm, time cycle, and physiological demands for one or another mediator during specific types or phases of activity.

It would be important for future studies to ascertain the factors that (1) regulate such cyclicity in neural mediators, (2) regulate the release of these substances, (3) determine whether the substances are released independently or concomitantly, and (4) determine the genetic composition of these neurones that ultimately directs their use of one or more neuroactive substance in communication. Finally, of course, one needs to know the precise connectivity of these special neurones. Where do their processes go, what paths do they take to get there, and what cells do they connect at their destinations (see figure 1.8)?

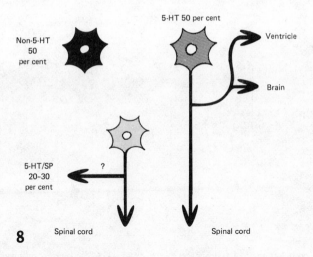

Figure 1.8 Schematic diagram to show that approximately 50 per cent of raphe pallidus neurones contain 5-HT and the remainder do not. Of the former, 20–30 per cent have substance P (SP) in coexistence.

## GABA/MOTILIN PURKINJE NEURONES

GABA is a major inhibitory neurotransmitter in the mammalian CNS, and deficits of GABA have been implicated in certain neurological and psychiatric disorders such as Huntington's chorea, Parkinson's disease and schizophrenia. Considerable interest has been attached in recent years to the identification of GABA-containing neurones, their possible inhibitory function, the identification of receptors, and the pharmacological manipulations of GABA-activated receptor sites. The cerebellum remains a major area in the CNS where the amino acid transmitters figure largely, and a considerable literature supports the identification of GABA as the inhibitory transmitter for many cerebellar neurones (figure 1.9). Among the approaches that have been used to support the localisation and role of GABA are (1) autoradiography following the uptake of $[^3H]$ - GABA (Hökfelt and Ljungdahl, 1970); (2) immunocytochemistry on tissue sections with antibodies directed against the enzyme GAD, responsible for the synthesis of GABA (McLaughlin *et al.*, 1974, 1975; Barber and Saito, 1976; Wood *et al.*, 1976) or with anti-GAD antibody injected directly into the live tissue to trace GABA specific pathways (Chan-Palay *et al.*, 1979); (3) immunocytochemistry with antibodies directed against the enzyme GABA-transaminase (GABA-T), the major metabolic enzyme for GABA (Barber and Saito 1976; Chan-Palay *et al.*, 1979); (4) autoradiographic demonstrations of various receptor-GABA binding sites with $[^3H]$-GABA analogues such as $[^3H]$-muscimol (Chan-Palay, 1978; Chan-Palay and Palay, 1978; Chan-Palay, 1979*c*). Of the cerebellar neurons in the cortex, a majority (though not all) of the small interneurones, for example, stellate, basket and Golgi cells are labelled by uptake of $[^3H]$-GABA,

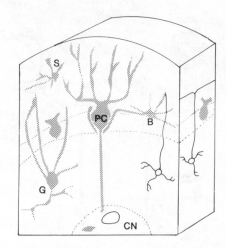

**9**

Figure 1.9 Cerebellar cortical and nuclear neurones with GAD immunoreactivity and uptake capacities for [$^3$H]-GABA are indicated by stipple. These are stellate (S), basket (B), Purkinje cells (PC), Golgi cells (G) of the cortex, and some small neurones in the deep cerebellar nuclei (CN).

anti-GAD antibody, GABA-T, and [$^3$H]-muscimol binding, indicating that GABA is a reasonably consistent constituent. In the deep cerebellar nuclei, the largest projection neurones are never marked by these GABA methods, whereas a population of smaller neurones are (Chan-Palay, 1977*b*; Mugnaini and Oertel, 1981). The present studies, however, are concerned with the Purkinje cells, the intracortical projection neurones responsible for the major relay of information from the complex cerebellar cortical network to the deep nuclear cells and to the lateral vestibular nucleus. Since the basic organisation, cytology, and connections of these cells are well known and have been the subject of major works (Ramon y Cajal, 1952; Palay and Chan-Palay, 1974; Eccles *et al.*, 1967), the details need not be repeated here. Only the pertinent facts will be drawn out to substantiate the case that coexistence of neuroactive substances occurs in Purkinje cells and that this opens up a frontier for advances in our understanding of the cerebellum.

Purkinje cells were demonstrated by a combination of pharmacological and physiological approaches to contain GABA and to have a postsynaptic inhibitory effect on Deiters neurones (Obata *et al.*, 1963; Obata, 1969). The presence of GABA has been confirmed by microdissection techniques (Obata, 1976). From these and subsequent findings it has been generally assumed that Purkinje cells are homogeneous, and that they all contain GABA and are inhibitory. Nevertheless, a critical analysis of the literature indicates that, in fact, whereas GABA could be localised to many cerebellar cortical structures reliably, the Purkinje cells remained the most inconsistent in this regard:

(1) Autoradiography with [$^3$H]-GABA uptake has produced evidence for

labelled cortical interneurones but did not reliably label Purkinje cells (Chan-Palay, 1977*b*; Hökfelt and Ljundahl, 1970; Sotelo *et al.*, 1972).

(2) Autoradiography with [$^3$H]-muscimol binding has consistently labelled intracortical interneurones but not Purkinje cells (Sotelo *et al.*, 1972).

(3) Immunocytochemical studies with anti-GAD antibodies have indicated that Purkinje cell somata are difficult to visualise unless colchicine is used to retard axoplasmic transport (Ribak *et al.*, 1978). A recent study (Oertel *et al.*, 1981) claims that all Purkinje cells can be labelled with the use of colchicine and a polyclonal antibody raised against a GAD preparation that is not the completely purified enzyme. However, closer examination of this material indicates that, in fact, unlabelled Purkinje cells are present.

(4) Other studies with anti-GABA-T have also indicated that not all Purkinje cells exhibit immunoreactivity to this serum even with the aid of colchicine (Barber and Saito, 1976; Chan-Palay, 1978). These reports were supported by other immunocytochemical studies in the literature indicating that positive labelling with anti-cyclic AMP (Bloom *et al.*, 1972; Chan-Palay and Palay, 1979) or with anti-cyclic GMP (Chan-Palay and Palay, 1979) was also patchy.

(5) *In vivo* injections of anti-GAD antibodies combined with anterograde and retrograde transport as a means of tracing chemically specific pathways indicated that although a large number of Purkinje cells contain GABA, some Purkinje cells contain only minor amounts and some contain none. The question was raised then whether or not this patchy labelling of Purkinje cells reflects cyclic changes in GABA content and fluctuating levels of GAD (Chan-Palay *et al.*, 1979; see figure 1.10).

The increasing concern that other neuroactive substances are likely to be present in Purkinje cells has resulted in a search in our laboratory for candidates among the growing catalogue of neuroactive peptides and amino acids (Chan-Palay *et al.*, 1982*a,c*; Chan-Palay *et al.*, 1981; 1982*b*). One successful candidate for this role is motilin, a 22-amino acid polypeptide isolated from porcine gut, which stimulates enteric smooth muscle (Brown, 1967; Brown *et al.*, 1971), has endocrine effects when administered systematically (Christofides *et al.*, 1979), and has an excitatory effect on neurones of the cerebral cortex and spinal cord (Phillips and Kirkpatrick, 1979).

Motilin-like immunoreactivity is detectable in peripheral nervous system (Chey *et al.*, 1980) and in the brain of a number of species, in the hypothalamus and pituitary (Jacobowitz *et al.*, 1981), and in the cerebellum (Nilaver *et al.*, 1981; Chan-Palay *et al.*, 1981). In the cerebellum, motilin-like immunoreactivity can be found almost exclusively in Purkinje cells; approximately 60–70 per cent of the Purkinje cells are motilin-positive and 30–40 per cent are not. These motilin cells occur mainly in the lateral cerebellum and the flocculonodular lobe with numerous terminals in the deep cerebellar nuclei and Deiters nucleus (see figures 1.11, 1.12, 1.13). GAD-immunoreactive Purkinje cells also form approximately 60–70 per cent of the population and 30–40 per cent of Purkinje cells are not GAD-positive. GAD Purkinje cells are found in the vermal and para-vermal regions with a large representative in the flocculonodular lobe (Chan-

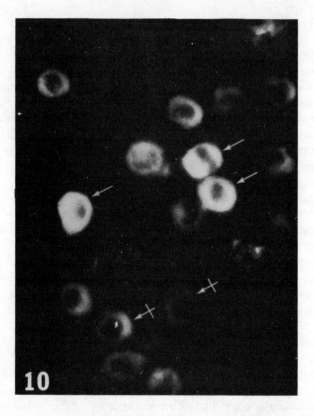

Figure 1.10 Photomicrograph showing GAD-immunoreactive Purkinje cell somata, excluding nuclei, after an *in vivo* injection with anti-GAD antibodies into the cerebellar cortex. Some cells are intensely labelled (arrows), others lightly labelled (crossed arrows), and still others not reactive at all, indicating that not all Purkinje cells have the capacity to bind anti-GAD antibodies and that not all Purkinje cells contain GAD. Rat cerebellum, immunofluorescence (×200).

Palay *et al.*, 1981), and numerous terminals occur in the deep cerebellar nuclei and Deiters nucleus. None of these results is numerically altered by the administration of colchicine. A combined double labelling study with anti-GAD and anti-motilin antibodies indicates that not only do some Purkinje cells contain either GAD- or motilin-immunoreactivity exclusively, but also certain cells, approximately 10–20 per cent, have both GAD and motilin (Chan-Palay *et al.*, 1981) and others have neither substances (figure 1.14). These findings call for a reassessment of present assumptions that Purkinje cells are a homogeneous population in structure, connections, and function. The existence of chemical heterogeneity in Purkinje cells requires that this assessment take place at the single neurone level and calls into question the present concept of how the cerebellum works.

Preliminary studies have been done with metabolically intact and viable peri-

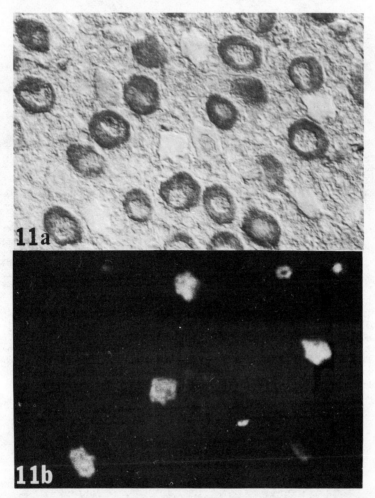

Figure 1.11  Purkinje cell field rich in motilin-immunoreactive cells. A pair of photomicrographs showing the same field of Purkinje cells in which 17 large neurones are labelled with
motilin antibodies (left) and five of the remaining Purkinje cells are labelled with GAD antibodies (right). Mouse cerebellum lobule V, vermis: (*a*) immunoperoxidase and (*b*) immunofluorescence (×200).

karya isolated from developing rat cerebellum at the sixth postnatal day according to previously described methods (Balazs *et al.*, 1977; Cohen *et al.*, 1978)
with the collaboration of Dr R. Balazs and his colleagues in London. The cells
display normal ultrastructure and metabolic activity as a result largely of the
gentle procedure used in cell dissociation: low trypsin concentration combined
with a trypsin inhibitor after a relatively short period of tissue digestion, the
use of isotonic conditions and physiological *p*H throughout the procedures, and
avoidance of high centrifugal forces. From these preparations several cell frac-

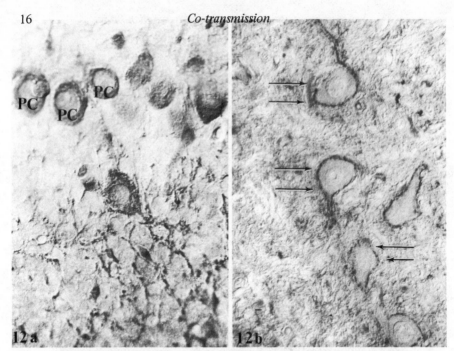

Figure 1.12  (*a*) Intense motilin-immunoreactivity demonstrated in a row of Purkinje cells (PC) and more rarely, in the cell body, dendritic and axonal processes of a Golgi cell in the granular layer. Rat cerebellar cortex, vibratome sections, peroxidase anti-peroxidase method (Chan-Palay and Nilaver, unpublished; ×350). (*b*) Motilin-immunoreactive terminals (arrows) on the somata and primary dendrites of large neurones in the dentate nucleus of the rat's cerebellum (×350).

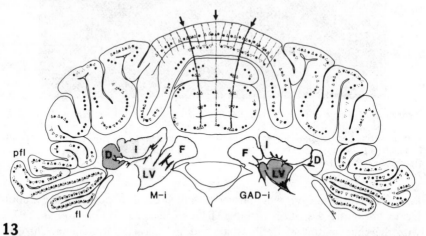

**13**

Figure 1.13  Schematic drawing of the distribution of motilin-immunoreactive Purkinje cells (triangles) and GAD-immunoreactive Purkinje cells (black dots) in a coronal section of the cerebellum. Both cell types are more concentrated in the flocculus (fl) and dorsal and ventral paraflocculus (pfl) than elsewhere, and in the vermis they participate in the formation of the sagittal microzones (arrows). Motilin-immunoreactive terminal axon projections in the deep cerebellar nuclei (D, dentate; I, interpositus; F, fastigial; LV, lateral vesitbular nucleus) are represented on the left; a comparable representation for GAD-immunoreactive terminal axon projections is shown on the right. Arrows indicate microbands formed by motilin and GAD cells.

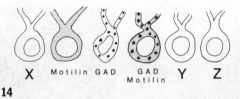

Figure 1.14 Schematic diagram showing the existence of immunoreactivity for motilin, GAD and GAD/motilin in coexistence in the Purkinje cells of the cerebellum. Other neurones labelled X, Y, and Z have none of these reactivities and are likely to contain other neuro-active substances.

tions could be obtained, one of which is of central interest to us, the "E" fraction consisting of the perikarya of large neurones, consisting mainly, though not exclusively, of Purkinje cells. In this fraction, electron microscopic studies have shown good structural preservation, continuous plasma membranes, and notably intact mitochondria. Viability of the cells is good, 80 per cent exclude trypan blue, and plating efficiency of these cells in tissue culture is very high (Cohen *et al.*, 1978).

Preparations of the "E" or Purkinje cell fractions were layered on to slides fixed with 4 per cent formaldehyde and 0.1 per cent glutaraldehyde in 0.12 M phosphate buffer (*p*H 7.3) for several hours and dried. The cells were then rinsed well in Tris buffer (*p*H 7.6) and allowed to react with a sequence of different antibodies, including anti-GAD antibody and anti-motilin antibody. Each set of Purkinje cells was exposed to a primary antibody, then the reaction was completed with peroxidase-conjugated goat-anti-rabbit serum and finally stained with DAB and $H_2O_2$. All cells were counted and their immunoreactivity intensities divided into three categories: high (++); medium (+); and absent (−).

| GAD-immunoreacted preparations | Motilin-immunoreacted preparations |
|---|---|
| 70.9 per cent cells had (++) reactions; | 68.3 per cent cells had (++) reactions |
| 18.1 per cent cells had (+) reactions; | 19.0 per cent cells had (+) reactions |
| 11.1 per cent cells had (−) reactions, | 12.4 per cent cells had (−) reactions |
| (*n* = 19,716) | (*n* = 27,268) |

When the GAD-stained preparations were restained with anti-motilin antibody or vice versa, the numbers of stained cells were equivalent. Double label experiments indicate that many (approximately 60 per cent) Purkinje cells contain both GAD and motilin immunoreactivities (see figure 1.15). These results indicate that: (1) Purkinje cell fractions provide a suitable model for testing the coexistence of GAD with motilin and other neuroactive substances; (2) the quantitative estimates obtained from Purkinje cell fractions correlates those made on tissue sections; (3) at 6 d postnatally Purkinje cells already express the definitive neuromediator profile; (4) and the model should enable us to study selected Purkinje cells with known content of single or multiple neuromediators under various experimental conditions.

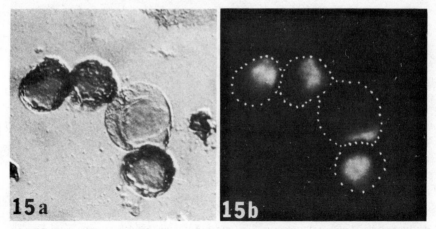

Figure 1.15  Four isolated Purkinje cells from 6-d-old developing rat cerebellum after reaction with anti-GAD antibody peroxidase (*a*) and antimotilin antibody with FITC (*b*). Note that only three of the four cells have GAD, but all four have motilin, and three have both substances coexisting (×350).

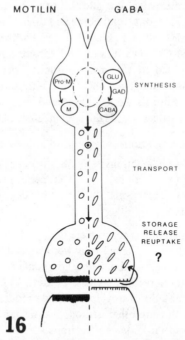

Figure 1.16  Schematic diagram of Purkinje cell with motilin and GABA coexisting in its soma and processes. Separate mechanisms for the synthesis, transport, storage and release of motilin and GABA are illustrated. A translation of promotilin (pro-M) to motilin (M) is suggested for motilin on the left, whereas the synthesis of GABA from glutamate through GAD is shown on the right. The diagram raises these issues: what are the sizes and shapes of synaptic vesicles and the physiological functions associated with each neuroactive compound?

Major questions remain to be addressed: (1) What are the cytological features of a pure GAD-immunoreactive, GABA-containing Purkinje cell, and what are its connections? (2) What are the cytological features of a pure motilin-immunoreactive Purkinje cell and what are its connections? (3) What are the similarities and differences between these cells and what can be learned about their separate chemical and physiological functions? (4) What are the ultrastructural correlates for dual neuroactive chemical content in the Purkinje cell? (5) Does the cell segregate the synthesis, transport, and release machinery for GABA and for motilin in different populations of such cellular organelles, or do they coexist? Can these compartments be distinguished immunocytochemically at the ultrastructural level and are synaptic vesicles involved (see figure 1.16)? (6) Are the pure motilin-immunoreactive, pure GAD-immunoreactive, and dual motilin/GAD-immunoreactive cells related in a cyclic manner so that they are not separate cell types but represent a single type of neurone in different phases fixed in time by an immunocytochemical experiment (see figure 1.17)? (7) Motilin and GAD cells occur in small foci. Can one trace the origins of these Purkinje cells to specific precursor cells very early in development and test these hypotheses of cyclicity and genetic regulations? (8) At least 30 per cent

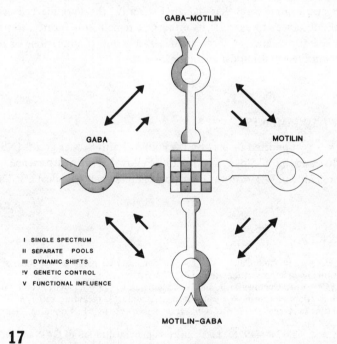

**17**

Figure 1.17 Schematic diagram to illustrate the concept of the dynamic relationships between GABA and motilin occurring in a single neurone. A neurone with both substances may have fluctuating levels of one or the other, depending on rhythm, cycle time and functional demands for one or another specific types or phases of activity.

of all cerebellar Purkinje cells have neither GAD- nor motilin-immunoreactivity. What neuroactive substances might they contain? There are indeed indications in the literature that enkephalin-like immunoreactivity occurs in some cerebellar Golgi cells and mossy fibres (Shulman *et al.*, 1981). Taurine has been demonstrated in cerebellar Purkinje, basket, stellate and Golgi neurones distributed in sagittal microzones and in deep cerebellar nuclease neurones (Chan-Palay *et al.*, 1982*a,c*). Somatostatin enkephalin and β-endorphin have also been localized to cerebellar neurones (Chan-Palay *et al.*, 1982*b*, and unpublished data).

In summary, we present the Purkinje cell, the familiar giant cell of the cerebellar cortex, as a model in which the phenomenon of coexistence of neuroactive substances can be readily studied. The other fundamental questions that need to be answered are functional ones. What neuromediative role does motilin have? Is it inhibitory, non-inhibitory, "modulatory" or excitatory?

Recent iontophoretic studies of motilin and other neuroactive substances indicate that motilin has an inhibitory effect on lateral vestibular nucleus neurones (Chan-Palay *et al.*, 1982*b*). Motilin inhibition has a rapid onset and recovery and when motilin and GABA are iontophoresed in tandem, their depressant effects summate. Thus these observations are consistent with earlier studies that indicated that Purkinje cells exert an inhibitory influence on the vestibular and central cerebellar nuclei. Evidently, the Purkinje cell can use a variety of substances to exercise its effects. It remains for future investigations to reveal the significance of these various agents and combinations of multiple messengers in their multimodal encoding.

## ACKNOWLEDGEMENTS

This work was supported in part by US Public Health Service grants (NS 03659; NS 14740) and by a Sloan Foundation Fellowship in neuroscience. I thank Mr H. Cook and Ms J. Barton for their photographic and technical assistance.

## REFERENCES

Andrezik, J. A. and Chan-Palay, V. (1977). The nucleus paragigantocellularis lateralis: Definition and afferents. *Anat. Rec.*, **184**, 524–525
Balazs, R., Cohen, J., Garthwaite, J. and Woodhams, P. L. (1977). Isolation and biochemical characterization of morphologically defined structures, including cell types, from the cerebellum. In *Amino Acids as Chemical Transmitters*. (ed. F. Fonnum), Plenum Press, New York pp. 629–651
Barber, R. and Saito, K. (1976). Light microscopic visualization of GAD and GABA-T in immunocytochemical preparations of rodent CNS. In *GABA in Nervous System Function* (ed. E. Roberts, T. N. Chase and D. B. Towers), Raven Press, New York pp. 113–131
Barber, R. P., Vaughn, J. E., Slemmon, J. R., Salvaterra, P. M., Roberts, E. and Leeman, S. E. (1979). The origin, distribution and synaptic relationships of substance P axons in rat spinal cord. *J. comp. Neurol.*, **184**, 331–352

Baumgarten, H. G. and Lachenmeyer, L. (1972). 5,7-dihydroxytryptamine: improvement in chemical lesioning of indolamine neurons in the mammalian brain. *Z. Zellforsch.*, 135, 399–414

Beaudet, A. and Descarries, L. (1979). Radioautographic characterization of a serotonin-accumulating nerve cell group in adult rat hypothalamus. *Brain Res.*, 160, 231–243

Beaudet, A., Pickel, V. M., Joh, T. H. Miller, R. J. and Cuenod, M. (1980). Simultaneous detection of serotonin and tyrosine hydroxylase or enkephalin-containing neurons by combined radioautography and immunocytochemistry in the central nervous system of the rat. *Soc. Neurosci., Abstr.*, 6, 353

Bjorklund, A., Lindvall, O. S. and Svensson, L.-A. (1972). Mechanisms of fluorophore formation in the histochemical glyoxylic acid method for monoamines. *Histochemie*, 32, 113–131

Bloom, F. E., Hoffer, B. J., Battenberg, E. F., Siggins, G. R., Steiner, A. L., Parker, C. W. and Wedner, H. J. (1972a). Adenosine 3',5'-monophosphate is localised in cerebellar neurons: immunofluorescence evidence. *Science*, 177, 436–438

Bloom, F. E., Hoffer, B. J., Siggins, G. R., Barker, J. L. and Nicoll, R. A. (1972b). Effects of serotonin on central neurons: Microiontophoretic administration. *Fedn Proc.*, 31, 97–106

Bogdansky, D. F., Fletcher, A., Borodie, B. B. and Udenfriend, S. (1956). Identification and assay of serotonin in brain. *J. Pharmac. exp. Ther.*, 117, 82–88

Brown, J. C. (1967). Presence of a gastric motor-stimulating property in duodenal extracts. *Gastroenterology*, 52, 225–229

Brown, J. C., Mutt, V. and Dryburgh, J. R. (1971). The further purification of motilin, a gastric motor activity stimulating polypeptide from the mucosa of the small intestine of hogs. *Can. J. Physiol. Pharmac.*, 49, 399–405

Burnstock, G. (1976). Do some nerve cells release more than one transmitter? *Neuroscience*, 1, 239–248

Ramon y Cajal, S. (1952). *Histologie du Systeme Nerveux de l'Homme et des Vertebres* (trans. L. Axoulay), 1 and 2, Maloine, Paris, reprinted 1952 and 1955, Consejo Superior de Investigaciones Cientificas, Madrid.

Chan-Palay, V. (1975). Fine structure of labelled axons in the cerebellar cortex and nuclei of rodents and primates after intraventricular infusions with tritiated serotonin. *Anat. Embryol.*, 148, 235–265

Chan-Palay, V. (1976). Serotonin axons in the suprea-and subependymal plexuses and in the leptomininges: their roles in local alterations of cerebrospinal fluid and vasomotor activity. *Brain Res.*, 102, 103–130

Chan-Palay, V. (1977a). Indoleamine neurones and their processes in the normal rat brain and in chronic diet-induced thiamine deficiency demonstrated by uptake of [3] H-serotonin. *J. comp. Neurol.*, 174, 467–493

Chan-Palay, V. (1977b). *Cerebellar Dentate Nucleus: Organisation, Cytology, and Transmitters*. Springer-Verlag, Berlin, Heidelberg and New York, p. 548

Chan-Palay, V. (1978a). Morphological correlates for transmitter synthesis, transport, release, uptake and catabolism: a study of serotonin neurons in the nucleus paragigantocellularis lateralis. In *Amino Acids as Chemical Transmitters*, NATO Advanced Study Symposium, Plenum Press, New York, pp. 1–29

Chan-Palay, V. (1978b). The paratrigeminal nucleus. I. Neurons and synaptic organization including axoaxonic and dendrodendritic interrelations in the neuropil. *J. Neurocytol.*, 7, 405–418

Chan-Palay, V. (1978c). The paratrigeminal nucleus. II. Identification and interrelations of catecholamine, indoleamine and substance P containing axons in the neuropil. *J. Neurocytol.*, 7, 419–422

Chan-Palay, V. (1978d). Autoradiographic localization of γ-aminobutyric acid receptors in the rat central nervous system using [3] H-muscimol. *Proc. natn. Acad. Sci. U.S.A.*, 75, 1024–1028

Chan-Palay, V. (1979a). Combined immunocytochemistry and autoradiography after *in vivo* injections of monoclonal antibody to substance P and [3] H-serotonin: Coexistence of two putative transmitters in single raphe cells and fibre plexuses. *Anat. Embryol.*, 156, 241–254

Chan-Palay, V. (1979*b*). Immunocytochemical detection of substance P neurons, their processes and connections by *in vivo* injections of monoclonal antibodies: light and electron microscopy. *Anat. Embryol.*, 156, 225–240

Chan-Palay, V. (1979*c*). Recent advances in the morphological localization of GABA receptors in the cerebellum by means of ³H-muscinol. *Progr. Brain Res.*, 51, 303–322

Chan-Palay, V. (1981). Evidence for coexistence of serotonin and substance P in single raphe cells and fiber plexuses: combined immunocytochemistry and autoradiography. In *Advances in Experimental Biology and Medicine*, 133 (ed. B. Haber, S. Gabay, M. Issidories and S. Allivisatos), Plenum Press, New York, pp. 81–100

Chan-Palay, V. and Palay, S. L. (1977*a*). Immunocytochemical identification of substance P cells and their processes in rat sensory ganglia and their terminals in the spinal cord: light microscopic studies. *Proc. natn. Acad. Sci. U.S.A.*, 74, 3597–3601

Chan-Palay, V. and Palay, S. L. (1977*b*). Ultrastructural identification of substance P cells and their processes in rat sensory ganglia and their terminals in the spinal cord by immuno-cytochemistry. *Proc. natn. Acad. Sci. U.S.A.*, 74, 4050–4054

Chan-Palay, V. and Palay, S. L. (1978). Ultrastructural localisation of gamma-aminobutyric acid receptors in the mammalian central nervous system by means of ³H-muscimol binding. *Proc. natn. Acad. Sci. U.S.A.*, 75, 2977–2980

Chan-Palay, V. and Palay, S. L. (1979). Light and electron microscope immunocytochemical localization of cyclic GMP: evidence for involvement of neuroglia. *Proc. natn. Acad. Sci. U.S.A.*, 76, 1485–1489

Chan-Palay, V., Jonsson, G. and Palay, S. L. (1978). Serotonin and substance P coexist in neurons of the rat's central nervous system. *Proc. natn. Acad. Sci. U.S.A.*, 75, 1582–1586

Chan-Palay, V., Palay, S. L. and Wu, J.-Y. (1979*a*). Gamma-aminobutyric acid pathways in the cerebellum studied by retrograde and anterograde transport of glutamic acid decar-boxylase antibody after *in vivo* injections. *Anat. Embryol.*, 157, 1–14

Chan-Palay, V., Wu, J.-Y. and Palay, S. L. (1979*b*). Immunocytochemical localization of GABA-transaminase at cellular and ultrastructural levels. *Proc. natn. Acad. Sci. U.S.A.*, 76, 2067–2071

Chan-Palay, V., Lin, C.-T., Palay, S. L., Yamamoto, M. and Wu, J.-Y. (1982*a*). Taurine in the mammalian cerebellum: Demonstration by autoradiography with [³H]-taurine and immunocytochemistry with antibodies against the taurine-synthesising enzyme, cysteine-sulfinic acid decarboxylase. *Proc. natn. Acad. Sci. U.S.A.*, 79, 2695–2699

Chan-Palay, V., Ito, M., Tongroach, P., Sakurai, M. and Palay, S. L. (1982*b*). Inhibitory effects of motilin, somatostatin, (Leu) enkephalin, (Met) enkephalin, and taurine on neurons of the lateral vestibular nucleus: Interactions with γ-aminobutyric acid. *Proc. natn. Acad. Sci. U.S.A.*, in press

Chan-Palay, V., Palay, S. L., Li, C. and Wu, J.-Y. (1982*c*). Sagittal cerebellar microbands of taurine neurons. Immunocytochemical demonstration by using antibodies against the taurine synthesising enzyme cysteine sulfinic acid decarboxylase. *Proc. natn. Acad. Sci. U.S.A.*, in press

Chan-Palay, V., Nilaver, G., Palay, S. L., Beinfeld, M. G., Zimmerman, E. A., Wu, J.-Y. and O'Donohue, T. L. (1981). Chemical heterogeneity in cerebellar Purkinje cells: Existence and coexistence of glutamic acid decarboxylase-like and motilin-like immunoreactivities. *Proc. natn. Acad. Sci. U.S.A.*, 78, in press

Chey, W. Y., Escoffery, R., Roth, F., Chang, T. M., You, C. H. and Yajima, H. (1980). Motilin-like immunoreactivity (MLI) in the gut and neurons of peripheral and central nervous system. *Regulatory Peptides*, suppl., 1, 19

Christofides, N. D., Modlin, I. M., Fitzpatrick, M. L. and Bloom, S. R. (1979). Effect of motilin on the rate of gastric emptying and gut hormone release during breakfast. *Gastro-enterology*, 76, 903–907

Cohen, J., Balazs, R., Hajos, F., Currie, D. W. and Dutton, G. R. (1978). Separation of cell types from developing cerebellum. *Brain Res.*, 148, 313–331

Consolazione, A. and Cuello, A. C. (1982). CNS serotonin pathways. In *Biology of Sero-tonergic Transmission*. (ed. N. N. Osborne), Wiley, Chichester, UK, pp. 29–61

Consolazione, A., Milstein, C., Wright, B. and Cuello, A. C. (1981). Immunocytochemical detection of serotonin with monoclonal antibodies. *J. Histochem. Cytochem*, in press

Coons, A. G. (1958). Fluorescent Antibody Methods. In *General Cytochemical Methods* (ed. J. F. Danielli), Academic Press, New York, pp. 399–422

Cuello, A. C., Jessell, T. M., Kanazawa, I. and Iversen, L. L. (1977). Substance P: localization in synaptic vesicles in rat central nervous system. *J. Neurochem.*, 29, 747–751

Cuello, A. C., Galfre, G. and Milstein, C. (1979). Detection of substance P in the central nervous system by a monoclonal antibody. *Proc. natn. Acad. Sci. U.S.A.*, 76, 3532–3536

Cuello, A. C., Milstein, C. and Priestley, J. V. (1981). Use of monoclonal antibodies in immunocytochemistry with special reference to the central nervous system. *Brain Res. Bull.*, 5, 575–587

Cuello, A. C. and Milstein, C. (1982). Use of internally labelled monoclonal antibodies. In *Radioimmunology.* (ed. Ch. A. Bizollon), Elsevier-North Holland, Amsterdam, pp. 293–305

Dahlstrom, A. and Fuxe, K. (1964). Evidence for the existence of monoamine-containing neurons in the central nervous system. *Acta Physiol. Scand.* suppl., 62, 1–55

Descarries, L., Beaudet, A. and Watkins, K. C. (1975). Serotonin nerve terminals in adult rat neocortex. *Brain Res.*, 100, 563–588

Eccles, J., Ito, M. and Szentagothai, J. (1976). *The Cerebellum as a Neuronal Machine.* Springer-Verlag, Berlin, Heidelberg and New York

Fuxe, K. and Jonsson, G. (1967). A modification of the histochemical fluorescence method for the improved localization of 5-hydroxytryptamine. *Histochemie*, 11, 161–166

Gamrani, H., Calas, A., Belin, M. F., Aguera, M. and Pujol, J. F. (1979). High resolution radioautographic identification of $^3$H-GABA labeled neurons in the rat nucleus raphe dorsalis. *Neurosci. Lett.*, 15, 43–48

Gershon, M. (1981). Properties and development of peripheral serotonergic neurons. *J. Physiol. Paris*, 77, 257–265

Glazer, E. J., Steinbusch, H., Verhofstad, A. and Basbaum, A. I. (1981). Serotonergic neurons of the cat nucleus raphe dorsalis and paragigantocellularis contain enkephalin. *J. Physiol. Paris*, 77, 241–245

Hökfelt, T. and Ljungdahl, A. (1970). Cellular localization of labelled gamma-aminobutyric acid ($^3$H-GABA) in rat cerebellar cortex: an autoradiographic study. *Brain Res.*, 22, 391–396

Hökfelt, T., Elde, R., Johansson, O., Luft, R., Nilsson, G. and Arimura, A. (1976). Immunohistochemical evidence for separate populations of somatostatin-containing and substance P-containing primary afferent neurons in the rat. *Neuroscience*, 1, 131–136

Hökfelt, T., Johansson, O., Kellerth, J.-O., Ljungdahl, A., Nilsson, G., Nygards, A. and Pernow, B. (1977). Immunohistochemical distribution of substance P. In *Substance P* (ed. Von Euler, U.S. and Pernow, B.), Raven Press, New York, pp. 117–143

Hökfelt, T., Ljungdahl, A, Steinbusch, H., Verhofstad, A., Nilsson, G., Brodin, E., Pernow, B. and Goldstein, M. (1978). Immunohistochemical evidence of substance P-like immunoreactivity in some 5-hydroxytryptamine-containing neurons in the rat central nervous system. *Neuroscience*, 3, 517–538

Jacobowitz, D. M., O'Donohue, T. L. and Chey, W. Y. (1981). Mapping of motilin-immunoreactive neurons of the rat brain. *Peptides*, in press

Joh, T. H., Shikimi, T., Pickel, V. M. and Reis, D. J. (1975). Brain tryptophan hydroxylase: Purification of, production of antibodies to, and cellular and ultrastructural localization in serotonergic neurons of rat midbrain. *Proc. natn. Acad. Sci. U.S.A.*, 72, 3575–3579

Köhler, G. and Milstein, C. (1975). Continuous culture of fused cells secreting antibody of predefined specificity. *Nature Lond.*, 256, 495–497

Massari, V. D., Tizabi, Y., Gottesfeld, Z. and Jacobowitz, D. M. (1978). A fluorescence histochemical and biochemical evaluation of the effect of p-chloro-amphetamine on individual serotonergic nuclei in the rat brain. *Neuroscience*, 3, 339–344

McLaughlin, B., Wood, J. G., Saito, K., Barber, R., Vaughn, J. E., Roberts, E. and Wu, J.-Y. (1974). The fine structural localization of glutamate decarboxylase in synaptic terminals of rodent cerebellum. *Brain Res.*, 76, 377–391

McLaughlin, B. J., Wood, J. G., Saito, K., Roberts, E. and Wu, J.-Y. (1975). The fine structural localization of glutamate decarboxylase in developing axonal processes and presynaptic terminals of rodent cerebellum. *Brain Res.*, 85, 355–371

Mouren-Mathieu, A. M., Leger, L. and Descarries, L. (1976). Radioautographic visualization of central monoamine neurons after local instillation of tritiated serotonin and norepinephrine in adult cat. *Soc. Neurosci. Abstr.*, **2**, part 1, 497.

Mugnaini, E. and Oertel, W. (1981). Distribution of GAD positive neurons in the rat cerebellar nuclei. *Soc. Neurosci. Abstr.*, **7**, 122

Nanopoulos, D., Belin, M. F., Maitre, M., Vincendon, G. and Pujol, J. F. (1981). Immunocytochemical evidence for the existence of GABAergic neurons in the nucleus raphe dorsalis. Possible existence of neurons containing serotonin and GABA. *Brain Res.*, in press

Nilaver, G., Zimmerman, E. A., Defendini, R., Beinfeld, M. C. and O'Donohue, T. L. (1981). Motilin in brain: immunocytochemical studies. *Soc. Neurosci. Abstr.*, in press

Obata, K. (1969). Gamma-aminobutyric acid in Purkinje cells and motor neurones. *Experentia Basel*, **25**, 1283

Obata, K. (1976). Association of GABA with cerebellar Purkinje cells: Single cell analysis. In *GABA in Nervous System Function*. (ed. E. Roberts, T. N. Chase and D. B. Tower), Raven Press, New York, pp. 113–131

Obata, K., Ito, M., Ochi, R. and Sato, N. (1967). Pharmacological properties of the postsynaptic inhibition by Purkinje cell axons and the action of gamma-aminobutyric acid on Deiters neurones. *Expl Brain Res.*, **4**, 43–57

Oertel, W. H., Mugnaini, E., Schmechel, D. E., Tappaz, M. L. and Kopin, I. J. (1982). The immunocytochemical demonstration of GABA-ergic neurons – methods and application. In *Cytochemical Methods in Neuroanatomy* (ed. V. Chan-Palay and S. L. Palay), Alan R. Liss. New York

Osborne, N. N. (1979). Is Dale's principle valid? *Trends in Neuroscience*, **2**, 73–75

Palay, S. L. and Chan-Palay, V. (1974). *Cerebellar Cortex, Cytology and Organization*. Springer-Verlag, Berlin, Heidelberg and New York

Panuia, P., Emson, P. and Wu, J.-Y. (1980). Demonstration of enkephalin, substance P and glutamate decarboxylase-like immunoreactivity in cultured cells derived from newborn rat neostriatum. *Histochemistry*, **69**, 169–179

Pearse, A. G. E. (1969). The cytochemistry and ultrastructure of polypeptide hormone-producing cells of the APUD series and the embryonic, physiologic and pathologic implications of the concept. *J. Histochem. Cytochem.*, **17**, 303–313

Phillip, J. W. and Kirkpatrick, J. R. (1979). Motilin excites neurons in the cerebral cortex and spinal cord. *Eur. J. Pharmac.*, **58**, 469–472

Pickel, V. M., Joh, T. H. and Reis, D. J. (1976). Monoamine synthesizing enzymes in central dopaminergic, noradrenergic and serotonergic neurons. Immunocytochemical localization by light and electron microscopy. *J. Histochem. Cytochem.*, **24**, 792–806

Pickel, V., Reis, D. J. and Leeman, S. E. (1977). Ultrastructural localization of substance P in neurons of rat spinal cord. *Brain Res.*, **122**, 534–540

Ribak, C. E., Vaughn, J. E. and Saito, K. (1978). Immunocytochemical localization of glutamic acid decarboxylase in neuronal somata following colchicine inhibition of axonal transport. *Brain Res.*, **140**, 315–332

Schulman, J. A., Finger, T. E., Brecha, N. and Karten, H. J. (1981). Enkephalin immunoreactivity in Golgi cells and mossy fibers of mammalian avian, amphibian and teleost cerebellum. *Neuroscience*, **6**, 2407–2416

Sotelo, C., Privat, A., and Drian, M. J. (1972). Localization of ($^3$H) GABA in tissue culture of rat cerebellum using electron microscopy radioautography. *Brain Res.*, **45**, 302–308

Steinbusch, H. W. M. (1981). Distribution of serotonin-immunoreactivity in the central nervous system of the rat cell bodies and terminals. *Neuroscience*, **4**, 557–618

Twarog, B. M. and Page, I. H. (1953). Serotonin content of some mammalian tissues and urine and a method for its determination. *J. Physiol. Lond.*, **175**, 157–161.

Wood, J. G., McLaughlin, B. J. and Vaughn, J. E. (1976). Immunocytochemical localization of GAD in electron microscopic preparations of rodent CNS. In *GABA in Nervous System Function* (ed. E. Roberts, N. Chase, D. B. Towers), Raven Press, New York, pp. 133–148

# 2
# Coexistence of putative neuromodulators in the same axon: pharmacological consequences at receptors

E. Costa (Laboratory of Preclinical Pharmacology, National Institute of Mental Health, Saint Elizabeths Hospital, Washington, D.C. 20032, USA)

## INTRODUCTION

With the discovery that two or more molecular species of neuromodulators coexist in the same axon (Kerkut et al., 1967; Brownstein et al., 1974; Hanley et al., 1974; Cottrell, 1977; Hokfelt et al., 1980), Dale's postulate that each neurone contains one and only one putative neurotransmitter can no longer be considered an acceptable generalisation. There are two versions of what has become to be known as Dale's principle stating that a neurone contains and releases the same transmitter(s) from its various axon terminals (Dale, 1935), and its re-interpretation stating that a neurone contains and secretes one and only one neuromodulator (Eccles et al., 1956). The coexistence of two or more neuromodulators in the same axon makes the molecular uniqueness of the neuromodulator present in any given neurone a principle with several exceptions. Since the number of neuronal systems in which more than one putative transmitter coexists in the same axon is continually increasing (Hokfelt et al., 1980; Lundberg, 1981), it seems likely that in the not too distant future the idealised neurone should be viewed as one containing more than one neuromodulator. Should the present trend continue, one might even predict that a neurone with only one putative neurotransmitter might become the exception.

The coexistence of two molecular species of neuromodulators in the same axon or in the same synaptic vesicle can affect synaptic function in a number of theoretical ways which are illustrated in figure 2.1. This drawing presupposes that the postsynaptic receptor is a supramolecular entity composed of several

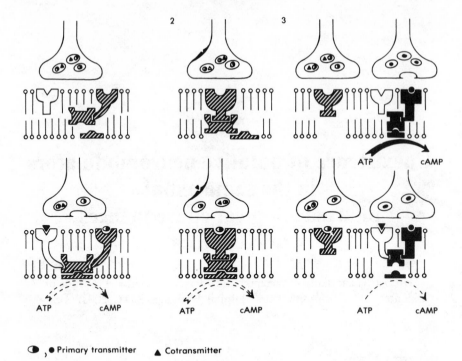

○ , ● Primary transmitter     ▲ Cotransmitter

Figure 2.1 Diagrammatic representation of three possible models of the interaction between primary transmitter and cotransmitter in the regulation of a receptor response transduced by cyclic AMP: (1) the transmitter and cotransmitter are released on the same postsynaptic receptors and the cotransmitter facilitates or disfacilitates the response elicited by the transmitter; (2) the cotransmitter is the presynaptic modulator for the release or synthesis of the cotransmitter; (3) the cotransmitter acts on the postsynaptic receptor of an adjacent neurone. This presentation deals only with case number 1, but cases 2 and 3 are also theoretically possible and may create interesting models to be considered for a complete study of the receptor consequences of the coexistence of two modulators.

membrane proteins functionally organised into three units: primary transmitter recognition sites, coupling device, and transducer system. When the primary transmitter recognition site is occupied, it causes an interaction between the coupler and transducer leading to an activation of the transducer function. This can be expressed as an activation of an enzyme regulating the formation of second messengers or the opening or closing of an ion gate. It seems that the receptor functions at a variable gain and that the gain is set by the co-transmitter which is co-released (discontinually?) with the primary transmitter. We have proposed that the cotransmitter acts on specific recognition sites which interact with one of the three functional units of the receptor and through this interaction determines the gain of the receptor function. Evidence has been obtained for co-secretion of noradrenaline or acetylcholine and a purine, possibly adenosine (Furshpan *et al.*, 1981).

Figure 2.1 presents some of the possible synaptic changes associated with the coexistence of a putative primary transmitter of the amine or amino acid class with a putative cotransmitter of the polypeptide class similar in some way to the model studied by Lundberg (1981; see also Hokfelt *et al.*, chapter 4). The neuromodulator (co-transmitter) that exists with the amine or amino acid transmitter (primary transmitter) may function as a trophic factor for either the same or a contiguous neurone. If it acts on the same neurone it could be either released extraneuronally and act on presynaptic recognition sites (figure 2.1b), or it could not be released extraneuronally but acts on mechanisms located intra-neuronally. The primary transmitter and the co-transmitter could act post-synaptically and when these two molecules are co-released the co-transmitter modulates the gain of the synaptic function that is activated by the primary transmitter. This interaction can occur with different modalities. As shown in figure 2.1, the interaction occurs via an intermediary action on the coupler which is located in the postsynaptic membrane and binds to both the recognition site for the primary transmitter and the co-transmitter and the regulatory site of the transducer function, usually an ion gate or an enzyme that synthesises a second messenger. Among many theoretical alternatives, figure 2.1 also depicts one in which the neuropeptide acts postsynaptically on an adjacent axon terminal (figure 2.1c), and finally the case (figure 2.1a), in which the neuropeptide modulates the response of a transmitter released from the axon terminal on a receptor facing this axon. Of course, these are just a few examples of the many hypothetical cases that can be operative if the synaptic transmission is modulated by two neuromodulators.

## RECEPTORS AS SUPRAMOLECULAR UNITS

The study of the regulatory components of adenylate cyclase has revealed the existence of a protein characterised by its capacity to bind guanine nucleotide that can be solubilised together with the catalytic moiety of adenylate cyclase (Ross and Gilman, 1980). As this protein contains sites that are operative in the activation of the enzyme by guanine nucleotides and fluoride, the protein has been termed G/F (Sternweis *et al.*, 1981). An important effector in the adenylate cyclase regulation by the G/F protein is GTP which seems to be metabolised by a GTPase located in a protein component of the receptor which is located in the membrane presumably very close to the G/F protein (Koski and Klee, 1981). This G/F protein is the target of several effectors of membrane bound adenylate cyclase, such as the recognition sites for a number of putative neurotransmitters. Presumably the occupancy of these recognition sites by specific ligands causes transitional modifications of the protein in which the recognition sites are located. We know very little about these changes and how they influence the mobility of the protein in the lipoid matrix of the membrane but it seems that some of the changes may modulate the G/F protein by changing the GTPase activity and, therefore, make available different amounts of GTP or GDP for saturation of the G/F protein. These and other interactions of membrane proteins have been instrumental in creating the basis for the current views on the organisation of postsynaptic receptors as described in the introduction.

Receptors are seen as supramolecular units that transform a chemical signal reaching the recognition site for the primary transmitter into a metabolic signal operating in the internal milieu of the postsynaptic cell. This takes the form of a change in either the flux of a specific ion or in the synthesis of an organic second messenger which by activating an intracellular metabolic step (protein kinase?) modifies the activity of the enzymes or of regulatory proteins inside the postsynaptic cells. Thus, the binding of a chemical signal to a specific recognition site brings about the internalisation of the stimulus in the postsynaptic cell. To appreciate the complexity of this process, one must consider the supramolecular organisation of the receptors for the neurotransmitters. Current concepts of membrane structure (Singer and Nicolson, 1972) have suggested that these units are located in the phospholipid bilayer of the postsynaptic membrane and are formed by a number of membrane-associated proteins. These are either integral proteins floating in the membrane phospholipids or peripheral proteins. The function of the receptor can be affected by modification of the phospholipid microenvironment where the protein floats (Hirata and Axelrod, 1980), or by modifications of the proteins. Both modifications may be receptor mediated and the endogenous ligand for these receptors may be one of the neuromodulators coexisting within the nerve terminal innervating the receptor.

We have neither an exact understanding of the way in which the cotransmitters interact to elicit this modulation, nor a complete understanding of the way in which the cotransmitters modulate the most extensively studied coupling mechanisms, the G/F binding protein (Ross and Gilman, 1980). The G/F binding protein has two binding sites for nucleotides, one for GTP and the other for GDP. When the GDP binds to the G/F protein the amplification capacity of the system operates at a minimum, whereas the binding of GTP to the G/F protein elicits maximal amplification of the system that is modulated by this protein. It seems that a GTPase activity is linked to the function of the G/F protein as there is preliminary evidence that occupancy of the recognition site of opiate receptors functioning as co-transmitters reduce the amplification of the receptor-regulated adenylate cyclase via an activation of the GTPase (Koski and Klee, 1981). The activation of this enzyme increases GDP availability and, therefore, makes available more GDP for the GDP binding site located in the G/F protein thereby diminishing the amplification of receptor mediated activation of the adenylate cyclase coupled to the G/F protein.

The functional state of G/F binding protein also influences the binding characteristics of the transmitter recognition site, this binding is down-regulated when the G/F protein binds GTP (Ross and Gilman, 1980). Since the GTPase activity is the effector in regulating the G/F protein, it is important to study the modalities of GTPase regulation. Some evidence indirectly supports the view that the G/F protein and, perhaps, other proteins functioning as receptor coupler devices

(Costa *et al.*, 1977; Costa, 1980) located in postsynaptic membranes, function as a part of the supramolecular structure of the receptor by harmonising receptor amplification to some properties of the postsynaptic membranes. Membrane polarity and resting potential may be factors that regulate the coupler function; for instance, the GTPase activity regulating G/F proteins might be modulated by the transmembrane potential and, therefore, the receptor response might be regulated by the degree of depolarisation or hyperpolarisation; two membrane characteristics that are eminently related to neuronal activity.

## REGULATION OF THE INTERACTIONS BETWEEN G/F COUPLER PROTEIN AND ADENYLATE CYCLASE BY TWO RECEPTORS FOR NEUROTRANS-MITTERS LOCATED IN THE SAME MEMBRANE

Before considering the co-transmitter model as it applies to synaptic mechanisms, it may be important to study how the gain of the activation of adenylate cyclase linked to a G/F protein can be modulated by neurotransmitter receptors located in a membrane that lacks innervation. Such an example can be found in the mammotrophs of pituitary where a non-innervated dopamine (DA) receptor (DA2) modulates the secretion of prolactin (MacLeod, 1976) and the adenylate cyclase activation elicited by the binding of vasoactive intestinal peptide (VIP) (Borghi *et al.*, 1979) to specific receptors (Onali *et al.*, 1981). It is important to note that the activation of VIP receptors elicits a prolactin secretion from mammotroph cells (Enjalbert *et al.*, 1980*a*), whereas the activation of DA2 receptors inhibits the prolactin secretion and the adenylate cyclase activity stimulated by VIP but fails to change the basal rate of adenylate cyclase activity or prolactin secretion (Onali *et al.*, 1981).

The pituitary recognition sites for DA have been termed DA2 to differentiate them from other DA recognition sites (DA1), located in the membranes of certain brain neurones and parathyroid cells. These DA1 recognition sites are directly coupled to adenylate cyclase while DA2 sites of pituitary, which were formerly considered completely dissociated from adenylate cyclase, seem to specifically inhibit the VIP-dependent stimulation of the enzyme (Onali *et al.*, 1981; Cote *et al.*, 1981). Occupancy of DA2 receptors fails to change the stimulation of the pituitary cyclase by prostaglandin (Onali *et al.*, 1981). This cylase stimulation is not associated with prolactin secretion and, because of this, the specificity of the subclass of the DA2 recognition sites that are negatively coupled to the cyclase are emphasised.

Recently, VIP, a polypeptide isolated from porcine duodenum (Said and Mutt, 1970) has been included among the endogenous hypothalamic releasing factors because when injected into male rats, it increases the plasma prolactin content (Enjalbert *et al.*, 1980*b*). *In vitro*, VIP activates pituitary adenylate cyclase and stimulates prolactin secretion selectively. Because of these considerations the VIP-sensitive adenylate cyclase was used as a model to study whether the inhibition of prolactin secretion from mammotrophs caused by DA results from the coupling of the DA2 recognition sites with adenylate cyclase. The adenylate cyclase of mammotrophs is stimulated by VIP in a concentration dependent manner, a concentration of $10^{-7}$M of VIP causes half-maximal activation (Onali *et al.*, 1981). DA in a concentration of $10^{-5}$M fails to change the basal adenylate cyclase activity, but it blocks or curtails the adenylate cyclase stimulation by various doses of VIP. The inhibitory action of DA on the VIP stimulated cyclase occurs without a lag phase and remains constant for about 15 minutes (Onali *et al.*, 1981).

Kinetically, the activation of DA2 receptors decreases primarily the maximal velocity of the adenylate cyclase activation by VIP, but it changes the apparent affinity of VIP for the recognition sites only slightly; hence, the DA inhibition of the adenylate cyclase activation by VIP could be considered noncompetitive. A pharmacological study of the characteristics of the DA2 receptors of mammotrophs was performed using pituitary cell membranes, a wide spectrum of DA2 and DA1 receptor agonists, and as an index of the response, the increase in cyclic AMP formation (Onali *et al.*, 1981). From this study, it was concluded that the inhibitory action of DA was not mimicked by ergot alkaloids endowed with high potency on DA2 recognition sites, such as lisuride and ergotril; hence, a DA2 receptor of mammotroph lacks a high affinity for ergot alkaloid derivatives (Onali *et al.*, 1981). At a concentration of $10^{-6}$M, a number of neuroleptics that block DA1 and DA2 receptors fail to change the basal activity of adenylate cyclase or the VIP stimulation of the enzyme but severely curtail the inhibition of VIP stimulation by DA in a dose related fashion. This action is stereoselective and is shared by (-)-sulpuride which selectively inhibits DA2 receptors (Trabucchi *et al.*, 1975).

Guanine nucleotides and the G/F protein that specifically bind these nucleotides play an important role in regulating the stimulation of adenylate cyclase by VIP (table 2.1) located in the membrane of mammotrophs. To investigate whether this regulatory protein was mediating the DA inhibition Onali *et al.* (1981) tested the effect of GTP on this inhibition. In the presence of $10^{-7}$ M GTP, DA was completely ineffective in inhibiting even a slight stimulation of

Table 2.1  GTP dependency of the VIP stimulation of rat anterior pituitary adenylate cyclase and of its inhibition by DA

| Addition | CyclicAMP formed basal ($-$ GTP) = 100 | | |
| --- | --- | --- | --- |
| | $-$ GTP | + GTP $10^{-7}$M | + GTP $10^{-5}$M |
| Basal | 100 | 140 | 341 |
| VIP $10^{-7}$M (A) | 186 | 421 | 1256 |
| Dopamine $10^{-5}$M (B) | 108 | 149 | 327 |
| A + B | 186 | 460 | 882 |

From Onali *et al.* (1981).

adenylate cyclase by VIP. Only when the concentration of GTP was raised to $10^{-5}$ M could the DA inhibition be detected (table 2.1). These results indicate that the cyclase inhibition by DA depends on the presence of GTP. One can surmise that the saturation of the G/F protein binding sites with GTP is important for the activation of adenylate cyclase by VIP while the saturation of the GDP binding sites located in the same G/F protein are important to express the inhibition of the VIP stimulation by DA.

Experiments in which the activity of DA was studied in the presence of GTP and in the presence of a non-hydrolysable GTP analogue show that DA inhibition is operative only in the presence of GTP (Onali *et al.*, 1981). This suggests that DA inhibition of VIP-stimulated adenylate cyclase requires a molecular form of GTP that can be hydrolysed, and indicates that the GDP binding to the G/F protein may be operative in mediating the inhibition by DA. As the hydrolysis of GTP is necessary for the DA inhibition to occur, one can propose that DA may accelerate GTP hydrolysis; therefore, it increases the amount of GDP formed favouring the persistance of the G/F protein configuration resulting from GDP binding which limits the coupling function of the G/F protein and subsequently reduces the VIP activation of adenylate cyclase.

In conclusion, these experiments exemplify that the putative transmitter, DA, may function as a cotransmitter. By acting on the coupler, it can set the gain of a receptor-linked transducer function activated by VIP, a polypeptide, which in this case, functions as the primary transmitter because it initiates the adenylate cyclase activation that causes the secretion of prolactin.

## INDEPENDENCE OF TWO RECEPTOR FUNCTIONS TRANSDUCED BY GUANYLATE CYCLASE AND LOCATED IN THE SAME MEMBRANE

The interaction of two receptors in regulating an adenylate cyclase that produces a given response as discussed above, raises the question of whether a similar interaction occurs always among receptors that are located in the same membrane and express their function by way of the same transducer system. To clarify this issue, $N_4TG_1$ neuroblastoma was used; this is a 6-thioguanine-resistant mutant derived from the N4 neuroblastoma clone (Gwynn and Costa, 1982), whose membrane contains recognition sites for acetylcholine, histamine and opioid, all these recognition sites being linked to guanylate cylase. The addition of opiate receptor agonists causes a rapid dose-related elevation of the cyclic GMP content in the $N_4TG_1$ neuroblastoma cell. This response shows pharmacological specificity and desensitisation. Cells completely desensitised showed no loss of high affinity recognition sites for opioids. To gain insight into the possible mechanisms underlying receptor interactions, we have examined whether cross-desensitisation develops between opioids and other receptor agonists which like opioids elevate the cyclic GMP content of $N_4TG_1$ cells.

No cross-desensitisation was observed between opioids, histamine and carbachol in the transmitter-mediated elevation of cyclic GMP. This finding indicates that the interaction between VIP and DA receptors that are located in the same membrane and use the same transducer, expresses a specialised type of inter-action and does not represent a common feature of all receptors that are con-tiguous and express their function through the same transducer.

## RECEPTORS INNERVATED BY AXON TERMINALS RELEASING TWO PUTATIVE NEUROMODULATORS

No definite information is available on the fine structure of the subcellular storage sites for a putative co-transmitter coexisting in the same axon terminals with a putative primary transmitter. In cholinergic neurones innervating salivary or other exocrine glands, in which VIP coexists with acetylcholine (ACh), it has been reported (Lundberg *et al.*, 1981) that acetylcholine is located in small clear vesicles, VIP resides in the large dense cored vesicles. In these neurones, VIP is synthesised in the karyoplasm, from there it travels to the nerve terminals by a facilitated axonal transport. VIP travels while stored in vesicles and moves at a speed of $9 \text{ m h}^{-1}$.

Usually, the large densed core granules that store neuropeptides contain pre-cursors and enzymes for the degradation of these precursors into those molecular forms of the neuropeptides that are optimal for the putative neurotransmitter function (Pickering *et al.*, 1975). However, the location of the primary trans-mitter in a different vesicle from that which stores the co-transmitter cannot be taken as a general rule; in fact, as reported by Viveros and Wilson (chapter 5), the enkephalins (Costa *et al.*, 1979) and catecholamines may coexist in the same granules of chromaffin cells. The question then arises: can nerve impulses selectively release transmitter or co-transmitter when the two neuromodulators are stored in the same vesicle?

To answer this question, we have directly measured the release of catechol-amines and opiate peptides into the blood effluent from adrenal medulla of anesthetised dogs during electrical stimulation of the distal part of a transected splanchnic nerve (Hanbauer *et al.*, 1982; Govoni *et al.*, 1981). By using stimuli of 10 V in which the frequency of nerve stimulation was increased step wise from 0.5 to 6 Hz, it was found that 1 Hz was about the threshold stimulus for the release of both opiates and catecholamines. The release increased progressively from 1 to 6 Hz and approached maximal rates at a frequency of about 5 Hz. These experiments show that if there is a mechanism that recruits selectively the release of primary transmitter (catecholamines) or co-transmitter (enke-phalins), such a mechanism does not seem to depend on the frequency of the stimulation (Hanbauer *et al.*, 1982). Although the stimulation of the splanchnic nerve and the assay of the blood effluent from the dog adrenal failed to help us in reaching a better understanding of how and whether poly-peptides or catecholamines can be preferentially released from the adrenal medulla by nerve impulses, by using this preparation, we could show that splanchnic nerve stimulation can release *in vivo* from chromaffin cells high and low molecular weight peptides endowed with cross-immunoreactivity against enkephalins (Govoni *et al.*, 1981; Hanbauer *et al.*, 1982).

In order to study whether these peptides elicit cardiocirculatory responses we have used reserpine-treated dogs with cannulated lumbar vein (Hanbauer *et al.*, 1982). In these dogs splanchnic nerve stimulation releases little or no catecholamines but the amount of opiate peptides released is normal. Using such a preparation one is in the position to study whether opiate peptides released by splanchnic nerve stimulation affect the blood pressure of dogs. Whereas in normal dogs the stimulation of the splanchnic nerve causes hypertension, in reserpine-treated dogs, it causes a hypotension that is reversed by naloxone. From these data, one could speculate that the opiate peptides coexisting in the same granule with catecholamines are still present in reserpine-treated dogs, although catecholamines are depleted.

These peptides are released by nerve stimulation and they act on specific sites to elicit a decrease in vascular tone, this action is blocked by naloxone. The tone of the cardiovascular system seems to be modified by an action of these peptides on opiate-like receptors. Thus, one could suggest that adrenal medulla represents an important model to study the peripheral action of opiate peptides and the physiological role of these cotransmitters in the modulation of factors regulating vascular tone, such as catecholamines. The importance of medullary opiate peptides in cardiovascular function seems to be emphasised by studies of spontaneously hypertensive rats (Wistar-Kyoto). In these rats, the content of opiate peptides in adrenal medulla is decreased early in life, before the onset of the spontaneous hypertension (Di Giulio *et al.*, 1979).

## ACETYCHOLINE AND OPIATE RECEPTOR INTERACTIONS IN THE MEMBRANE OF CHROMAFFIN CELLS

Enkephalin-like peptides seem to coexist with ACh in many axons such as the cholinergic splanchnic axons innervating the chromaffin cells of adrenal medulla (Schultzberg *et al.*, 1978). If these enkephalin-like peptides were to act as co-transmitters (Costa *et al.*, 1980) or neuromodulators of ACh, which in these axons is considered a classic primary transmitter, the following should be expected: (1) chromaffin cells should contain opiate recognition sites; (2) the action of ACh should be modified by opiates; (3) this modification should correlate with the modifications in the ACh binding. The coupling and transducer systems operated by ACh, the primary transmitter, may also be modified by opiates. Using primary cultures of medullary chromaffin cells, these three aspects of the modulatory role of opiates on cholinergic transmission have been studied.

Adrenal homogenates contain high affinity recognition sites for opiates (Chavkin *et al.*, 1979). These sites are located on the chromaffin cell membranes and possess a certain degree of stereoselectivity (Saiani and Guidotti, 1982), but their pharmacological profile cannot be classified in any of the four categories of opiate receptors ($\mu$, $\delta$, K and 6), (Robson and Kosterlitz, 1979; Adler, 1981). We should bear in mind that this classification was initiated to characterise opiate receptor agonists when morphine analogues were considered drugs; at that time no consideration was given to the function of opiate receptors and to their relationship to other transmitter functions. It is not surprising, therefore, that we find that there are opiate receptors that do not qualify as typical binding sites for the four categories of opiate drugs. This peculiarity would be particularly appropriate for receptors that (similarly to those of the adrenal) are almost insensitive to morphine, which when the classification was initiated was the drug of choice to study opiate receptors. We are aware of only a single attempt made to classify opiate receptors according to functional characteristics.

Viewing opiate receptors as the modulatory sites for the amplication of the response of primary transmitter receptors, it was proposed that there are two classes of opiate receptors, type A or B, modulating catecholamines and ACh receptors, respectively (Knoll, 1977). We believe that a such a classification has some merit and, albeit too restrictive, can be taken as a basis for further experimentation. The present experiments are a step in this direction. Saiani and Guidotti (1982) have shown that the opiate receptor of adrenal medulla is located in the membrane of bovine chromaffin cells; it has a high affinity for etorphine, $\beta$-endorphin and diprenorphin; and it seems to be coupled with the nicotinic receptor of chromaffin cells (Kumakura *et al.*, 1980). Since this receptor can be distinguished from the classic $\mu$, $\delta$, 6 and K receptors, it may qualify for a special type of functional classification.

The data presented in table 2.2 show that the displacement of [³H]-etorphine from chromaffin cell receptor as a Ki for beta-endorphin that is 3 to 20 times smaller than that for classic agonists of the $\mu$, $\delta$, 6 and K classes. As shown, the ranking order of the potency of various opiates to inhibit the release of catechol-

Table 2.2   $K_i$ for displacement of [³H]-etorphine binding and $IC_{30}$ for antagonism of catecholamine release elicited by ACh* in cultured chromaffin cells

| Opiate receptor agonist | $K_i$ (nM) | $IC_{30}$ ($\mu$M) |
|---|---|---|
| Etorphine | 1 | 0.2 |
| $\beta$-endorphin | 15 | 0.3 |
| (D-Ala²-Me Phe, Met(O)⁵01)-enkephalin | 30 | 0.6 |
| N-allylnormetazocine (6) | 45 | 10 |
| Ethylketazocine (K) | 100 | 60 |
| D-Ala²-D-Leu⁵-enkephalin ($\delta$) | 400 | 80 |
| Morphine ($\mu$) | 300 | 200 |

*ACh $5 \times 10^6$ M and $10^6$ cells.
From Saiani and Guidotti (1982), modified.

amines by ACh is in keeping with their ranking order for the displacement of [$^3$H]-etorphine. Thus, there is evidence of a ranking order and a chemical specificity of opiate ligands linked to their capacity to inhibit the release of catecholamines elicited by ACh. It should be noted that although the ranking order is the same, every compound is about 100-fold more potent in displacing [$^3$H]-etorphine than in antagonising the catecholamine depletion caused by ACh. Although we cannot explain the reason for this difference, it has been pointed out (Saiani and Guidotti, 1982) that it is almost impossible to replicate the same conditions when one measures function and binding capacity of the recognition site for a neurotransmitter, and these difficulties may account for part of the discrepancy. In fact, there are a number of factors operative in maximising the binding of a ligand to its recognition site but these factors do not affect to the same extent the gain of receptor responsiveness. One should also keep in mind that as shown by Shultzberg *et al.* (1978) not every splanchnic axon contains opiate peptides; because the $B_{max}$ of opiate receptors is higher than that of ACh receptors, there may be a number of opiate receptors involved in other actions of chromaffin cells, some of which may be opposing the antisecretory activity toward the ACh-induced release of catecholamine.

A possible reason for the abnormal behaviour of the opiate receptor located in the membranes of chromaffin cells is that it selectively responds to either blood-borne β-endorphin or to a specific opiate peptide of a yet unknown structure which is stored in the splanchnic nerve. In fact, ten to twelve Met-enkephalin-containing polypeptides have been isolated from acid extracts of bovine adrenal medulla ranging from about 0.5 to 12 kilodaltons (Gubler *et al.*, 1982). Many have been completely sequenced and others partially so. These peptides were suggested to be the intermediates in the biosynthetic pathway of enkephalin and to be metabolites of proenkephalin (Gubler *et al.*, 1982). So far, this protein has not been purified to homogeneity; however, it has been shown to be about 40 to 50 kilodaltons in size and to contain one Leu- and six or seven Met-enkephalin sequences. The information on the primary structure of most of the proenkephalin molecules has been deduced from nucleotide sequences of cDNA clones (Gubler *et al.*, 1982).

It is debatable whether all the proenkephalin fragments isolated from adrenal medulla (Jones *et al.*, 1982; Yang *et al.*, 1980) express steps in the pathway for the biosynthesis of Met[5]-and Leu[5]-enkephalin; perhaps, some of these peptides are not enkephalin precursors but have a function of their own. In fact, stimulation of the splanchnic nerve causes the release of high molecular weight enkephalin-like immunoreactivity (Hanbauer *et al.*, 1982). We also know that there are heptapeptides which are enkephalins with the carboxyl terminus extended, that are known to have much greater biological activity than the enkephalins. These are dynorphin, α-neoendorphin and the heptapeptide, Met[5]-enkephalin-Arg[6]-Phe[7].

Although the origin of the heptapeptide is still undetermined, it seems that chromaffin cells in adrenal and brain neurones store this heptapeptide and high molecular weight heptapeptide-like activity, in addition to proenkephalin (Yang and Costa, 1982). Dynorphin and α-neoendorphin are likely to be products of the metabolism of precursors different from proenkephalin; in fact, they show no apparent homology with any region of the proenkephalin that has been so far analysed. Finally, β-endorphin, which is synthesised from pro-opiocortin represents a possible agonist for the opiate receptors of the medulla and it is secreted from anterior pituitary gland. Like the heptapeptide, β-endorphin also has a greater biological activity than $Met^5$-enkephalin. Indeed, the carboxyl extensions that distinguish β-endorphin, the heptapeptide, and other medullary peptides may stabilise these polypeptides and target them for specific receptors.

To probe the molecular nature of the interaction between ACh and opiate receptors, we have used α-bungarotoxin, which is known to be a high affinity ligand for nicotinic receptors in the neuromuscular cholinergic synapse (Kumakura *et al.*, 1981). It is debatable whether this compound is a good antagonist of the nicotinic receptors present in brain, ganglia and in the membrane of chromaffin cells. We have found that the compound is a good ligand and a potent antagonist of the ACh-induced release of catecholamines from chromaffin cells (Saiani *et al.*, 1982). In addition, we have found that in the presence of opiate agonists the binding of α-bungarotoxin to the membranes of cells of adrenal medulla is impaired because of a reduction in the $B_{max}$; the kinetics of this interaction suggest that occupancy of the opiate receptors located on the membrane of chromaffin cells allosterically decreases the number of ACh recognition sites that are available. As all the preparations of α-bungarotoxin contain impurities, we are presently ascertaining whether some of the above mentioned interactions between α-bungarotoxin and ACh receptors that function in the membrane of chromaffin cells can be attributed to the contaminants that are present.

## REGULATION OF GABAERGIC SYNAPSES

Like many other putative neurotransmitters, γ-aminobutyric acid (GABA) also coexists in the same axon with neuropeptide(s) that in the periphery function as neuromodulators. For instance, it is known that about 25 per cent of the cerebellar Purkinje cells that contain glutamic acid decarboxylase (the specific maker of GABAergic synapses) also contain motilin-like immunoreactivity (Chan-Palay *et al.*, 1982; see also Chan-Palay, chapter one). This evidence for the coexistence of two neuromodulators in the GABAergic axons is associated with the presence in GABAergic synapses (Mohler *et al.*, 1980; 1981) of specific recognition sites which are presumed to bind an endogenous ligand and are marked by benzodiazepines (Braestrup and Squires, 1978; Mohler and Okada, 1977). Since occupancy of the benzodiazepine recognition sites can bring about either potentiation (Costa and Guidotti, 1979; Haefely *et al.*, 1979) or inhibition of GABAergic synaptic function (Cowen *et al.*, 1981; Tenen and Hirsch, 1980), depending on the ligand used, one can surmise that benzodiazepines mark a recognition site for an endogenous cotransmitter operative in GABAergic transmission (Costa *et al.*, 1975; Costa *et al.*, 1978). Thus, the regulation of the $Cl^-$ gate opening, which is the transducer function coupled with GABAergic transmission, is amplified or restricted according to the chemical nature of the ligand occupying the so-called benzodiazepine recognition site. Taking the facilitation of GABA-ergic synapses caused by benzodiazepines as an index, and assuming that benzo-diazepines antagonise the action of a physiological ligand, we can surmise that the physiological agonist of the benzodiazepine recognition site acts by reducing the $B_{max}$ for GABA binding of specific high affinity recognition sites (Massotti *et al.*, 1981a;b).

Direct studies have been carried out to verify such and other similar inter-actions between GABA and benzodiazepine recognition sites (Tallman *et al.*, 1978; Guidotti *et al.*, 1978a;b), and the results obtained are summarised in table 2.3. As shown, the stimulation of GABA recognition sites by agonists

Table 2.3   Modulation of GABA and benzodiazepine (BZD) recognition sites by specific ligands

| Kinetic parameter | Modulation of BZD by GABA | Modulation of $\beta$-carboline binding by GABA | Modulation of GABA binding by BZD |
|---|---|---|---|
| $B_{max}$ | Unchanged | Unchanged | Increased |
| KD | Decreased | Increased | Unchanged |

From Tallman *et al.* (1978), Guidotti *et al.*, 1978a,b), and Braestrup and Nielsen (1981).

facilitates the binding of benzodiazepines but disfacilitates the binding of other high affinity ligands of benzodiazepine recognition sites, such as the $\beta$-carboline derivatives (Braestrup and Nielsen, 1981). Since in several aspects, $\beta$-carboline derivatives act like the endogenous ligand, one can surmise that GABA decreases the binding of the endogenous ligand to its recognition site. In contrast, the occupancy of the benzodiazepine recognition site by a benzodiazepine derivative increases the number of binding sites for GABA (Tallman *et al.*, 1978; Baraldi *et al.*, 1979), a decrease in GABA binding occurring when the benzodiazepine recognition sites are occupied by $\beta$-carboline derivatives (Costa, unpublished observations). Presumably, these changes in the characteristics of the recognition sites for the various ligands that modulate GABAergic synapses are due to con-formational changes in the recognition sites.

That conformational changes can occur in GABA recognition sites could be inferred from a report by Enna and Snyder (1977) showing that crude synaptic membranes contain two populations of recognition sites with different affinities for GABA. Moreover, these authors have shown that the kinetic properties of a certain proportion of GABA recognition sites located in crude synaptic mem-brane preparations can change according to the procedure used to prepare the membranes and the amounts of endogenous modulators of GABA binding that remain associated with the postsynaptic membranes. Massotti *et al.*, (1981a;b), Guidotti *et al.*, (1978a), Costa *et al.* (1978) and Toffano *et al.* (1978) have confirmed Enna and Snyder's report (1977) and have studied whether the two populations of GABA recognition sites that were defined by these studies have different physiological significance. Investigations of GABA recognition sites present in the substantia nigra of rats have shown that the high affinity GABA recognition sites increase following denervation (Guidotti *et al.*, 1979). Perhaps the gain in the transduction operated by GABA recognition sites is modulated by changing the ratio between the number of high and low affinity binding sites for GABA.

Current evidence suggests that in GABAergic synapses there may be endogenous modulators, which are located in postsynaptic membranes and harmonise the number of high affinity binding sites for GABA with the changes in the characteristics of the postsynaptic membranes (Costa *et al.*, 1978; Costa and Guidotti, 1979). One such regulatory substance could be the protein termed GABA-modulin (Baraldi *et al.*, 1979), which has been found in membranes of neuroblastoma cells containing GABA receptors. This will be discussed later in this chapter.

### Benzodiazepine and GABAergic transmission

Data supporting the idea that benzodiazepines specifically enhance GABAergic transmission have been obtained in experiments concerned with (1) presynaptic inhibition in the spinal cord; (2) pre- and postsynaptic inhibition in the dorsal column nuclei; (3) recurrent inhibition in the hippocampus, hypothalamus, cerebral and cerebellar cortex; and (4) synaptic inhibition produced by directly stimulating long axons of GABAergic projection pathways (Haefely *et al.*, 1981). It must be specified that benzodiazepines enhance GABAergic transmission in long axons only when the GABAergic transmission is partially impaired either by depletion of GABA or by partial inhibition of GABA receptors. Although the facilitating action on GABA transmission by benzodiazepines is no longer in doubt (Costa *et al.*, 1975), present efforts are directed at understanding the molecular mechanisms that are operative. One of the mechanisms investigated first was whether this facilitation depended on an action of GABA on cyclic nucleotide content.

Several investigators have found that benzodiazepines increase cyclic AMP content in various preparations but the action of these drugs occurs at doses several orders of magnitude greater than those operative in the mediation of the central actions of benzodiazepines (Haefely *et al.*, 1981). Benzodiazepines, given in therapeutic doses, consistently lower the cerebellar cyclic GMP content, and their relative potency seems to be related to their potency as sedatives and anxiolytics (Biggio *et al.*, 1977a;b). This lowering of cyclic GMP content by the benzodiazepines occurs only in the cerebellum, depends on the GABA content, and is believed to reflect an action of benzodiazepines on the balance between excitatory (glutamate) and inhibitory (GABAergic) inputs (Biggio *et al.*, 1977a). In agreement with this interpretation, the action of benzodiazepines on cerebellar cyclic GMP content could be mimicked by GABA mimetics injected into the cerebellar cortex (Biggio *et al.*, 1977a). Immunocytochemical studies have shown that cyclic GMP is also located in neuroglial cells and that the relationship between glutamatergic transmission and the increases in cyclic GMP content may be more complicated than anticipated when it was believed that glutamate was the single mediator operative in increasing cyclic GMP content (Haefely *et al.*, 1981).

## Benzodiazepine recognition sites

The presence of specific and high affinity binding sites for benzodiazepines was first demonstrated in crude synaptic membrane of CNS prepared from various species, including man (Mohler and Okada, 1977; Braestrup and Squires, 1978; Nielsen *et al.*, 1978; Speth *et al.*, 1978). The binding characteristics and relative affinity of the various benzodiazepines are compatible with the view that these binding sites mediate the specific pharmacological effects of benzodiazepines (see Haefely *et al.*, 1981). Enantiomers of benzodiazepines with a chirality centre in position 3 differ in their potency in displacing [$^3$H]-flunitrazepam from specific binding sites, this potency agrees with the different potencies in the pharmacological activity of the stereoisomers.

The radioautographic localisation of the benzodiazepine recognition sites has been made possible by the covalent bonding of [$^3$H]-flunitrazepam with specific recognition sites that occur following exposure to ultraviolet light (Mohler *et al.*, 1980). By combining this technique with electromicroscopic autoradiography, it has been possible to visualise the fine structure of the sites where benzodiazepines bind. Rats were injected intravenously with [$^3$H]-flunitrazepam and some time after, their brain areas were dissected and illuminated *in vitro* with near ultraviolet light to cause the covalent binding of the radioactive probe. Successive electromicroscopic studies indicated that this radioactive ligand was selectively bound to regions of synaptic contacts (Mohler *et al.*, 1981). These were characterised as part of GABAergic synapses by combining radioautography to locate [$^3$H]-flunitrazepam with immunohistochemical detection of glutamic acid decarboxylase, the neurochemical marker for GABAergic axons.

These findings clearly indicate that the location of benzodiazepine recognition sites resides in GABAergic synapses; however, there are still some doubts on whether all the benzodiazepine recognition sites are located on the GABAergic synapses; some of them could well be on the GABAergic axons or on other receptors (Braestrup and Nielsen, 1980). There was no indication that benzodiazepines bind covalently to glial cells.

One method of testing whether a ligand binds to a recognition site as an agonist is to investigate whether on chronic administration, it causes down regu-

lation of the recognition site. Braestrup *et al.* (1979) treated rats for 8 weeks
with extremely high daily doses of diazepam (90 mg/kg); there were no signs
of down regulation of the benzodiazepine recognition site, suggesting that as
for opiates, benzodiazepine recognition sites also do not show down regulation.
Although slight changes in $B_{max}$ (15 per cent) were detected after benzodiazepines 60 to 150 mg/kg daily for 7 to 10 d, one could generalise that benzodiazepines do not down regulate their recognition site and presumably bind as
antagonists (Haefely *et al.*, 1981). Hence, if the binding of benzodiazepines to
these recognition sites located in GABAergic synapses relieves anxiety the
binding of endogenous agonists to the benzodiazepine recognition site may
facilitate the onset of anxiety. It could be debated that a certain level of anxiety
has physiological importance and has a survival value.

### Endogenous ligands for benzodiazepine recognition sites

The concept that drugs which modify brain function and bind with high affinity
to selective sites act as exogenous competitors for endogenous ligands at functional receptors lead various investigators to search for endogenous ligands for
benzodiazepine recognition sites. Mohler *et al.* (1979), while performing a
chromatographic separation of various components present in brain extracts,
found three peaks which inhibited [³H]-diazepam binding. When this material
was identified, it was found to contain derivatives of inosine, hypoxanthine, and
nicotinamide. As their affinities for the benzodiazepine recognition site were
lower than those expected for an endogenous ligand, it was considered unlikely
that they would act as physiological ligands. In addition, systemic administration
of high doses of these compounds suggested that the only one that could be
regarded as a potential endogenous ligand of physiological relevance was nicotinamide. However, even this compound did not seem to possess the characteristics necessary to support its role as an endogenous ligand.

Other groups of investigators (Skolnick *et al.*, 1978; 1979*a;b;c*; Marangos
*et al.*, 1978; 1979*a*) have come to the conclusion that purine but not pyrimidine
derivatives could be considered as endogenous ligands for benzodiazepine
binding. However, after a number of pertinent experiments, it is now accepted
that purines also do not fulfill all the requirements for being endogenous ligands
of benzodiazepine recognition sites.

An endogenous compound that binds with high affinity to benzodiazepine
recognition sites has been isolated from human urine and was found to be the
ethyl ester of β-carboline-3-carboxylate (Nielsen *et al.*, 1979; 1981). A study of
the structure-activity relationship of chemical analogues of this β-carboline
derivative shows that the potency of various compounds changes drastically
with small structural variations (Nielsen *et al.*, 1981). The esters are all active in
antagonising [³H]-diazepam binding but the carboxylic derivative is not
(Marangos and Patel, 1981). Unfortunately, there are no esters of the carbolines

in tissues, suggesting that the active $\beta$-carboline derivative extracted from urine could be artifactual in nature.

A large molecular weight protein (40 to 70 kilodaltons) isolated from bovine brain by Collello *et al.* (1978), competitively displaces [$^3$H]-diazepam from its specific binding site and was termed benzodiazepine competitive factor I. Competitive inhibitory activity was found in fractions containing entities between 1 and 2 kilodaltons and this fraction was termed benzodiazepine competitive factor II. Factor I was five times more potent than factor II; it was heat stable, but destroyed with trypsin digestion, suggesting a polypeptide nature. Karobath *et al.* (1978; 1979) have described a diazepam binding inhibitory factor (DIF) in partially purified acetone extracts of brain. The highest levels of DIF were found in skeletal muscle and myocardium of rats while the brain of rats, mice, cows and man contained less activity. Tissues within the brain, cortex, and hippocampus, were richest in DIF.

Woolf and Nixon (1981), using as a reference bioassay the displacement of [$^3$H]-diazepam band to rat synaptosomes and working with extracts of rat bile ducts, have isolated and characterised a protein that at low concentrations competitively inhibits [$^3$H]-diazepam binding to specific CNS recognition sites. This protein was termed nephentin, has a molecular weight of 16 kilodaltons, is cationic at neutral $pH$ and has a good thermal stability. The $K_i$ for [$^3$H]-diazepam displacement is $4.6 \times 10^{-8}$ M. Since its biological activity is stable after tryptic digestion, if the preparation possessed a high degree of purity, it is possible that a fragment generated by trypsinisation possesses the same activity as nephentin. Thus, one might speculate that the activity present in the brain could be due to a nephentin fragment, and that the large nephentin fragment present in the periphery could somehow be the ligand for the peripheral benzodiazepine receptors. Histoimmunofluorescence experiments, carried out using an antibody to a partially purified preparation of nephentin, revealed the presence of nephentin-like immunofluorescence in neurones of deep cortical layers of rat brain.

In a preceding report, we inferred that a partially purified preparation of a brain basic protein, termed GABA-modulin, displaced [$^3$H]-diazepam competitively and therefore could function as an endogenous agonist of benzodiazepine binding sites (Guidotti *et al.*, 1978*b*). However, successive studies clarified that this preparation of GABA-modulin contained an impurity that was responsible for the competitive displacement of [$^3$H]-diazepam from its binding site in crude synaptic membrane preparations. This impurity can be eliminated from GABA-modulin preparations following their precipitation with 40 to 60 per cent ammonium sulphate. The impurity was purified to homogeneity with column chromatography, reverse phase HPLC and polyacrylamide gel electrophoresis (Costa *et al.*, 1982). It is present in brain but not in liver or spleen. It has a molecular weight of 9.5 kilodaltons and displaces [$^3$H]-flunitrazepam with a $K_i$ in the $\mu$M range. The data of table 2.4 summarise the properties of this endogenous ligand for the benzodiazepine recognition site.

Table 2.4   Characteristics of an endogenous putative
ligand for diazepam binding sites

| | |
|---|---|
| Molecular weight | ~ 9500 |
| Thermostability | Yes |
| Resistance to tryptic digestion (2 h at 37°C) | No |
| Resistance to pronase digestion (2 h at 37°C) | No |
| $K_i$ for competitive inhibition of [$^3$H]-diazepam binding | 0.5 $\mu$M |
| Inhibitor of GABA binding | No |
| Binds GABA | No |
| Binds [$^3$H]-diazepam | No |
| Degradation by phospholipase (A, B, C) | No |
| Dialysable | No |
| N-terminal free | No |
| Carboxyterminal free | Yes |
| Precipitated by $(NH_4)_2SO_4$ | No |

From Costa *et al.* (1982), modified.

As shown in table 2.4, the endogenous ligand is thermostable, its biological activity is destroyed by trypsin and pronase digestion, and it inhibits competitively the specific binding of [$^3$H]-flunitrazepam to crude synaptic membranes without altering [$^3$H]-GABA binding. As the endogenous peptide also fails to bind diazepam or flunitrazepam or GABA, it is important now to know whether it is located in GABA neurones and whether it is co-released with GABA, by depolarisation. It remains to be understood how the occupancy of the benzodiazepine recognition sites brings about those conformational changes in GABA recognition sites which we assume are operative in causing the increase in the binding capacity of this site. The binding characteristics of this endogenous ligand resemble those of a β-choline derivative (Braestrup and Nielsen, 1981) with regard to preferential action in certain brain structures and decrease affinity binding in presence of GABA (Costa *et al.*, 1981).

We have carried out preliminary experiments on the biological activity of this endogenous ligand, by injecting this peptide intraventricularly into rats and comparing its activity with that of benzodiazepines in a conflict situation, electric shock, or inhibition of drinking in thirsty rats. In this test, benzodiazepines elicit punishment behaviour while the endogenous polypeptide that displaces benzodiazepines from their specific binding site does not. Actually, it seems that it may antagonise the punishment behaviour elicited by benzodiazepines. From the amino acid composition of this endogenous ligand for the benzodiazepine binding site shown in table 2.5, we know that the amino terminus is blocked.

Table 2.5 Amino acid composition of
an endogenous putative ligand
for diazepam binding purified
from rat brain

| Amino acid | Number of residues |
|---|---|
| Lys | 19 |
| His | 3 |
| Arg | 3 |
| Asx | 10 |
| Thr | 7 |
| Ser | 10 |
| Glx | 12 |
| Pro | 3 |
| Gly | 6 |
| Ala | 8 |
| Cys | 0 |
| Val | 4 |
| Met | 2 |
| Ile | 3 |
| Leu | 7 |
| Tyr | 4 |
| Phe | 3 |
| Total | 104 |

Asx = Asp + Asn.
Glx = Glu + Gln.
TRP is destroyed in this analysis.

## Molecular changes in GABA receptor characteristics triggered by the occupancy of benzodiazepine recognition sites

An impressive amount of studies have been carried out in the past two years to determine how temperature, $pH$, ion, and various transmitters affect the benzodiazepine binding (see Haefely *et al.*, 1981). The information derived from these experiments has been structured to support the view that there are multiple forms of benzodiazepine receptors. It is interesting to note the obsession of those people interested in ligand binding to interpret a variability of binding to crude synaptic membrane preparations as evidence for the existence of multiple receptors. In the case of benzodiazepine receptors, this tendency complicates the issue prematurely because it not only creates the nomenclature of benzodiazepine receptors types I or II without a corresponding different function, but it also switches the focus from studies of molecular mechanisms to descriptive studies of binding.

Our studies of the molecular mechanisms involved in the action of benzodiazepines has suggested that the putative endogenous cotransmitter that regulates the receptors marked by the binding of benzodiazepines, down-regulates the high affinity binding sites for GABA by acting on a coupler device that links the GABA recognition sites with the chloride ion gate. Perhaps a brain protein which has been purified to homogeneity in our laboratory and termed GABA-modulin (see tables 2.6 and 2.7) functions as a coupler device (Guidotti *et al.*, 1982). Our current working hypothesis is that GABA-modulin is an integral

Table 2.6   Characteristics of GABA-modulin

| | |
|---|---|
| Molecular weight | 19000 |
| Thermostability | Moderate |
| Is the activity resistant to tryptic digestion 10 min at $30^{\circ}$C? | Yes |
| Is the activity resistant to tryptic digestion 1 h at $30^{\circ}$? | No |
| Is the activity resistant to thrombine digestion 2 h at $30^{\circ}$? | Yes |
| Non-competitive inhibitor of [$^3$H]-GABA binding | Yes |
| Inhibition of [$^3$H]-diazepam binding | No |
| Binds GABA or diazepam? | No |
| Dialysable | No |
| Phosphorylated by a protein kinase (cyclicAMP dependent) | Yes |
| Binds to synaptic membranes | Yes |
| N-terminus blocked by pyroglutamyl | Yes |
| Carboxyterminus free | Yes |
| GABA content | $< 1$ pmol/10 nmol |
| Phospholipid content | $< 10$ nmol/10 $\mu$mol |
| Precipitated by | $(NH_4)_2SO_4$ |

From Costa *et al.* (1982) modified.

protein of the membrane facing the GABAergic terminals which when coupled to the GABA recognition site, decreases its affinity for the endogenous ligand. As indicated in table 2.6, a mild digestion with trypsin does not decrease the activity, suggesting that some fragments of GABA-modulin could function as the effector in the down regulation of GABA binding. GABA-modulin can also be phosphorylated by cyclic AMP-dependent protein kinase, but we do not know the biological significance of such phosphorylation.

We are now exploring whether the tryptic formation of active fragments of GABA-modulin is regulated by phosphorylation and whether these are the molecular events that mediate the modulation of GABA recognition sites when the endogenous agonist occupies the recognition sites for benzodiazepines. Thus, GABA-modulin may be a sensing device located in the membrane of the post-synaptic cells innervated by GABAergic axons, that harmonises the responsiveness of GABA receptors to the value of the potential of the postsynaptic membrane and therefore ultimately harmonises GABA receptor function with the

Table 2.7   Amino acid composition of
GABA-modulin purified from
rat brain

| Amino acid | Number of residues |
|------------|:------------------:|
| Asx | 10 |
| Thr | 8 |
| Ser | 14 |
| Glx | 11 |
| Pro | 11 |
| Gly | 16 |
| Ala | 2 |
| Cys | 0 |
| Val | 4 |
| Met | 3 |
| Ile | 3 |
| Leu | 7 |
| Tyr | 2 |
| Phe | 6 |
| His | 7 |
| Lys | 9 |
| Arg | 17 |
| | 135 |

Asx = Asp + Asn.
Glx = Glu + Gln.
TRP is destroyed in this analysis.

activity of the postsynaptic cell in which the GABA receptor is located. It is important to note that in this harmonising action an important element is represented by the endogenous agonist of the benzodiazepine receptor which presumably is a secretory product of the GABAergic axon. Hence, the co-transmitter regulates GABA receptor as a feed forward inhibitor, whereas GABA-modulin regulates GABA receptor as a feedback inhibitor.

In preliminary experiments to determine whether a partially purified preparation of GABA-modulin was endowed with biological activity, we have injected this preparation into the ventricles of rats receiving isoniazid in doses that decreased the biosynthesis of GABA and therefore lowered GABA content. We observed that GABA-modulin increased the number of rats with recurrent convulsions from 5 to 100 per cent and the number of deaths elicited by isoniazid from 3 to 75 per cent. Indeed, this proconvulsant action indicates that GABA-modulin can change GABA-modulated responses. We are now investigating whether this proconvulsant action derives from GABA-modulin's ability to down-regulate GABA receptors *in vivo*. This pharmacological experiment suggests that GABA-modulin can change GABAergic transmission and encourages the continuation of the current line of investigation. Preliminary experiments on the binding of purified GABA-modulin labelled with $^{125}$I show a specific binding of GABA-modulin to crude synaptic membrane preparations. Thus, the results of *in vivo* studies suggest that it should be investigated whether, following the decrease in GABA content elicited by isoniazid, either the number of binding sites for GABA-modulin or the number of high affinity GABA recognition sites have changed.

## CONCLUSIONS

The preliminary evidence marshalled in this chapter supports the view that coexistence of two or more neuromodulators in the same axon can be associated with a new model of synaptic function, in which the responses elicited by each of the two modulators are integrated in the overall regulation of the synaptic response. Considering receptors as supramolecular units where function is determined by the participation of three basic elements (transmitter recognition site, coupler and transducer), we view one of the two synaptic modulators as the cotransmitter that sets the gain of the synaptic response and the other as the primary transmitter responsible for triggering the chain of events leading to the internalisation of the stimulus. This is initiated by the release of a chemical signal in the extracellular milieu, which by activating receptor function, transforms this extracellular signal into a metabolic signal that reaches specific intracellular receptors in the postsynaptic cells. Thus, the signal is internalised and transformed from a chemical into a metabolic signal. This transformation is operated by the transducer subunit of the receptor.

We know of two types of transducers: one of them operates by regulating the rates of specific ion fluxes across the membrane, the other activates specialised enzyme systems that produce metabolic second messengers inside the postsynaptic cell. The opening of the ion gates or the formation of second messengers operate with a variable gain which could be determined by the interaction of the cotransmitter with the coupling device. This device senses conditions in the postsynaptic membrane which vary as a result of activity of the cell, and reacts to the message of the cotransmitter by amplifying or reducing the intensity of the response triggered by the primary transmitter.

Viewing the transducer as the pivot unit in the internalisation of the stimulus, we can suggest that cotransmitters modulate receptor function according to information derived from activity in the innervating axon; the coupler system instead feedbacks into the transducer information derived from activity in the postsynaptic cell. Examples for an integrated response elicited by the transmitter and cotransmitter were given using non-innervated VIP receptors of pituitary and innervated cholinergic receptors of chromaffin cells. Moreover, this model was extended as a working model to study the molecular function operative in GABA transmission. In this synapse, the action of benzodiazepines is seen as that of a specific antagonist to an endogenous cotransmitter that down-regulates high-affinity recognition sites for GABA.

# REFERENCES

Adler, M. W. (1981). The *in vivo* differentiation of opiate receptors. *Life Sci.*, 28, 1543–1545

Baraldi, M., Guidotti, A., Schwartz, J. P. and Costa, E. (1979). GABA receptors in cloned cell lines: a model for study of benzodiazepine action at the molecular level. *Science*, 205, 821–823

Biggio, G., Brodie, B. B., Costa, E. and Guidotti, A. (1977a). Mechanism by which diazepam, muscimol, and other drugs change the content of cGMP in cerebellar cortex. *Proc. natn. Acad. Sci. U.S.A.*, 74, 3592–3596

Biggio, G., Costa, E. and Guidotti, A. (1977b). Pharmacologically-induced changes in the 3',5'-cyclic guanosine monophosphate content of rat cerebellar cortex: differences between apomorphine, haloperidol and harmaline. *J. Pharmac. exp. Ther.*, 200, 207–215

Borghi, C., Nicosia, S., Giachetti, A. and Said, S. I. (1979). Adenylate cyclase of rat pituitary gland: stimulation by vasoactive intestinal polypeptide (VIP). *FEBS Lett.*, 108, 403–406

Braestrup, C. and Nielsen, M. (1980). Multiple benzodiazepine receptors *Trends in Neuroscience*, 3, 301–303

Braestrup, C. and Nielsen, M. (1981). GABA reduces binding of $^3$H-methyl-beta-carboline-3-carboxylate to brain benzodiazepine receptors. *Nature London*, 294, 472–474

Braestrup, C., Nielsen, M. and Squires, F. (1979). No changes in benzodiazepine receptors after withdrawal from continuous treatment with lorazepam and diazepam. *Life Sci.*, 24, 347–350

Braestrup, C. and Squires, R. F. (1978). Benzodiazepine receptors in brain *Nature London*, 266, 732–734

Brownstein, M. J., Saavedra, J. M., Axelrod, J. and Carpenter, D. O. (1974). Coexistence of several putative neurotransmitters in single identified neurons of aplysia. *Proc. natn. Acad. Sci. U.S.A.*, 71, 4662–4665

Burnstock, G. (1980). Purinergic modulation of cholinergic transmission. *Gen. Pharmac.*, 11, 15–18

Burnstock, G. (1976). Do some nerve cells release more than one transmitter? *Neuroscience*, I, 239–248

Chan-Palay, V., Nilaver, G., Palay, S. L., Beinfeld, M. D., Zimmerman, E. A., Wu, J-Y. and O'Donohue, T. L. (1982). Chemical heterogeneity in cerebellar Purkinje cells: existence and coexistence of glutamic acid decarboxylase like and motilin like immunoreactivities. *Proc. natn. Acad. Sci. U.S.A.*, 78, 7787–7791

Chavkin, C., Cox, B. M. and Goldstein, A. (1979). Stereospecific opiate binding in bovine adrenal medulla. *Molec. Pharmac.*, 15, 751–753

Colello, G. D., Hockenbery, D. M., Bosman, H. B., Fuchs, S., Folkers, K. (1978). Competitive inhibition of benzodiazepine binding by fractions from porcine brain. *Proc. natn. Acad. Sci. U.S.A.*, 75, 6319–6323

Costa, E. (1980). Receptor plasticity: biochemical correlates and pharmacological significance. *Adv. biochem. Psychopharmac.*, 24, 363–377

Costa, E., Corda, M. G., Forchetti, C., Ebstein, B. and Guidotti, A. (1982). GABA/Benzodiazepine interactions. Presented at the Third World Congress of Biological Psychiatry, held in Stockholm, June 1981

Costa, E., Di Giulio, A., Fratta, W., Hong, J. and Yang, Y.-Y. T. (1979). Interactions of enkephalinergic and catecholaminergic neurons in CNS and periphery. In *Catecholamines; Basic and Clinical Frontiers*, (ed. E. Usdin, I. J. Kopin and J. Barchas), Pergamon Press, Oxford, pp. 1020–1025

Costa, E., Gnegy, M., Revuelta, A. and Uzunov, P. (1977). Regulation of dopamine-dependent adenylate cyclase by a $Ca^{2+}$ binding protein stored in synaptic membranes. *Adv. Biochem. Psychopharmac.*, 16, 403–408

Costa, E. and Guidotti, A. (1979). Molecular mechanisms in the receptor action of benzodiazepines. *A. Rev. Pharmac. Toxicol.*, 19, 531–545

Costa, E., Guidotti, A., Mao, C. C. and Suria, A. (1975). New concepts on the mechanism of action of benzodiazepines. *Life Sci.*, 17, 167–186

Costa, E., Guidotti, A. and Saiani, L. (1980). Opiate receptors and adrenal medullary function. *Nature London*, 288, 303–304

Costa, E., Guidotti, A. and Toffano, G. (1978). Molecular mechanisms mediating the action of benzodiazepines on GABA receptors. *Br. J. Psychiat.*, 133, 239–248

Cote, T. E., Grewe, C. W. and Kebabian, J. W. (1981). Stimulation of D-2 dopamine receptor in the intermediate lobe of rat pituitary gland decreases the responsiveness of the beta-adrenoceptor: biochemical mechanism. *Endocrinology*, 108, 420–426

Cottrell, G. A. (1977). Identified amine containing neurons and their synaptic connections. *Neuroscience*, 2, 1–18

Cowen, P. J., Green, A. R., Nutt, D. J., Martin, I. L. (1981). Ethyl-beta-carboline carboxylate lowers seizure threshold and antagonises fluzazepam induced sedation in rats. *Nature London*, 290, 54–55

Dale, H. H. (1935). Pharmacology and nerve endings. *Proc. R. Soc. Med.*, 28, 319–332

Di Giulio, A. M., Majane, E. M., Yang, H.-Y. T. (1979). Decreased content of immuno-reactive enkephalin like peptides in peripheral tissues of spontaneous hypertensive rats. *Nature London*, 278, 646–647

Eccles, J. C., Fatt, P. and Landgren, S. (1956). Central pathway for direct inhibitory action of impulses in largest afferent nerve fibers to muscle. *J. Neurophysiol.*, 19, 75–98

Enjalbert, A., Arancibia, S., Ruberg, M., Priam, M., Bluet-Pajot, M. T., Rotsztejn, W. H. and Kordon, C. (1980a). Stimulation of *in vitro* prolactin release by vasoactive intestinal peptide. *Neuroendocrinology*, 31, 200–204

Enjalbert, A., Ruberg, M., Arancibia, S., Priam, M. and Kordon, C. (1980b). In *Synthesis and Release of Adenohypophyseal Hormones*, (ed. M. Jutiss, and K. W. McKerns), Plenum Press, New York, pp. 525–542

Enna, S. J., Snyder, S. H. (1977). Influences of ions, enzymes and detergents on gamma-aminobutyric acid: receptor binding in synaptic membranes of rat brain. *Molec. Pharmac.*, 13, 442–453

Furshpan, E. J., Potter, D. D. and Landis, S. C. (1981). On the transmitter repertoire of sympathetic neurons in culture. In *The Harvey Lecture Series*, Academic Press, New York

Govoni, S., Hanbauer, I., Hexum, T. D., Yang, H.-Y. T., Kelly, G. D. and Costa, E. (1981). *In vivo* characterisation of the mechanisms that secrete enkephalin like peptides stored in dog adrenal medulla. *Neuropharmacology*, 20, 639–645

Gubler, V., Seeburg, P., Hoffman, B. J., Gage, L. P. and Undenfried, S. (1982). Molecular cloning establishes proenkephalin as precursor of enkephalin containing peptides. *Nature London*, in press

Guidotti, A., Gale, K., Suria, A., Toffano, G. (1979). Biochemical evidence for two classes of GABA receptors in rat brain. *Brain Res.*, 172, 566–571

Guidotti, A., Konkel, D. R., Ebstein, B., Corda, M. G., Krutzsch, H., Meek, J. L. and Costa, E. (1982). Isolation and characterisation of GABA modulin from rat brain. *Proc. natn. Acad. Sci. U.S.A.*, in press

Guidotti, A., Toffano, G. Grandison, L. and Costa, E. (1978a). Second messenger responses and the regulation of high affinity receptor binding to study pharmacological modification of GABAergic transmission. In *Amino Acid as Chemical Transmitters*, (ed. F. Fonnum), Plenum, New York, pp. 517–530

Guidotti, A., Toffano, G. and Costa, E. (1978b). An endogenous protein modulates the affinity of GABA and benzodiazepine receptors in rat brain. *Nature London*, 257, 553–555

Gwynn, G. and Costa, E. (1982). Opioids regulate cyclic GMP formation in cloned neuro-blastoma cells. *Proc. natn. Acad. Sci. U.S.A.*, in press

Haefely, W., Pieri, L., Polc, P. and Schaffmer, R. (1981). General Pharmacology and neuro-pharmacology of benzodiazepine derivatives. In *Handbook of Experimental Pharmacology*, volume 55, Springer, Berlin, pp. 13–262

Haefely, W., Polc, P., Schaffner, R., Keller, H. H., Pieri, L. and Mohler, H. (1979). Facili-tation of GABAergic transmission by drugs. In *GABA-Neurotransmitters* (ed. P. Krogsgaard-Larsen, J. Scheel-Krueger and H. Kofod), Munksgaard, Copenhagen, pp. 357–375

Hanbauer, I., Govoni, S., Majane, E. A., Yang, H.-Y. T. and Costa, E. (1982). *In vivo* regu-lation of the release of met enkephalin like peptides from dog adrenal medulla. *Adv. Biochem. Psychopharmac.*, 31, in press

Hanley, M. R., Cottrell, G. A., Emson, P. C. and Fonnum, F. (1974). Enzymatic synthesis of acetylcholine by a serotonin containing neuron from Helix. *Nature London*, 251, 631–633

Hirata, F. and Axelrod, J. (1980). Phospholipid methylation and biological signal transmission. *Science*, 209, 1082–1090

Hokfelt, T., Lundberg, J. M., Schultzberg, M., Johansson, O., Ljungdahl, A. and Rehfeld, J. (1980). Coexistence of peptides and putative transmitters in neurons. *Adv. Biochem. Psychopharmac.*, 22, 1–23

Jones, B. N., Shivaly, J. E., Kilpatrick, D. L., Stern, A. S., Lewis, R. V., Kojuna, K. and Udenfriend, S. (1982). Two adrenal opioid proteins of 8600 and 12600 daltons: intermediates in the processing of proenkephalin. *Proc. natn. Acad. Sci. U.S.A.*, in press

Karobath, M., Sperk, G. (1978). Evidence for an endogenous factor interfering with $^3$H-diazepam binding to rat brain membranes. *Eur. J. Pharmac.*, 49, 323–326

Karobath, M., Sperk, G. and Schonbeck, G. (1979). Evidence for an endogenous compound interfering with $^3$H-diazepam binding to rat brain membranes. In *Biological Psychiatry Today*, Holland Biochemical Press, pp. 114–118

Kerkut, G. A., Sedden, C. L. and Walker, R. T. (1967). Uptake of Dopa and 5-hydroxytryptophan by monoamine forming neurons in the brain of Helix asparsa. *Comp. Biochem. Physiol.*, 23, 157–162

Knoll, J. (1977). Two kinds of opiate receptors. *Pol. J. Pharmac. Pharm.*, 29, 165–175

Koski, G. and Klee, W. A. (1981). Opiates inhibit adenylate cyclase by stimulating GTP hydrolysis. *Proc. natn. Acad. Sci. U.S.A.*, 78, 4185–4189

Kumakura, K., Guidotti, A., Yang, H.-Y. T., Saiani, L. and Costa, E. (1980). A role for the opiate peptides that presumably coexist with acetylcholine in the splanchnic nerves. *Adv. Biochem. Psychopharmac.*, 22, 571–580

Kumakura, K., Karoum, F., Guidotti, A. and Costa, E. (1980). Modulation of nicotinic receptors by opiate receptor agonists in cultured adrenal chromaffin cells. *Nature London*, 283, 489–492

Lundberg, J. M. (1981). Evidence for coexistence of vasoactive intestinal polypeptide (VIP) and acetylcholine in neurons of cat exocrine glands, morphological, biochemical and functional studies. *Acta. Physiol. Scand.* suppl. 496, 1–57

MacLeod, R. M. (1976). In *Frontiers in Neuroendocrinology* (ed. L. Martini and G. Ganong), Raven Press, New York, pp. 169–194

Marangos, P. J. and Patel, J. (1981). Properties of 3H-beta-carboline-3-carboxylate ethyl ester binding to the benzodiazepine receptor. *Life Sci.*, 29, 1705–1714

Marangos, P. S., Paul, S. M., Goodwin, F. K. and Skolnick, P. (1979). Putative endogenous ligands for the benzodiazepine receptor. *Life Sci.*, 25, 1093–1102

Marangos, P. J., Paul, S. M., Greenlaw, P., Goodwin, F. K. and Skolnick, P. (1978). Denervation of an endogenous competitive inhibitor(s) of $^3$H-diazepam binding in bovine brain. *Life Sci.*, 22, 1893–1900

Massotti, M., Guidotti, A. and Costa, E. (1981a). Characterization of benzodiazepine and gamma-aminobutyric recognition sites and their endogenous modulators. *J. Neurosci.*, 1, 409–418

Massotti, M., Mazzari, S., Schmidt, R., Guidotti, A. and Costa, E. (1981b). Endogenous inhibitors of Na= independent $^3$H-GABA binding to crude synaptic membranes. *Neurochem. Res.*, 6, 551–566

Mohler, H., Battersby, M. K. and Richards, J. G. (1980). Benzodiazepine receptor protein identified and visualized in brain tissue by a photoaffinity label. *Proc. natn. Acad. Sci. U.S.A.*, 77, 1666–1670

Mohler, H. and Okada, T. (1977). Benzodiazepine receptor: demonstration in the central nervous system. *Science*, 198, 849–851

Mohler, H., Polc, P., Cumin, R., Pieri, L. and Kettler, R. (1979). Nicotinamide in a brain constituent with benzodiazepine like actions. *Nature London*, 278, 563–565

Mohler, H., Wu, J-Y. and Richards, J. G. (1981). Benzodiazepine receptors: autoradiographic and immunocytochemical evidence for their localization in regions of GABA-ergic synaptic contacts. In *GABA and Benzodiazepine Receptors*, (ed. E. Costa, G. DiChiara and G. L. Gessa), Raven Press, New York, pp. 139–146

Nielsen, M., Braestrup, C. and Squires, R. F. (1978). Evidence for a late evolutionary appearance of brain specific benzodiazepine receptors: an investigation of 18 vertebrate and 5 invertebrate species. *Brain. Res.*, 141, 342–346

Nielsen, M., Gredal, D. and Braestrup, C. (1979). Some properties of $^3$H-diazepam displacing activity from human urine. *Life Sci.*, 25, 679–686

Nielsen, M., Schoul, Braestrup, C. (1981). [3]H-propyl-beta-carboline-3-carboxylate binds specifically to brain benzodiazepine receptors. *J. Neurochem.*, 36, 276–285

Onali, P. L., Schwartz, J. P. and Costa, E. (1981). Dopaminergic modulation of adenylate cyclase stimulation by vasoactive intestinal peptides (VIP) in anterior pituitary. *Proc. natn. Acad. Sci. U.S.A.*, 78, 6531–6534

Pickering, B. T., Jones, C. W., Burford, C. D., McPherson, M., Swam, R. W., Heap, P. F. and Morris, J. F. (1975). The role of neurophysin proteins: suggestions from the study of their transport and turnover. *Ann. N.Y. Acad. Sci.*, 248, 15–35

Robson, L. E. and Kosterlitz, H. W. (1979). Specific protection of the binding sites of D-Ala$^2$-D-Leu$^5$-enkephalin ($\delta$-receptor) and dihydromorphine ($\mu$ receptor). *Proc. R. Soc. Lond.*, 205, 425–432

Ross, E. M. and Gilman, A. G. (1980). Biochemical properties of hormone sensitive adenylate cyclase. *A. Rev. Biochem.*, 49, 533–564

Saiani, L. and Guidotti, A. (1982). Opiate receptor-mediated inhibition of catecholamine release in primary cultures of bovine adrenal chromaffin cells. *J. Neurochem.*, in press

Saiani, L., Guidotti, A. and Costa, E. (1982). Interaction between alpha-bungarotoxin, nicotinic and opiate receptors in bovine adrenal medulla. *Fedn. Proc.*, in press

Schultzberg, M., Lundberg, J. M., Hökfelt, T., Terenius, L., Brandt, J., Elde, R. P. and Goldstein, M. (1978). Enkephalin like immunoreactivity in gland cells and nerve terminals of adrenal medulla. *Neuroscience*, 3, 1169–1186

Singer, S. J. and Nicolson, G. L. (1972). The fluid mosaic model of the structure of cell membranes. *Science*, 175, 720–731

Skolnick, P., Marangos, P. J., Goodwin, F. K., Edwards, M. and Paul, S. (1978). Identification of inosine and hypoxantine as endogenous inhibitors of $^3$H-diazepam binding in the central nervous system. *Life Sci.*, 23, 1473–1480

Skolnick, P., Syapin, P. J. and Pangh, B. A. (1979a). Reduction in benzodiazepine receptors associated with Purkinge cell degeneration in nervous mutant mice. *Nature London*, 277, 397–399

Skolnick, P., Marangos, P. J., Syapin, P., Goodwin, F. K. and Paul, S. (1979b). CNS benzodiazepine receptors. Physiological studies and putative endogenous ligands. *Pharmac. Biochem. Behav.*, 10, 815–823

Skolnick, P., Syapin, J. P., Pangh, B. A., Moncade, V., Marangos, P. J. and Paul, S. M. (1979c). Inosine an endogenous ligand of the brain benzodiazepine receptor, antagonizes pentyl enetetrazole evoked seizures. *Proc. natn. Acad. Sci. U.S.A.*, 76, 1515–1518

Speth, R. C., Wastek, G. T. and Johnson, H. I. (1978). Benzodiazepine binding in human brain. Characterization using $^3$H-flunitrazepam. *Life Sci.*, 22, 859–866

Sternweis, P. C., Northrup, J. K., Smigel, M. D. and Gilman, A. G. (1981). The regulatory component of adenylate cyclase: purification and properties *J. biol. Chem.*, 256, 11517–11526

Tallman, J. F., Thomas, J. W. and Gallager, D. W. (1978). GABAergic modulation of benzodiazepine binding sites sensitivity. *Nature London*, 24, 383–385

Tenen, S. E. and Hirsch, J. D. (1980). Beta-carboline-3-carboxylic acid ethyl ester antagonizes diazepam activity. *Nature London*, 288, 609–610

Toffano, G., Guidotti, A. and Costa, E. (1978). Purification of an endogenous protein inhibitor for the high affinity binding of gamma aminobutyric acid to synaptic membranes of rat brain. *Proc. natn. Acad. Sci. U.S.A.*, 75, 4024–4028

Trabucchi, M., Longoni, R., Rresia, P. and Spano, P. F. (1975). Sulpiride: a study of the effects on dopamine receptors in rat neostriatum and limbic forebrain. *Life Sci.*, 17, 1551–1556

Woolf, J. H. and Nixon, J. C. (1981). Endogenous effector of the benzodiazepine binding site: purification and characterization. *Biochemistry*, 20, 4263–4269

Yang, H.-Y. T. and Costa, E. (1982). Regional distribution of met$^5$-enkephalin-Arg$^6$-Phe$^7$ immunoreactivity in rat brain. *Fedn. Proc.*, in press

Yang, Y. T., Di Giulio, A. M., Fratta, W., Hong, J. S., Majane, E. A. and Costa, E. (1980). Enkephalin in bovine adrenal gland: multiple molecular forms of [met$^5$]-enkephalin immunoreactive peptides. *Neuropharmacology*, 19, 209–216

# 3

# Neuronal coexistence of putative transmitters in the spinal cord and brainstem of the rat

R. F. T. Gilbert, P. C. Emson and S. Hunt (MRC Neurochemical Pharmacology Unit, MRC Centre, Medical School, Hills Road, Cambridge, UK)
G. W. Bennett and C. A. Marsden (Department of Physiology and Pharmacology, Queen's Medical Centre, Clifton Boulevard, Nottingham, UK)

## INTRODUCTION

Neuronal coexistence of a biogenic amine transmitter with a biologically-active peptide was first reported in the CNS in descending serotonergic pathways to the spinal cord. Some serotonin (5-hydroxytryptamine)-containing cell bodies in the medullary raphe nuclei and other adjacent cell groups were shown to contain substance P (SP)-like immunoreactivity (Chan-Palay *et al.*, 1978; Hökfelt *et al.*, 1978; Chan-Palay, 1979), and subsequently also thyrotropin-releasing hormone (TRH)-like immunoreactivity (Hökfelt *et al.*, 1980; Johansson *et al.*, 1981). The first part of this chapter describes combined immunocytochemical and biochemical studies which further characterise the coexistence of SP and TRH in bulbospinal serotonergic neurones of the rat.

The second part of the chapter concerns recent studies on a novel peptide immunoreactivity in the rat brainstem and spinal cord. An antiserum raised against avian pancreatic polypeptide (APP) can be used immunocytochemically to label neuronal populations which also contain catecholamines or enkephalins.

## GENERAL METHODS

Immunocytochemical staining of tissue sections was performed using the unlabelled antibody peroxidase-antiperoxidase (PAP) method of Sternberger (1974) as described by Hunt *et al.* (1981*a*). All antisera used were raised in rabbits and details of their sources and dilutions used are given in table 3.1. For each of the antisera, specific staining could be abolished by preabsorption with excess antigen (100 μg/ml diluted antiserum).

The peptide contents of tissue extracts were measured by specific radio-immunoassays as previously described for SP (Kanazawa and Jessell, 1976), somatostatin (Gilbert *et al.*, 1981*a*), methionine-enkephalin (MET) (Clement-Jones *et al.*, 1980) and thyrotropin-releasing hormone (Bennett *et al.*, 1981). High affinity uptake of [³H]-serotonin into spinal cord homogenates was measured using the method of Horn (1973), and the serotonin content of spinal cord tissue was measured using a high pressure liquid chromatographic assay with electrochemical detection (Marsden, 1981).

Table 3.1   Antisera used for immunocytochemistry

| Antiserum | Source | Final dilution | Reference |
|---|---|---|---|
| Substance P (R8) | Dr P. C. Emson, Cambridge | 1:1000 | Gilbert *et al.* (1981*a*) |
| Thyrotropin-releasing hormone (V4619) | Dr T. J. Visser, Rotterdam | 1:300 | Gilbert *et al.* (1981*a*) |
| Serotonin | Dr H. W. M. Steinbusch, Nijmegen | 1:400 | Steinbusch *et al.* (1978) |
| Avian pancreatic polypeptide | Dr J. R. Kimmel, Kansas City | 1:500 | Lorén *et al.* (1979) |
| Tyrosine hydroxylase | Professor M. Goldstein New York | 1:500 | Park and Goldstein (1976) |
| Methionine-enkephalin | Dr P. C. Emson, Cambridge | 1:1000 | Hunt *et al.* (1980) |

## SP AND TRH IN BULBOSPINAL PATHWAYS

### Characterisation of peptide immunoreactivities

SP-, TRH-, MET- and SRIF-immunoreactivities in spinal cord extracts all diluted in parallel to the synthetic peptides in the respective radioimmunoassays. In the case of SP, this occurred using antisera which selectively recognise the amino- and carboxy-terminal regions of the SP sequence (R140 and GP-1 respectively) (Lee *et al.*, 1980). In addition, using either of these two antisera the apparent SP content of spinal cord extracts was the same (Gilbert *et al.*, 1981*a*).

Previous reports have shown that SP-like bioactivity in extracts of bovine dorsal root (Takahashi *et al.*, 1974) and cat spinal cord (Takahashi and Otsuka, 1975) is identical to synthetic SP by the criteria of gel chromatography and high voltage electrophoresis. We have since further shown that the SP-like immunoreactive material in acetic acid extracts of dorsal and ventral rat spinal cord elutes in the same position as synthetic SP after gel chromatography and reverse phase high pressure liquid chromatography (figure 3.1) (Gilbert *et al.*, 1981*a*). Thus, SP-like material present in both primary afferent fibres and in descending fibres to the spinal cord is indistinguishable from authentic SP.

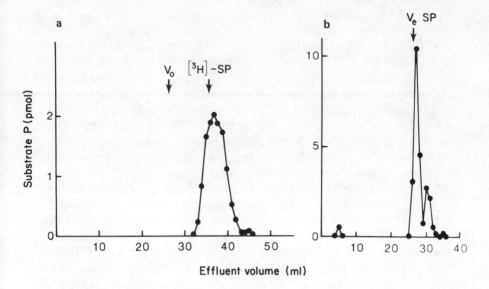

Figure 3.1 (*a*) Gel filtration of an acetic acid extract of rat ventral spinal cord on a 1.5 × 20 cm Biogel P-2 column using 0.1 M ammonium acetate buffer (*p*H 5.4) as solvent. Arrows denote the void volume of the column ($V_0$) and the position at which $[^3H]$-$[Phe]_8$-SP elutes.
(*b*) Reverse phase high pressure liquid chromatography of the peak fractions of SP-like material obtained from gel filtration of a rat ventral spinal cord extract. A μ-Bondapak $C_{18}$ column (0.39 × 30 cm) was used, and the sample eluted using a 20 min linear gradient from 5–65 per cent acetonitrile in 10 mM ammonium acetate (*p*H 4.0). The arrow denotes the position at which synthetic SP elutes ($V_e$ SP). For both (*a*) and (*b*), the content of SP-like material in each fraction was measured in a specific SP radioimmunoassay using a carboxy-terminal directed antiserum (GP-1).

The identity of TRH-like material in the spinal cord wth synthetic TRH was cast in some doubt by the work of Youngblood *et al.* (1978). However, subsequently, high pressure liquid chromatographic separation of spinal cord TRH-like immunoreactivity has confirmed that the bulk of it is identical with authentic TRH (Gilbert, Hanley and Bennett, unpublished; Jackson, 1980; Spindel and Wurtman, 1980).

These characterisation studies demonstrate that authentic SP and TRH are found in the ventral horn of the spinal cord, and show that the results obtained with radioimmunoassays and immunocytochemistry do not represent cross-reactivity of the antisera used with other peptide sequences within the descending serotonergic fibres.

## Effects of serotonin neurotoxins

Serotonergic neurones in the medullary raphe nuclei are known to project to the spinal cord (Dahlström and Fuxe, 1965; Bowker *et al.*, 1981). After lesioning of these descending fibres with the serotonin neurotoxins 5,6- or 5,7-dihydroxytryptamine (5,6- or 5,7-DHT) (Baumgarten *et al.*, 1971, 1973), serotonin-, SP- and TRH-immunoreactive fibres disappeared from the ventral horn at all levels of the spinal cord (Hökfelt *et al.*, 1978; Gilbert *et al.*, 1981a; Johansson *et al.*, 1981) and from the thoracic sympathetic lateral column (SLC) (Gilbert *et al.*, 1981a) (figure 3.2). The loss of positively-stained fibres from the ventral horn 3 weeks after 5,7-DHT (200 μg free base) was almost complete, but in the SLC, some residual damaged fibres were still visible.

The immunocytochemical results were paralleled by biochemical determinations of the serotonin and peptide contents of ventral spinal cord extracts. Serotonin, SP and TRH were each depleted by more than 70 per cent from the ventral horn of cervical and lumbar regions of spinal cord following neurotoxin treatment (Björklund *et al.*, 1979; Gilbert *et al.*, 1981a) (figure 3.3). In addition, serotonin was almost totally depleted from the dorsal spinal cord, and a small (20–30 per cent) depletion of SP could be detected from this region (figure 3.4) (Gilbert *et al.*, 1981a). The amount of SP in the dorsal horn is several times greater than that in the ventral horn because of the termination of SP-containing small-diameter primary afferent fibres in the substantia gelatinosa (Hökfelt *et al.*, 1975). The SP-containing primary afferent fibres are not lesioned by 5,7-DHT, and thus the partial SP depletion from the dorsal horn is consistent with the presence of SP in serotonergic fibres innervating the dorsal horn. In contrast to the fibres innervating the ventral horn, this population of fibres do not also appear to contain TRH since no TRH-positive fibres can be seen in the dorsal horn.

The specificity of the depletions of SP and TRH from the spinal cord after 5,7-DHT was demonstrated by the lack of depletion of two other neuropeptides, MET and SRIF from either the dorsal or ventral cord (Gilbert *et al.*, 1981a). In addition, treatment with the catecholamine neurotoxin 6-hydroxydopamine (Thoenen and Tranzer, 1968; Ungerstedt, 1968; Uretsky and Iversen, 1969), did not deplete SP, MET or SRIF from any region of the spinal cord despite an 84 per cent loss of the spinal cord noradrenaline content (Gilbert *et al.*, 1981a).

Immunocytochemical staining of the spinal cord and lower medulla oblongata at different times after 5,7-DHT treatment revealed a characteristic pattern of loss of serotonin-, SP- and TRH-containing fibres. One day after drug treatment, damaged and intensely immunoreactive axons staining for the three substances could be seen in the ventral medulla oblongata. At this time, all positive terminals in the cervical ventral horn had disappeared, whereas those in the lower sacral ventral horn did not disappear for at least one week after 5,7-DHT. Comparison of the SP content of the ventral horn at cervical and lumbar levels with high affinity uptake of [³H]-serotonin by homogenates of the same regions (as a

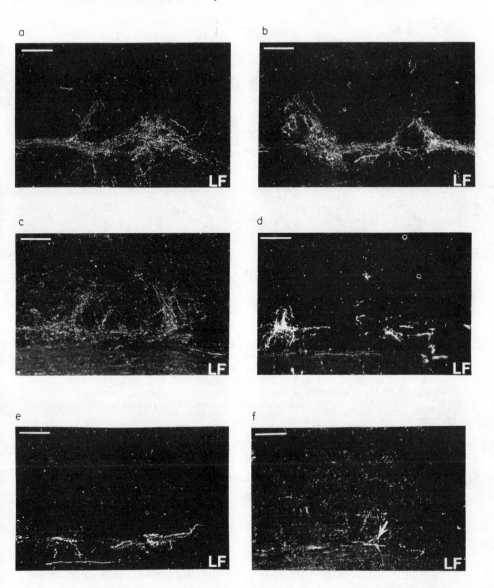

Figure 3.2 Photomicrographs of longitudinal horizontal sections of rat thoracic spinal cord stained for serotonin (*a,d*), TRH (*b,e*) and SP (*c,f*) by the PAP method and viewed under darkfield illumination. In sections from a control animal (*a-c*), fine varicose immunoreactive fibres can be seen around neurones of the sympathetic lateral column (SLC), whereas in sections taken from an animal pretreated 3 weeks previously with intracerebroventricular 5,7-DHT (200 μg free base) swollen degenerating fibres can be seen in the vicinity of the SLC. The sections stained for SP show that there are other SP-positive fibres in the thoracic intermediolateral grey matter which are not affected by 5,7-DHT; however, some swollen, degenerating SP fibres can be seen in the SLC after 5,7-DHT (arrow). Scale bars represent 100 μm (LF = lateral funiculus).

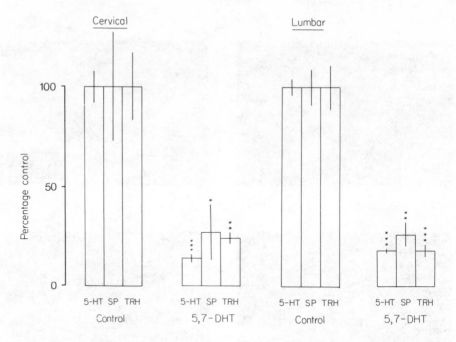

Figure 3.3 Histogram showing the serotonin (5-HT), SP and TRH contents of cervical and lumbar rat ventral spinal cord 2 weeks after intracerebroventricular 5,7-DHT (200 μg free base). Values are mean ± s.e.m. for determinations on 5–11 animals, and are expressed as a percentage of the mean content measured in control sham-operated animals. *$P < 0.05$; **$P < 0.01$; ***$P < 0.001$ by Student's $t$ test (two-tailed) (compared with sham-operated animals).

marker for intact serotonergic terminals) confirmed the rostrocaudal gradient of degeneration of the peptide-containing serotonergic fibres (Emson and Gilbert, 1980; Gilbert *et al.*, 1981*a*) (figure 3.5).

Extensive immunocytochemical studies have confirmed that SP- and TRH-like immunoreactivities are present in some medullary raphe serotonergic neurones which are known to project to the spinal cord (Chan-Palay *et al.*, 1978; Hökfelt *et al.*, 1978; Chan-Palay, 1979; Johansson *et al.*, 1981). Those findings together with the detailed results of ourselves and others (Hökfelt *et al.*, 1978; Singer *et al.*, 1980; Johansson *et al.*, 1981) on peptide and serotonin depletion from the spinal cord after serotonin neurotoxin treatment provide very strong evidence for the coexistence of SP and TRH in bulbospinal serotonergic neurones.

### Effects of other monoamine-depleting drugs

The neurotoxins 5,6- and 5,7-DHT deplete spinal cord serotonin by causing degeneration of the serotonergic axons and terminals. However, other drugs are able to deplete serotonin from neurones without damaging the neuronal elements

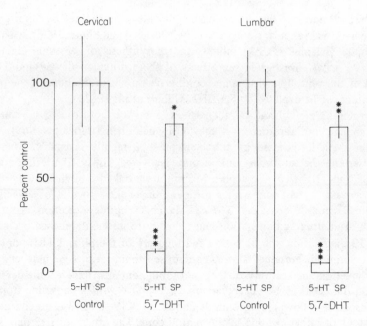

Figure 3.4 Histogram showing serotonin (5-HT) and SP contents of cervical and lumbar rat dorsal spinal cord 2 weeks after intracerebroventricular 5,7-DHT (200 μg free base). Values are mean ± s.e.m. for determinations on 5–11 animals, and are expressed as a percentage of the mean content measured in control sham-operated animals. *P < 0.05; **P < 0.02; ***P < 0.001 by Student's t-test (two-tailed) (compared with sham-operated animals).

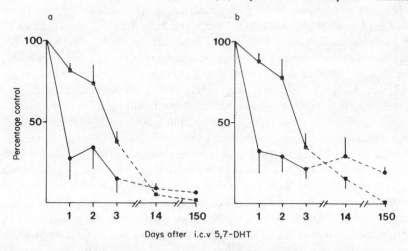

Figure 3.5 Time course of (a) [³H]-serotonin uptake capacity of whole spinal cord and (b) SP in ventral spinal cord after intracerebroventricular 5,7-DHT (200 μg free base). Both parameters were determined in tissue samples from the same animals. Values for each time after 5,7-DHT are mean ± s.e.m. for 3–10 animals and are expressed as a percentage of the mean values measured in control sham-operated animals. •, Cervical spinal cord; ■, lumbar spinal cord.

themselves. Reserpine and tetrabenazine deplete monoamines by interfering with the neuronal vesicular storage capacity (Giachetti and Shore, 1978), whereas *p*-chlorophenylalanine (PCPA) inhibits the biosynthesis of serotonin (Jequier *et al.*, 1967). We investigated the effects of these drugs on the SP and TRH content of the ventral cervical spinal cord, a region where the bulk of the peptide content can be depleted by 5,7-DHT (Gilbert *et al.*, 1981*b*).

Reserpine (2 mg/kg) and tetrabenazine (75 mg/kg) both caused substantial loss of spinal cord serotonin. As previously described (Carlsson, 1965), the serotonin depletion caused by tetrabenazine was rapidly reversible, whereas after reserpine the serotonin content only recovered slowly (figures 3.6*a* and 3.7*a*). SP and TRH were also depleted from the ventral cord by these two drugs, but to a lesser extent and with a different time-course to that observed for serotonin (figures 3.6*b,c* and 3.7*b,c*). Maximal peptide depletion occurred 24–28 h after drug administration and recovery to normal levels had occurred within 10 days. Thus, the depletion and recovery of the SP and TRH content of nerve terminals presumed also to contain serotonin seem to be independent of the depletion and recovery of their serotonin content. However, the peptide depletion did seem to be dependent on interference with monoamine storage functions, since following serotonin depletion by PCPA there was no change in the content of either peptide in the ventral cord. The effects of reserpine and tetrabenazine on SP and TRH were not non-specific, since the SP content of various forebrain regions and peripheral organs was not altered by high doses of reserpine, and two other peptides, MET and SRIF, were not depleted by reserpine from the ventral spinal cord.

The effects of reserpine and tetrabenazine on SP and TRH in the ventral spinal cord may be due to a direct action of these drugs on vesicles in which the peptides are co-stored with serotonin. Proof for such co-storage of SP, TRH and serotonin has not yet been obtained, however in other coexistence situations, enkephalins and noradrenaline in bovine splenic nerve (Wilson *et al.*, 1980) and vasoactive intestinal polypeptide and acetylcholine in secretomotor nerve terminals in salivary glands (Johansson and Lundberg, 1981) are co-stored in large dense core vesicles (LDVs) (80–120 nm in diameter), whereas the many small vesicles (30–50 nm in diameter) in the same nerves seem to contain only the amine. Terminals with such a heterogeneous vesicle population containing serotonin (Segu and Calas, 1978; Aghajanian and McCall, 1980; Ruda and Gobel, 1980) and TRH (Johansson *et al.*, 1980) have been seen around motor neurones in the ventral horn of the spinal cord and in the facial motor nucleus. Thus, although it is not possible to state conclusively that the two peptides and serotonin are co-stored in the same vesicles, it does seem likely that this does occur at least in the LDVs.

Reserpine can deplete monoamines from both large and small storage vesicles (Hökfelt, 1966, Tranzer and Thoenen, 1968; Jaim-Etcheverry and Zieher, 1974; Till and Banks, 1976). However, it seems unlikely that the peptide depletion produced by reserpine and tetrabenazine can be explained by the direct action

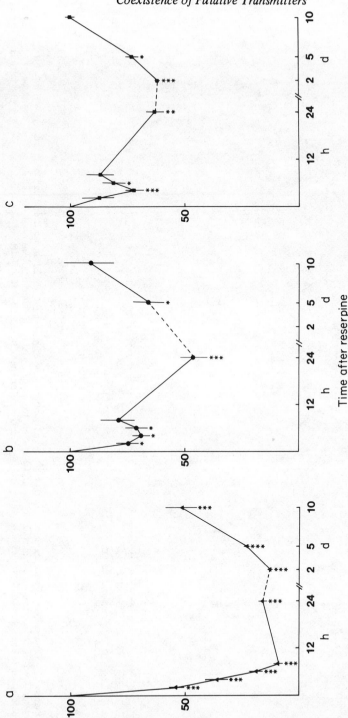

Figure 3.6  Time course of changes in the content of (*a*) serotonin in whole spinal cord, (*b*) SP in ventral spinal cord, and (*c*) TRH in ventral spinal cord after injection of reserpine 2 mg/kg. Values are mean ± s.e.m. for determinations on 4–8 animals, and are expressed as a percentage of the mean content of tissue from vehicle-injected animals. *$P < 0.05$; **$P < 0.01$; ***$P < 0.001$ (compared with controls).

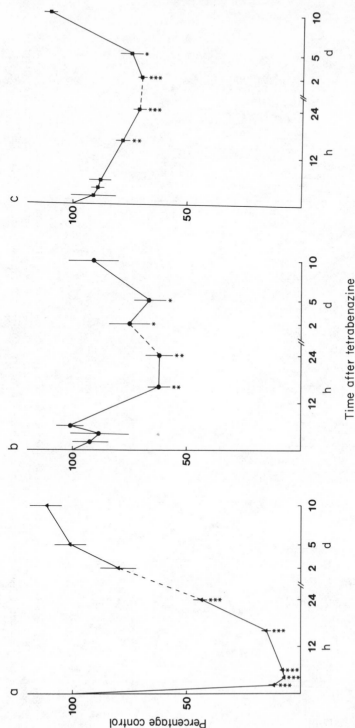

Figure 3.7 Time course of changes in the content of (*a*) serotonin in whole spinal cord, (*b*) SP in ventral spinal cord, and (*c*) TRH in ventral spinal cord after injection of tetrabenazine 75 mg/kg. Values are mean ± s.e.m. for determinations on 4–8 animals, and are expressed as a percentage of the mean content of tissue from vehicle-injected control animals. *$P < 0.05$; **$P < 0.01$; ***$P < 0.001$ (compared with controls).

of these drugs on the vesicular amine storage capacity. The two drugs are not known to affect the structural integrity of storage vesicles or to deplete their other soluble components besides monoamines. Also, since the rate of SP and TRH depletion is slower than that of serotonin after reserpine and tetrabenazine, this suggests that the peptide depletion is not a direct result of the inhibition of monoamine storage.

An alternative explanation for the SP and TRH depletion after reserpine and tetrabenazine may be that it occurs as a secondary phenomenon following the depletion of serotonin or other monoamines. For example, monoamine depletion in the CNS could lead to increased firing of the medullary raphe neurones causing prolonged release of the vesicular contents and leading to the depletion of terminal stores of SP and TRH as observed. Such depletion of soluble, non-monoamine contents of storage vesicles has been observed in the adrenal medulla after high doses of reserpine. In this case, depletion of dopamine -$\beta$-hydroxylase occurred due to secondary reflex neurogenic stimulation of the adrenomedullary cells (Viveros *et al.*, 1969).

Although the mechanism of SP and TRH depletion from the ventral spinal cord following interference with monoamine storage functions is far from clear, the specificity of this effect for these two peptides in a region where they are known to coexist with serotonin in the same nerve terminals, provides evidence for a close interplay between the amine and peptide contents of such multiple-transmitter neurones.

### Functional aspects

Descending serotonergic pathways to the spinal cord have been implicated in the control of pain transmission neurones in the dorsal horn (Messing and Lytle, 1977; Fields and Basbaum, 1978) and modulation of preganglionic sympathetic neurones in the thoracic intermediolateral column (Wing and Chalmers, 1974; Cabot *et al.*, 1979). However it is in the ventral horn, where fibres containing serotonin, SP and TRH can be seen around somatic motor neurones, that there is most information available regarding the functional significance of these multiple-transmitter neurones.

Systemic administration of serotonin precursors increases the amplitude of monosynaptic spinal reflexes (Anderson and Shibuya, 1966; Clineschmidt *et al.*, 1971; Barasi and Roberts, 1974), and increases the discharge of $\alpha$- and $\gamma$-motor neurones (Myslinski and Anderson, 1978). These results are difficult to interpret, since the effects observed may result from actions on interneurones as well as on motor neurones; however, iontophoresis provides a way in which the effects of serotonin can be studied on individual motor neurones. Early reports gave inconsistent results. Usually serotonin depressed the activity of motor neurones or had no effect at all, although occasional excitatory effects were observed (Curtis *et al.*, 1961; Engberg and Ryall, 1966; Phillis *et al.*, 1968). More recently, a number of studies have demonstrated that iontophoretically-applied serotonin does not induce direct excitation of motor neurones, but does enhance the effects of other excitatory synaptic inputs, and also facilitates excitation produced by iontophoresis of L-glutamate (McCall and Aghajanian, 1979; White and Neuman, 1980). These actions of serotonin are blocked by the antagonists methysergide and metergoline. Intracellular recording from facial motor neurones has shown that the increase in excitability produced by serotonin is associated with slow depolarisation and an increase in input resistance of the neuronal membrane which may be mediated by a decrease in potassium conductance (Vandermaelen and Aghajanian, 1980). Thus, by a postsynaptic action, serotonin seems to be able to act as a "gain-setter' to modulate the effects of other excitatory inputs to motor neurones.

The effects of SP and TRH on motor neurones are remarkably similar to those reported for serotonin. Both peptides cause depolarisation of motor neurones in the frog and neonatal rat spinal cord (Konishi and Otsuka, 1974*a,b*; Otsuka and Konishi, 1976; Nicoll, 1977, 1978). This depolarisation was slow in onset and long in duration, but was rarely sufficient to pass the firing threshold of the cells. However, such subthreshold depolarisation increases the excitability of motor neurones as demonstrated by increased amplitude of monosynaptic reflex responses (Otsuka and Konishi, 1976; Krivoy *et al.*, 1980), and increased cell firing in response to subthreshold depolarising current pulses (Nicoll, 1977, 1978). The reported increase in spontaneous motor neurone activity following systemic TRH administration is also consistent with an increase in motor neurone excitability (Cooper and Boyer, 1978).

Thus, the three substances which coexist in nerve terminals around motor neurones in the ventral horn all have similar actions on the presumed postsynaptic neurones. Release of each of the substances would be expected to increase the background level of excitability of motor neurones. The slow onset, long duration and small magnitude of the effects of all three substances contrast with those of L-glutamate, which produces rapid, large depolarisations resulting in intense firing of motor neurones (Nicoll, 1978). In terms of neuronal economy, it is not clear why the same neurone should synthesise and store three substances which appear to have the same postsynaptic actions. However, it is quite possible that there may be interactions between their effects which are not yet known. For example, a recent report has provided evidence that TRH may interact with postsynaptic 5-HT receptors, and potentiate serotonin release (Barbeau and Bedard, 1981).

## AVIAN PANCREATIC POLYPEPTIDE-LIKE IMMUNOREACTIVITY IN THE RAT CNS

Avian pancreatic polypeptide (APP) is a 36 amino acid polypeptide first isolated from chicken pancreas as a by-product of insulin purification (Kimmel *et al.*, 1971, 1975). Homologous polypeptides are found in mammalian species (Lin and Chance, 1974), and are localised in a subpopulation of pancreatic islet cells as well as in endocrine cells in other parts of the gastrointestinal tract (Larsson *et al.*, 1974). In the rat CNS, immunocytochemistry with antisera raised against APP demonstrates specific neuronal populations with an overall distribution different from that for other known putative neurotransmitters (Lorén *et al.*, 1979). The identity of the immunoreactive material is not yet known. It is clear, however, that the mammalian CNS contains peptides with sequence homologies to APP (Tatemoto and Mutt, 1980), one of which may represent the APP-like immunoreactive material.

## Coexistence of APP-like immunoreactivity with catecholamines in the brain

We and others have recently reported the distribution of APP-LI in the brainstem of the rat (Lundberg *et al.*, 1980; Hunt *et al.*, 1981*a*). After colchicine pretreatment, APP-positive cell bodies were observed in the locus coeruleus, the lateral reticular formation and the vagal nucleus/nucleus tractus solitarius region. These regions are all known to contain catecholaminergic (noradrenaline and/or adrenaline) cell bodies (Dahlström and Fuxe, 1964; Hökfelt *et al.*, 1974), and correspond to the cell groups A6, A1/A3 and A2, respectively, of Dahlström and Fuxe (1964). Using staining of single sections with two different antisera either successively with elution of the first antibody (Tramu *et al.*, 1978) or simultaneously using different coloured peroxidase substrates (Nilaver *et al.*, 1979), it was possible to show the presence of APP-LI in some tyrosine-hydroxylase (TH)-positive neurones in these cell groups (Hunt *et al.*, 1981*a*) (figure 3.8*a,b,e,f*). Not all TH-positive neurones stained for APP and *vice-versa*, suggesting that mixed populations of single- and dual-transmitter-containing neurones may exist.

## APP-like immunoreactivity in the spinal cord

In the rat spinal cord, APP-positive fibres and terminals were seen in the dorsal horn (especially the substantia gelatinosa), around neurones of the thoracic sympathetic intermediolateral nucleus and adjacent lateral funiculus. The latter fibres were found medially in the dorsal grey commissure and around the central canal, and from here extended laterally to the region of the parasympathetic intermediolateral nucleus and adjacent lateral funiculus (figure 3.9). The laterally-orientated fibres did not form a continuous column, but formed bundles which became increasingly dense and organised in more caudal sacral segments (figure 3.10). A further striking feature of the distribution of APP-positive fibres in the lumbosacral region was the innervation of Onuf's nucleus and a dorsomedial nucleus in the ventral horn of segments L6 and S1, which are motor nuclei supplying perineal muscles (Onufrowicz, 1901; Schroder, 1980) (figure 3.11).

After local colchicine injection, APP-positive cells could be seen in the substantia gelatinosa; however, these could be distinguished morphologically from other known peptide-containing neurones in this region (Hunt *et al.*,

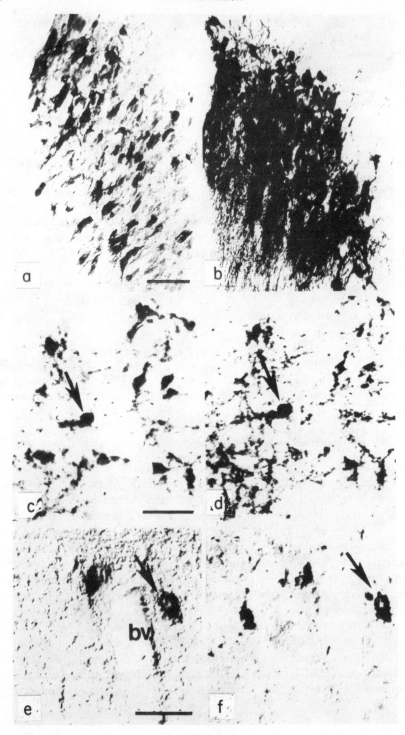

Figure 3.8 Photomicrographs of sections of rat spinal cord and brainstem stained for APP-(*a,c,e*), Met- (*d*) and tyrosine hydroxylase(TH)-like immunoreactivity (*b,f*) by the PAP technique and viewed under brightfield illumination. (*a*) and (*b*) are serial parasagittal sections through the locus coeruleus; (*c*) and (*d*): sequential staining of the same section of sacral spinal cord; (*e*) and (*f*): sequential staining of the same section of the A1 cell group. In (*c–f*) some double-labelled cells are labelled (arrows). A neurone containing only TH is indicated by an asterisk. Scale bars denote 100 μm (*a–d*) and 50 μm (*e,f*). bv, blood vessel.

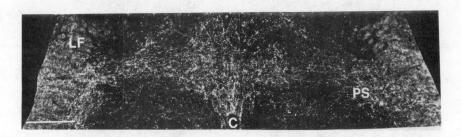

Figure 3.9 Photomicrograph of a transverse section of lumbar spinal cord (L6) stained for APP-like immunoreactivity by the PAP method and viewed under darkfield illumination. There is a dense aggregation of APP-positive fibres dorsal to the central canal (*c*) and these are continuous laterally with fibres in the region of the parasympathetic intermediolateral nucleus (PS). Many fibres can be seen crossing between the grey matter and the laterial funiculus (LF). Scale bar represents 100 μm.

1981*b*). Without use of colchicine, numerous APP-positive cell bodies were seen associated with the extensive fibre networks already described in lower lumbar and all sacral spinal cord segments (figure 3.12). These neurones were 15–25 μm in diameter, polygonal in shape with multiple processes extending from the perikaryon. They were themselves surrounded by many APP-positive fibres. The same population of neurones also stained for Met (Hunt *et al.*, 1981*a*) (figure 3.8*c,d*). Similar, although less intense Met-positive fibre networks were observed in the lumbosacral cord as were seen for APP. Glazer *et al.* (1980) have reported the presence of leucine-enkephalin (Leu)-like immunoreactivity in sacral parasympathetic neurones of the cat, and in terminals around Onuf's nucleus. It is not clear whether some of the APP/Met-positive neurones that we have identified correspond to these same preganglionic parasympathetic neurones.

### Origin of APP-like immunoreactivity in spinal cord

Since catecholaminergic neurones in the brainstem are known to give rise to descending as well as ascending projections (Dahlström and Fuxe, 1965; Lindvall and Björklund, 1978), it seemed possible that some of the APP-positive fibres in the spinal cord might be supraspinal in origin. However, no change in spinal cord APP-LI was observed below a cervical spinal cord hemitransection (S. P. Hunt, unpublished) even in regions known to receive a dense catecholaminergic

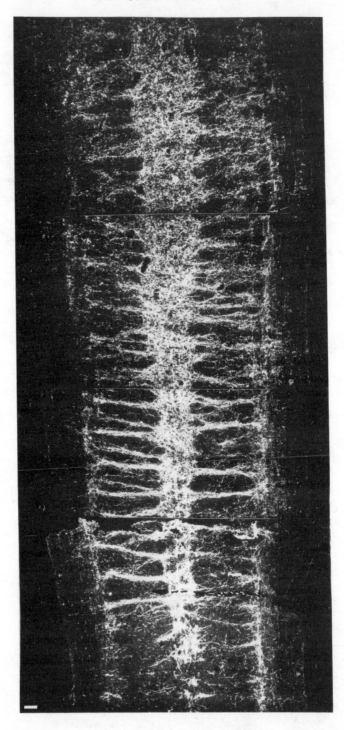

Figure 3.10 Photomicrograph of a longitudinal horizontal section through the lumbosacral spinal cord from L5 (top) to S4 (bottom) stained for APP-like immunoreactivity and viewed under darkfield illumination. The plane of section is at the level dorsoventrally of the mediolaterally-directed bands of fibres and the parasympathetic nucleus seen in figure 3.9. There is a dense network of APP-positive fibres on the midline, and laterally extending bands of fibres can be seen to become more densely organised in more caudal segments. Scale bar represents 100 $\mu$m.

innervation such as the sympathetic lateral column. Furthermore, APP-positive cells in the brainstem were retrogradely labelled following injection of a fluorescent dye (True Blue) into the hypothalamus, but not after injection into the cervical spinal cord (S. P. Hunt and D. van der Kooy, unpublished). Thus, it seems likely that most APP-positive cells in the brainstem project within the brainstem or to rostral structures.

These results imply that APP-like material in the spinal cord is derived from intrinsic or afferent neurones. The latter is unlikely since dorsal rhizotomy had no effect on APP-positive staining in the dorsal horn (Hunt *et al.*, 1981*a*). In view of the similar distribution of APP- and Met-positive fibres in the lumbosacral spinal cord, and the presence of numerous cell bodies containing both these peptide immunoreactivities in the same region, it can be postulated that the fibre networks derive from the observed neurones. It is also possible that some of these APP/Met-positive neurones may send efferent fibres out of the spinal cord via the ventral roots as has been demonstrated for Leu-positive cells in the cat sacral cord (Glazer *et al.*, 1980). Neither of these possibilities have yet been proved.

## Functional aspects

The intense innervation of Onuf's nucleus and the nearby dorsomedial nucleus in the sixth lumbar segment by APP-positive fibres is striking, and quite different from the pattern observed for other peptides such as SP, TRH and SRIF. The somatic motor neurones in these two nuclei innervate perineal muscles including the urethral sphincter, the anal sphincter, ischiocavernosus and bulbocavernous (Schroder, 1980). These striated muscles are somewhat unusual since although they are under voluntary control, they are functionally closely coupled with smooth muscles supplied by the sacral parasympathetic outflow. It is thus of interest to find that APP-positive fibres innervate the lumbosacral neurones which supply both these sets of muscles. This common afferent input may be a means by which the functions of the two types of muscle are integrated. However, since the APP-positive fibre network is not confined just to segments L6 and S1, but extends the whole length of the sacral spinal cord, it is probable that APP-positive neurones have additional functions in this region of the spinal cord.

a

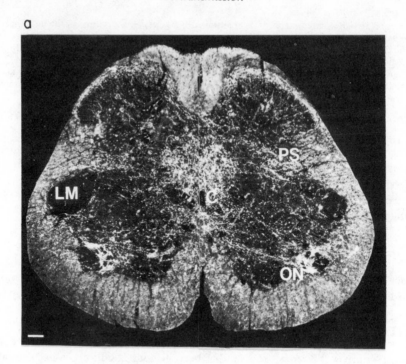

b

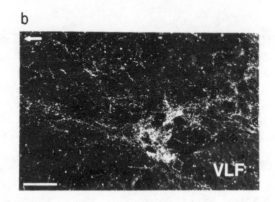

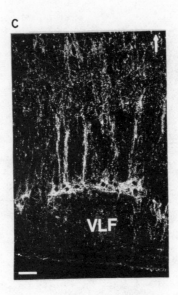

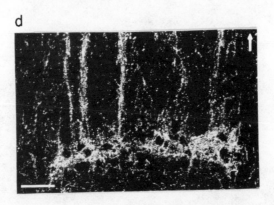

Figure 3.11 Photomicrographs of sections of rat spinal cord stained for APP-like immuno-reactivity with the PAP technique and viewed under darkfield illumination. (*a*) Montage showing APP-like immunoreactivity in a transverse section of lumbar spinal cord (L6). There is dense APP-positive staining in the substantia gelatinosa of the dorsal horn, around neurones of the parasympathetic intermediolateral nucleus (PS), dorsal to the central canal (C) and around neurones in Onuf's nucleus (ON). Note the absence of staining in a dorsolateral motor nucleus in the ventral horn (LM). (*b*) Higher power of Onuf's nucleus in transverse section. (*c*) and (*d*), APP-positive fibres in Onuf's nucleus seen in longitudinal horizontal section showing medially-directed strands of positive fibres, and positive fibres surrounding motor neurones in the nucleus. Arrows in one corner of (*b*), (*c*) and (*d*) indicate the medial direction. Scale bars denote 100 μm. VLF, ventrolateral funiculus.

*Co-transmission*

a

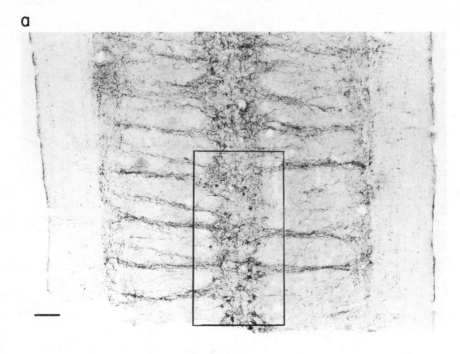

b

c

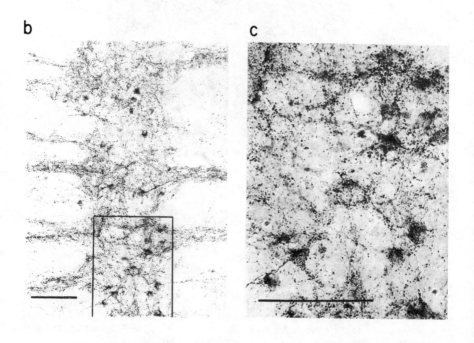

Figure 3.12 Photomicrographs of part of the section of rat lumbosacral spinal cord shown in figure 4.10. The section is stained for APP-like immunoreactivity using the PAP technique and is viewed under bright-field illumination. (*b*) Higher magnification of the region indicated on (*a*); (*c*) higher magnification of the region indicated on (*b*). Numerous APP-positive cell bodies can be seen near to the midline, and are themselves surrounded by many APP-immunoreactive fibres. Scale bars represent 100 μm.

## ACKNOWLEDGEMENTS

We thank Mrs J. Gallagher, Miss J. Irons and Mr P. Horsfield for excellent technical assistance. R. F. T. G was an MRC scholar.

## REFERENCES

Aghajanian, G. K. and McCall, R. B. (1980). Serotonergic input to facial motoneurones: localisation by electron-microscopic autoradiography. *Neuroscience*, **5**, 2155–62

Anderson, E. G. and Shibuya, T. (1966). The effects of 5-hydroxytryptophan and L-tryptophan on spinal synaptic activity. *J. Pharmac. exp. Ther.*, **153**, 352–60

Barasi, S. and Roberts, M. H. T. (1974). The modification of lumbar motoneurone excitability by stimulation of a putative 5-hydroxytryptamine pathway. *Br. J. Pharmac.*, **52**, 339–48

Barbeau, H. and Bedard, P. (1981). Similar motor effects of 5-HT and TRH in rats following chronic spinal transection and 5,7-dihydroxytryptamine injection. *Neuropharmacology*, **20**, 477–81

Baumgarten, H. G., Björklund, A., Lachenmayer, L., Nobin, A. and Stenevi, U. (1971). Long-lasting, selective depletion of brain serotonin by 5,6-dihydroxytryptamine. *Acta Physiol. Scand.*, suppl., **373**, 1–15

Baumgarten, H. G., Björklund, A., Lachenmayer, L. and Nobin, A. (1973). Evaluation of the effects of 5,7-dihydroxytryptamine on serotonin and catecholamine neurones in the rat CNS. *Acta Physiol. Scand.*, suppl., **391**, 1–19

Bennett, G. W., Balls, M., Clothier, R. M., Marsden, C. A., Robinson, G. and Wemyss-Holden, G. D. (1981). Location and release of TRH and 5-HT from amphibian skin. *Cell Biol. Int. Repts.*, **5**, 151–8

Björklund, A. J., Emson, P. C., Gilbert, R. F. T. and Skagerberg, G. (1979). Further evidence for the possible coexistence of 5-hydroxytryptamine and substance P in medullary raphe neurones of rat brain. *Br. J. Pharmac.*, **63**, 112P–3P

Bowker, R. M., Steinbusch, H. W. M. and Coulter, J. D. (1981). Serotonergic and peptidergic projections to the spinal cord demonstrated by a combined retrograde HRP histochemical and immunocytochemical staining method. *Brain Res.*, **211**, 412–7

Cabot, J. C., Wild, J. M. and Cohen, D. H. (1979). Raphe inhibition of sympathetic preganglionic neurones. *Science*, **203**, 184–6

Carlsson, A. (1965). Drugs which block the storage of 5-hydroxytryptamine and related amines. In *Handbuch der experimental Pharmacologie*, **19** (ed. V. Erspamer), Springer, Berlin, pp. 529–92

Chan-Palay, V., Jonsson, G. and Palay, S. L. (1978). Serotonin and substance P coexist in neurons of the rat's central nervous system. *Proc. natn. Acad. Sci. U.S.A.*, **75**, 1582–86

Chan-Palay, V. (1979). Combined immunocytochemistry and autoradiography after in vivo injections of monoclonal antibody to substance P and ³H-serotonin: Coexistence of two putative transmitters in single raphe cells and fibre plexuses. *Anat. Embryol.*, **156**, 241–54

Cooper, B. R. and Boyer, C. E. (1978). Stimulant action of thyrotropin releasing hormone on cat spinal cord. *Neuropharmacology*, **17**, 153–6

Clement-Jones, V., Lowry, P. J., Rees, L. H. and Besser, G. M. (1980). Development of a specific extracted radioimmunoassay for methionine-enkephalin in human plasma and cerebrospinal fluid. *J. Endocrinol.*, **86**, 231–43

Clineschmidt, B. V., Pierce, J. E. and Sjoerdsma, A. (1971). Interactions of tricyclic anti-depressants and 5-hydroxyindolealkylamine precursors on spinal monosynaptic reflex transmission. *J. Pharmac. exp. Ther.*, 179, 312–23

Curtis, D. R., Phillis, J. W. and Watkins, J. C. (1961). Cholinergic and non-cholinergic transmission in the mammalian spinal cord. *J. Physiol. Lond.*, 158, 296–323

Dahlström, A. and Fuxe, K. (1964). Evidence for the existence of monoamine-containing neurons in the central nervous system I. Demonstration of monoamines in the cell bodies of brain stem neurones. *Acta Physiol. Scand.*, suppl., 232, 1–55

Dahlström, A. and Fuxe, K. (1965). Evidence for the existence of monoamine neurons in the central nervous system. II. Experimentally-induced changes in the intraneuronal amine levels of bulbospinal neuron systems. *Acta Physiol. Scand.*, suppl., 247, 5–36

Emson, P. C. and Gilbert, R. F. T. (1980). Time course of degeneration of bulbo-spinal 5-HT/SP neurones after 5,7-dihydroxytryptamine. *Br. J. Pharmac.*, 69, 279P–80P

Engberg, I. and Ryall, R. W. (1966). The inhibitory action of noradrenaline and other monoamines on spinal neurones. *J. Physiol. Lond.*, 185, 298–322

Fields, H. L. and Basbaum, A. I. (1978). Brainstem control of spinal pain transmission neurones. *A. Rev. Physiol.*, 40, 193–221

Giachetti, A. and Shore, P. A. (1978). The reserpine receptor. *Life Sci.*, 23, 89–92

Gilbert, R. F. T., Emson, P. C., Hunt, S. P., Bennett, G. W., Marsden, C. A., Sandberg, B. E. B. and Steinbusch, H. W. (1981a). The effects of monoamine neurotoxins on peptides in the rat spinal cord. *Neuroscience*, in the press

Gilbert, R. F. T., Bennett, G. W., Marsden, C. A. and Emson, P. C. (1981b). The effects of 5-hydroxytryptamine-depleting drugs on peptides in the ventral spinal cord. *Eur. J. Pharmac.*, in the press

Glazer, E. J. and Basbaum, A. I. (1980). Leucine enkephalin: localisation in and axoplasmic transport by sacral parasympathetic preganglionic neurons. *Science*, 208, 1479–81

Hökfelt, T. (1966). The effect of reserpine on the intraneuronal vesicles of the rat vas deferens. *Experientia Basel*, 22, 56–7

Hökfelt, T., Kellerth, J.-O., Nilsson, G. and Pernow, B. (1975). Experimental immunohisto-chemical studies on the localisation and distribution of substance P in cat primary sensory neurons. *Brain Res.*, 100, 235–252

Hökfelt, T., Fuxe, K., Goldstein, M. and Johansson, O. (1974). Immunohistochemical evidence for the existence of adrenaline neurons in the rat brain. *Brain Res.*, 66, 235–251

Hökfelt, T., Ljungdahl, Å., Steinbusch, H., Verhofstad, A., Nilsson, G., Brodin, E., Pernow, B. and Goldstein, M. (1978). Immunohistochemical evidence of substance P-like immuno-reactivity in some 5-hydroxytryptamine-containing neurons in the rat central nervous system. *Neuroscience*, 3, 517–38

Hökfelt, T., Lundberg, J., Schultzberg, M., Johansson, O., Ljungdahl, Å. and Rehfeld, J. (1980). *Neural Peptides and Neuronal Communication* (ed. E. Costa and M. Trabucchi), Raven Press, New York, pp. 1–23

Horn, A. S. (1973). Structure activity relations for the inhibition of 5-HT uptake into rat hypothalamic homogenates by serotonin and tryptamine analogues. *J. Neurochem.*, 21, 883–8

Hunt, S. P., Emson, P. C., Gilbert, R., Goldstein, M. and Kimmell, J. R. (1981a). Presence of avian pancreatic polypeptide-like immunoreactivity in catecholamine- and methionine-enkephalin-containing neurones within the central nervous system. *Neurosci. Lett.*, 21, 125–30

Hunt, S. P., Kelly, J. S. and Emson, P. C. (1980). The electron microscopic localisation of methionine-enkephalin within the superficial layers (I and II) of the spinal cord. *Neuro-science*, 5, 1871–1890

Hunt, S. P., Kelly, J. S., Emson, P. C., Kimmel, J. R., Miller, R. J. and Wu, J. Y. (1981b). An immunohistochemical study of neuronal populations containing neuropeptides or GABA within the superficial layers of the rat dorsal horn. *Neuroscience*, submitted

Jackson, I. M. D. (1980). TRH in the rat nervous system: identity with synthetic TRH on high performance liquid chromatography following affinity chromatography. *Brain Res.*, 201, 245–8

Jaim-Etcheverry, G. and Zieher, L. M. (1974). Localising serotonin in central and peripheral nerves. In *The Neurosciences: Third Study Program* (ed. F. O. Schmitt and F. G. Worden), MIT Press, Cambridge, Massachusetts, pp. 917–24

Jequier, E., Lovenberg, W. and Sjoerdsma, A. (1967). Tryptophan hydroxylase inhibition: the mechanism by which p-CPA depletes rat brain serotonin. *Molec. Pharmac.*, 3, 274–8

Johansson, O. and Lundberg, J. M. (1981). Ultrastructural localisation of VIP-like immuno-reactivity in large dense-core vesicles of "cholinergic-type" nerve terminals in cat exocrine glands. *Neuroscience*, 6, 847–62

Johansson, O., Hökfelt, T., Jeffcoate, S. L., White, N. and Sternberger, L. A. (1980). Ultra-structural localisation of immunoreactive TRH. *Expl Brain Res.*, 38, 1–10

Johansson, O., Hökfelt, T., Pernow, B., Jeffcoate, S. L., White, N., Steinbusch, H. W. M., Verhofstad, A. A. J., Emson, P. C. and Spindel, E. (1981). Immunohistochemical support for three putative transmitters in one neuron: coexistence of 5-hydroxytryptamine, substance P- and TRH-like immunoreactivity in medullary neurons projecting to the spinal cord. *Neuroscience*, 6, 1857–81

Kanazawa, I. and Jessell, T. M. (1976). Post mortem changes and regional distribution of substance P in the rat and mouse nervous system. *Brain Res.*, 117, 362–7

Kimmel, J. R., Pollock, H. G. and Hazelwood, R. L. (1971). A new pancreatic polypeptide hormone. *Fedn Proc.*, 30, 1318 (abstract)

Kimmel, J. R., Hayden, L. J. and Pollock, H. G. (1975). Isolation and characterisation of a new pancreatic polypeptide hormone. *J. biol. Chem.*, 250, 9369–76

Konishi, S. and Otsuka, M. (1974a). The effects of substance P and other peptides on spinal neurones of the frog. *Brain Res.*, 65, 387–410

Konishi, S. and Otsuka, M. (1974b). Excitatory action of hypothalamic substance P on spinal motoneurones of newborn rats. *Nature Lond.*, 252, 734–5

Krivoy, W. A., Couch, J. R., Stewart, J. M. and Zimmerman, E. (1980). Modulation of cat monosynaptic reflexes by substance P. *Brain Res.*, 202, 365–72

Larsson, L.-I., Sundler, F., Håkanson, R., Pollock, H. G. and Kimmel, J. R. (1974). Locali-sation of APP, a postulated new hormone to a pancreatic endocrine cell type. *Histo-chemistry*, 42, 377–82

Lee, C. M., Emson, P. C. and Iversen, L. L. (1980). The development and application of a novel N-terminal directed substance P antiserum. *Life Sci.*, 27, 535–43

Lin, T.-M. and Chance, R. E. (1974). Gastrointestinal actions of a new bovine pancreatic polypeptide (BPP). In *Endocrinology of the Gut* (ed. W. Y. Chey and F. P. Brooks) Charles B. Slack, Thorofare, New Jersey, pp. 143–5

Lindvall, O. and Björklund, A. (1978). Organisation of catecholamine neurons in the rat central nervous system. *Handbook of Psychopharmacology*, vol. 9 (ed. L. L. Iversen, S. D. Iversen and S. H. Snyder, Plenum Press, New York, pp. 139–232

Loren, I., Alumets, J., Håkanson, R. and Sundler, F. (1979). Immunoreactive pancreatic polypeptide (PP) occurs in the central and peripheral nervous system: preliminary immunocytochemical observations. *Cell Tissue Res.*, 200, 179–86

Lundberg, J. M., Hökfelt, T., Anggård, A., Kimmel, J., Goldstein, M. and Markey, K. (1980). Coexistence of an avian pancreatic polypeptide (APP) immunoreactive sub-stance catecholamines in some peripheral and central neurones. *Acta Physiol. Scand.*, 110, 107–9

Marsden, C. A. (1981). Effect of L-tryptophan on mouse brain 5-hydroxytryptamine: comparison of values obtained using a fluoreimetric assay and a liquid chromatographic assay with electrochemical detection. *J. Neurochem.*, in press

McCall, R. B. and Aghajanian, G. K. (1979). Serotonergic facilitation of facial motoneuron excitation. *Brain Res.*, 169, 11–27

Messing, R. B. and Lytle, L. D. (1977). Serotonin-containing neurons: their possible role in pain and analgesia. *Pain*, 4, 1–21

Myslinski, N. R. and Anderson, E. G. (1978). The effects of serotonin precursors on α- and γ-motoneurone activity. *J. Pharmac. exp. Ther.*, 204, 19–26

Nicoll, R. A. (1977). Excitatory action of TRH on spinal motoneurones *Nature Lond.*, 265, 242–43

Nicoll, R. A. (1978). The action of thyrotropin-releasing hormone, substance P and related peptides on frog spinal motoneurones. *J. Pharmac. exp. Ther.*, 207, 817–824

Nilaver, G., Zimmerman, E. A., Defendini, R., Liotta, A. S., Krieger, D. T. and Brownstein, M. J. (1979). Adrenocorticotrophin and β-lipotropin in the hypothalamus. *J. cell. Biol.*, 81, 50-8

Onufrowicz, B. (1902). On the arrangement and function of the cell groups of the sacral region of the spinal cord in man. *Arch. Neurol. Psychopathol.*, 3, 387-412

Otsuka, M. and Konishi, S. (1976). Substance P and sensory transmitter. *Cold Spring Harb. Symp. quant. Biol.*, 40, 135-43

Park, D. H. and Goldstein, M. (1976). Purification of tyrosine hydroxylase from pheochromocytoma tumors. *Life Sci.*, 18, 55-60

Phillis, J. W., Tebecis, A. K. and York, D. H. (1968). Depression of spinal motoneurones by noradrenaline, 5-hydroxytryptamine and histamine. *Eur. J. Pharmac.*, 4, 471-5

Ruda, M. A. and Gobel, S. (1980). Ultrastructural characterisation of axonal endings in the substantia gelatinosa which take up $^3$H-serotonin. *Brain Res.*, 184, 57-83

Schroder, H. D. (1980). Organisation of the motoneurones innervating the pelvic muscles of the male rat. *J. comp. Neurol.*, 192, 567-87

Segu, I. and Calas, A. (1978). The topographical distribution of serotonergic terminals in the spinal cord of the cat: quantitative radio-autographic studies. *Brain Res.*, 153, 449-464

Singer, E., Sperk, G., Placheta, P. and Leeman, S. E. (1979). Reduction of substance P levels in the ventral cervical spinal cord of the rat after intracisternal 5,7-dihydroxytryptamine injection. *Brain Res.*, 174, 362-5

Spindel, E. and Wurtman, R. J. (1980). TRH immunoreactivity in rat brain regions, spinal cord and pancreas: validation by high-pressure liquid chromatography and thin-layer chromatography. *Brain Res.*, 201, 279-88

Steinbusch, H. W. M., Verhofstad, A. A. J. and Joosten, H. W. J. (1978). Localisation of serotonin in the central nervous system by immunohistochemistry: description of a specific and sensitive technique and some applications. *Neuroscience*, 3, 811-9

Sternberger, L. A. (1974). *Immunocytochemistry*, first edition, Prentice-Hall, Englewood Cliffs, New Jersey

Takahashi, T., Konishi, S., Powell, D., Leeman, S. E. and Otsuka, M. (1974). Identification of the motoneurone-depolarising peptide in bovine dorsal root as hypothalamic substance P. *Brain Res.*, 73, 59-69

Takahashi, T. and Otsuka, M. (1975). Regional distribution of substance P in the spinal cord and nerve roots of the cat and the effect of dorsal root section. *Brain Res.*, 87, 1-11

Tatemoto, K. and Mutt, V. (1980). Isolation of two novel candidate hormones using a chemical method for finding naturally-occurring polypeptides. *Nature Lond.*, 285, 417-8

Till, R. and Banks, P. (1976). Pharmacological and ultrastructural studies on the electron dense cores of the vesicles that accumulate in noradrenergic axons constricted *in vitro*. *Neuroscience*, 1, 49-55

Thoenen, H. and Tranzer, J. P. (1968). Chemical sympathectomy by selective destruction of adrenergic nerve endings with 6-hydroxydopamine. *Naunyn Schmied. Arch. Pharmac.*, 261, 271-88

Tramu, G., Pillez, A. and Leonardelli, J. (1978). An effective method of antibody elution for the successive or simultaneous localisation of two antigens by immunocytochemistry. *J. Histochem. Cytochem.*, 26, 322-4

Tranzer, J. P. and Thoenen, H. (1968). Various types of amine-storing vesicles in peripheral adrenergic nerve terminals. *Experientia Basel*, 24, 484-6

Ungerstedt, U. (1968). 6-hydroxydopamine induced degeneration of central monoamine neurons. *Eur. J. Pharmac.*, 5, 107-10

Uretsky, N. J. and Iversen, L. L. (1969). Effects of 6-hydroxydopamine on noradrenaline containing neurones in the rat brain. *Nature Lond.*, 221, 557-9

Vandermaelen, C. P. and Aghajanian, G. K. (1980). Intracellular studies showing modulation of facial motoneurone excitability by serotonin. *Nature Lond.*, 287, 346-7

Viveros, O. H., Arqueros, L., Connett, R. J. and Kirschner, N. (1969). Mechanism of secretion from the adrenal medulla. IV. The fate of the storage vesicles following insulin and reserpine administration. *Molec. Pharmac.*, 5, 69-82

White, S. R. and Neuman, R. S. (1980). Facilitation of spinal motoneurone excitability by 5-hydroxytryptamine and noradrenaline. *Brain Res.*, 188, 119-27

Wilson, S. P., Klein, R. L., Chang, K.-J., Gasparis, M. S., Viveros, O. H. and Yang, W. H. (1980). Are opioid peptides co-transmitters in noradrenergic vesicles of sympathetic nerves? *Nature Lond.*, **288**, 707–9 (1980a?)

Wing, L. M. H. and Chalmers, J. P. (1974). Participation of central serotonergic neurons in the control of the circulation of the unanesthetised rabbit. *Circulat. Res.*, **35**, 504–13

Youngblood, W. W., Lipton, M. A. and Kizer, J. S. (1978). TRH-like immunoreactivity in urine, serum and extrahypothalamic brain: non-identity with synthetic pyroglu-his-pro-NH$_2$. *Brain Res.*, **151**, 99–116

# 4

# Coexistence of classical transmitters and peptides in neurones

T. Hökfelt, J. M. Lundberg, L. Skirboll, O. Johansson, M. Schultzberg and
S. R. Vincent (Departments of Histology and Pharmacology, Karolinska
Institutet, S-104 01 Stockholm, Sweden, and Neuroendocrine Unit, Laboratory
of Clinical Sciences and Biology Psychiatry Branch, National Insitute of Mental
Health and Fogarty International Center, Bethesda, Maryland 20205, USA)

## INTRODUCTION

The term "coexistence" in the context of the occurrence of several putative
transmitter substances in a single neurone was perhaps first used by Brownstein
et al. (1974). The authors studied neurones isolated from invertebrate ganglia
and some of these cells contained 5-hydroxytryptamine (5-HT), octopamine
and acetylcholine. Similar types of neurones have also been investigated in other
laboratories and shown to contain more than one transmitter candidate (Kerkut
et al., 1967; Hanley and Cottrell, 1974; Cottrell, 1976; Osborne, 1977). However, as discussed by Osborne (1979), in no case has evidence been presented
that, if two (or more) transmitter candidates coexist in an invertebrate neurone,
both (all of them), in fact, fulfil a transmitter role in that particular neurone. A
different type of coexistence situation has been observed in developing autonomic neurones. Thus, such neurones may, at least under *in vitro* conditions,
switch from a cholinergic to an adrenergic transmitter and may during a certain
phase contain both acetylcholine and noradrenaline. Whether or not such a coexistence also occur in adults will still have to be established, but the reader is
reminded of early views held by Burn and Rand (1965) on the occurrence of
acetylcholine in noradrenergic neurones and the control of noradrenaline release
by acetylcholine. For an extensive treatment of this field the reader is referred
to some recent review articles by Patterson (1978) and Potter et al., (1981).

Other coexistence situations have also been discussed, for example, the occurrence of a putative nucleotide (ATP, adenosine) transmitter together with noradrenaline or acetylcholine (see Burnstock, 1976; and chapter 6). The coexistence
of noradrenaline and 5-HT in sympathetic nerves in the pineal gland represents
another interesting case (Owman, 1964; Jaim-Etcheverry and Zieher, 1971;
Jaim-Etcheverry and Zieher, chapter 8).

Here we concentrate on the occurrence of biologically active peptides in
neurones containing a classical transmitter such as noradrenaline. This situation
is an extension of the occurrence of amines and polypeptide hormones in
endocrine cells, for example, in the gastro-intestinal tract as described by several
groups (Pearse, 1969; Owman *et al.*, 1973; Larsson *et al.*, 1975; Solcia *et al.*, 1975;
Pearse and Takor, 1979). Pearse and his collaborators (Pearse, 1969; Pearse and
Takor, 1979; and chapter 10) have referred to these cells as the APUD (Amine
content and/or amine Precursor Uptake and Decarboxylation) system. We will
also describe a number of cases in which more than one peptide occur in a
neurone, mostly without the concomitant occurrence of a classical transmitter,
but in single cases also with such a compound. This work has in part been reviewed
earlier (see Hökfelt *et al.*, 1980*a* and *b*).

Isolation of numerous peptides in the 1970s and earlier, and the subsequent production of antisera to these compounds opened up possibilities to map
neurones containing small biologically active peptides in the brain, spinal cord
and periphery. The initial findings indicated that several peptide systems, such as
those containing substance P and enkephalin, were very widespread but represented unique systems. Thus, both substance P and enkephalin systems were
found to be at least as widespread as the monoamine systems described by
Dahlström and Fuxe (1964). Although overlapping in many brain areas, these
particular substances seemed to occur in separate neurones. In contrast, analysis
of the peripheral nervous system revealed that numerous sympathetic noradrenergic neurones in the prevertebral ganglia of the guinea-pig contain a
somatostatin-like peptide (Hökfelt *et al.*, 1977*a*). Similarly, coexistence was subsequently shown in the central nervous system. Thus, a substance P-like peptide
was present in many 5-HT neurones in the lower medulla oblongata, that is, in
the cell groups described as B1-B3 by Dahlström and Fuxe (1964). A growing
number of examples of coexistence have since been observed suggesting that
coexistence may, in fact, be a common phenomenon in the nervous system.
Although the functional significance of coexistence of a classical transmitter and
a peptide is still not well understood, there are studies in the periphery suggesting important interactions between the two such compounds. We present here a
brief review of this topic.

The presence of more than one peptide in a neurone was first described in
certain hypothalamic neurones containing both β-endorphin and adrenocorticotrophic hormone (ACTH) (Bloch *et al.*, 1978; Nilaver *et al.*, 1979; Watson
*et al.*, 1978). The explanation for these findings is the presence of a common
precursor for the two compounds (and some additional peptides) from which

β-endorphin and ACTH are processed by enzymatic cleavage (Mains *et al.*, 1977; Roberts and Herbert, 1977; Nakanishi *et al.*, 1979). More recently, however, numerous other examples of coexistence of two peptides have been demonstrated, in which there is no evidence, so far that common precursors exist, as will be discussed in this paper.

## METHODS

Nerve cells in the mammalian nervous system are in most instances too small to allow biochemical measurements of different compounds in one single cell. Furthermore, difficulties exist to dissect out single cells without nerve endings in close (synaptic) contact with the nerve cell and without glial processes. As mentioned above, however, such studies can and have been performed on single cells isolated from ganglia of invertebrates, such as *Aplysia*, which have large neurones (up to 200 μm in diameter). To provide evidence of coexistence in the comparatively small cells of the mammalian nervous system, biochemical techniques seem less well suited and, at least at the moment, morphology seems to represent a promising alternative. Of the various histochemical techniques available for this purpose, immunohistochemistry offers considerable advantages. The main reason for this is that almost any substance can be traced with this technique, provided that an antiserum can be raised against it and provided that it can be retained in the tissue section during processing for immunohistochemistry without loss of antigenicity.

Immunohistochemistry was introduced by Coons and his collaborators (Coons, 1958) about 40 years ago. Initially a direct immunofluorescence method was used, but subsequently an indirect technique with a higher sensitivity was developed. It is this technique, which has been used in our many other studies. More recently valuable modifications have been introduced, for example, the use of horseradish peroxidase as marker (Nakane and Pierce, 1967; Avrameas, 1969) instead of fluorescent dyes. The probably most frequently used technique today is the peroxidase-antiperoxidase (PAP) method of Sternberger and his collaborators (Sternberger *et al.*, 1970; Sternberger, 1979), which offers an extremely high degree of sensitivity as well as the possibility to carry out studies both at the light and electron microscopic level.

To retain antigens during the immunohistochemical procedure, tissues have to be exposed to fixation solutions such as alcohols, formalin or glutaraldehyde. As all these fixatives more or less destroy antigenicity, the fixation protocol has to be modified so that an acceptable retention and morphology are combined with an acceptable degree of antigen destruction. Ordinary formalin fixation, preferably carried out by perfusion of the experimental animals, has emerged as a suitable approach for studies of many antigens such as enzymes, peptides and even small molecules, such as 5-HT and noradrenaline (Hökfelt *et al.*, 1973; 1975). Immersion fixation in para-benzoquinone (Pearse and Polak, 1975), with or without formalin, is a useful alternative in many cases (Lundberg *et al.*, 1982*a*).

Principally, two approaches may be taken to identify two or more compounds within the same cell body (figure 4.1). First, thin adjacent sections may be incubated with different antisera. Single cell bodies will then be divided into two halves, which in fortunate conditions can be identified in the sections as belonging to the same cell. If sufficiently thin sections can be made, it is possible to follow the same cell through even more sections. Second, elution and restaining can be used as described, for example, by Tramu *et al.*, (1978). Briefly a section is incubated with an antiserum to the first antigen to be analysed and, after

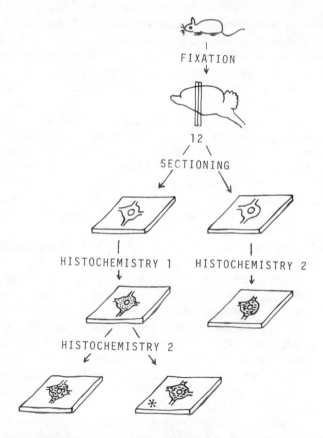

Figure 4.1 Schematic illustration of the histochemical approach for identifying two compounds in one cell. Thin adjacent sections are incubated with two different antibodies (or processed for two different histochemical techniques). In favourable conditions one and the same cell will be cut into two halves, which can be identified in the sections. Alternatively, the same section will first be processed for visualisation of one compound and subsequently for a second one. If immunohistochemistry is used, two main techniques can be used: Elution only of the antibody with retention of the marker (fluorophore) (lower left) allowing concomitant visualisation also of the second marker (dye with different colour), or elution of both antibody and marker (lower right, asterisk). With the latter approach, it is necessary to photograph the first marker before elution and restaining. For further details see text.

photography of the staining pattern, the antiserum is eluted with acidic potassium permanganate ($KMnO_4$) (Tramu *et al.*, 1978). To establish the complete elution of the first antiserum, the section is then incubated again with fluoresceinisothiocyanate (FITC)-conjugated antiserum, and if no staining is observed, indicating a complete elution, the section is reincubated with the antiserum to the second antigen to be studied, followed by FITC conjugated antibodies. The new staining pattern is photographed and compared with the previous one.

Both approaches offer advantages and disadvantages. Although the elution-restaining technique presents no problems in determining, whether or not the same cell has been restained with the second antibody, this procedure may damage antigenicity of the second compound and thus give rise to a false negative result. Therefore, the elution procedure has to be kept as short and mild as possible. In fact there are cases where the antigens are so sensitive that the acidic $KMnO_4$ cannot be used. This elution procedure seems to destroy, for example, 5-HT and thyrotropin releasing hormone (TRH), whereas substance P, enkephalin and somatostatin seem to survive this procedure fairly well. Therefore, if one wants to establish coexistence of 5-HT and substance P, the sequence of application has to be first 5-HT antiserum and then substance P antiserum. Nevertheless, it is our experience that the restaining mainly will result in a lower number of stained cells as compared to application of the same antiserum to a fresh section.

Negative results should therefore be interpreted with a very high degree of caution. The "adjacent section" procedure will not be hampered by this type of antigenic destruction. On the other hand, if the sections are not sufficiently thin, it may be difficult to establish beyond doubt identity of cell profiles in adjacent sections. Vandesande and Dierickx (1975) applied the peroxidase-antiperoxidase technique using first diaminobenzidine to obtain a brown reaction product for the first antibody, and after elution of this antibody and incubation with a new antibody, 4-Cl-1-naphthol as the second marker, which gives a bluish reaction product (see also Sternberger, 1979). Vandesande and Dierickx have also developed an electrophoresis procedure to remove the first antibody, which may be a valuable alternative.

A problem often encountered with any elution-restaining procedure is that different antisera are eluted to varying degrees. Each antiserum has to be tested individually, which can be done by varying the strength of the elution solution or by varying the time of incubation. We have used the latter procedure with times between 15 and 90 s. In fact, optimal conditions have to be established for each individual experiment.

A further possibility is to use antisera raised in different species combined with antisera labelled with different fluorescent dyes (see Sternberger, 1979). For example, one antigen may be traced by antiserum raised in a rabbit followed by FITC-conjugated sheep antirabbit antibodies. The other antibody may be a monoclonal antibody raised in a mouse, and followed with a rhodamine-conjugated pig anti-mouse antibody. This approach has been taken rarely because the majority of antisera in use up till now have all been raised in the same species, that is, the rabbit. Using appropriate filter combinations, which can be rapidly switched, the same section can then be analysed for the presence of two antigens (fluorophores), in the same cells. It may be noted that black and white films are often differentially sensitive to different colours. We therefore use Scopix Rl or Kodak Tri-X for FITC-induced fluorescence and Agfa professional 400 for rhodamine-induced fluorescence.

Finally, two major problems with immunohistochemistry should be discussed: specificity and sensitivity. It cannot be excluded that an antiserum raised to a certain peptide also reacts with one or more peptides which have structural similarities, that is, contain similar amino acid sequences. Against this background we will use terms such as "like-immunoreactivity", "immunoreactive" and sometimes "positive", although the latter term may be less suitable.

Sensitivity is a major problem with histochemical techniques in general. We have, for example, during the past 15 years experienced how the original formaldehyde-induced fluorescence technique (Falck, 1962; Falck *et al.*, 1962) has been followed by modifications and new developments, which have increased the sensitivity for visualising catecholamines leading to discovery of novel neuronal systems (for references, see Hökfelt *et al.*, 1982). In a similar way it is obvious that immunohistochemistry often is not sufficiently sensitive to visualise, for example, peptides in cell somata. This can be improved by colchicine administration (Dahlström, 1971), as has been shown and been discussed in several studies (see, for example, Ljungdahl *et al.*, 1978). But even then it may not be certain that the antibodies can "detect" all cells containing the peptide, and negative results should be interpreted with caution. Nevertheless, if strongly immunoreactive cells are seen together with immunonegative cells in the same sections, it may be concluded that considerable differences in antigen concentrations exist. (For further discussion on methodological aspects, see Priestley and Cuello, chapter 7.)

## TRANSMITTER-PEPTIDE COEXISTENCE

During the past few years numerous situations have been encountered where a classical transmitter substance and a peptide coexist. A summary of these findings can be found in Table 4.1.

### Occurrence in the central nervous system

In the raphe nuclei of the rat medulla oblongata and in adjacent areas around the pyramidal tract, numerous neuronal cell bodies contain 5-HT and a substance P-like peptide (Chan-Palay *et al.*, 1978; Hökfelt *et al.*, 1978; Chan-Palay, 1979; Johansson *et al.*, 1981). This was observed by combining the formaldehyde-induced fluorescence (Falck-Hillarp) technique for demonstration of 5-HT with immunohistochemical visualization of substance P (Chan-Palay *et al.*, 1978) or by combining autoradiography for 5-HT neurones and immunohistochemical

Table 4.1 Coexistence of classical transmitters and peptides*

| Classical transmitter | Peptide[†] | Tissue/region (species) |
|---|---|---|
| Dopamine | Enkephalin | Carotid body (cat) |
| | CCK | Ventral tegmental area (rat, human) |
| Noradrenaline | Somatostatin | Sympathetic ganglia (guinea-pig) |
| | | Adrenal medulla (man) |
| | | SIF cells (cat) |
| | Enkephalin | Sympathetic ganglia (rat, bovine) |
| | | Adrenal medulla (several species) |
| | | SIF cells (guinea-pig, cat) |
| | Neurotensin | Adrenal medulla (cat) |
| | APP | Sympathetic ganglia (rat, cat) |
| | | Locus coeruleus (rat) |
| Adrenaline | Enkephalin | Adrenal medulla (several species) |
| | APP | Medulla oblongata (rat) |
| 5-HT | Substance P | Medulla oblongata (rat) |
| | TRH | Medulla oblongata (rat) |
| | Substance P + TRH | Medulla oblongata (rat) |
| Acetylcholine[‡] | VIP | Autonomic ganglia (cat) |
| | Enkephalin | Preganglionic nerves (cat) |
| | Neurotensin | Preganglionic nerves (cat) |
| GABA | Somatostatin | Thalamus (cat) |

*For references, see text.
[†]In this column the peptide is indicated against which the antiserum used was raised. In view of the possibility of cross-reactivity, the exact nature of the peptide visualised with the immunohistochemical technique is uncertain.
[‡]The identification of acetylcholine-containing neurones is based on indirect evidence, for example, acetylcholinesterase staining, measurement of choline acetyltransferase, and so on (see Lundberg, 1981), as no reliable marker, such as antibodies to choline acetyltransferase, has been available for studies of coexistence.

demonstration of substance P neurones (Chan-Palay, 1979). In the latter study monoclonal substance P antiserum was injected into the raphe region and, after uptake of the antiserum into substance P neurones, the antiserum could be visualised by application of a second, peroxidase-labelled antibody. Finally, this coexistence situation was also demonstrated by incubating adjacent sections with substance P and 5-HT antiserum, respectively, and, in addition, using antiserum to aromatic 1-amino acid decarboxylase as a marker for 5-HT neurones (see Hökfelt *et al.*, 1978) or by incubation of the same section with 5-HT antiserum, followed by elution and restaining with substance P antiserum (Hökfelt *et al.*, 1980a; Johansson *et al.*, 1981).

The studies sited above all give evidence only for coexistence confined to the cell somata, but do not indicate if this is also true for the nerve endings arising from those cell bodies. This is a crucial question for advancing the hypothesis that two compounds are released together at synapses. Initial attempts to resolve this problem included treatment of rats with neurotoxins, such as 5, 6- and 5, 7-dihydroxytryptamine (5,6-DHT and 5,7-DHT, respectively), which were assumed to specifically destroy 5-HT neurones (Baumgarten et al., 1971; 1973; Daly et al., 1973; 1974), as well as cholchicine treatment and transection of the spinal cord (Hökfelt et al., 1978). These studies demonstrated that, after neurotoxin treatment and after transection of the spinal cord, there was a parallel disappearance of 5-HT and substance P immunoreactive nerve endings in the ventral horns of the spinal cord, suggesting that these fibres had a supraspinal origin and that substance P and 5-HT in fact were transported out from the cell bodies through the same axon to be stored in the same nerve ending. The effect of such neurotoxins could also be established by biochemical measurements (Björklund et al., 1979; Singer et al., 1979; Gilbert, 1981; see Gilbert et al., chapter 3). After colchicine and neurotoxin treatment accumulation of both substance P and 5-HT-like immunoreactivities in dilated axons could be observed in the same areas in the medulla oblongata with overlapping distribution patterns. Again, the neurotoxin and transection experiments are no proof for coexistence in nerve endings, as it may be argued that substance P is present in a separate population of neurones, which is, in contrast to previous assumptions, sensitive to the neurotoxins, or that these neurotoxins cause unspecific damage affecting substance P neurones. Such unspecific damage has in fact been demonstrated in certain cases for neurotoxins (see Jonsson, 1981). Further evidence for descending substance P/5-HT fibres has been obtained by combined retrograde tracing-immunofluorescence studies. Thus, after injection of the retrogradely transported dye Fast Blue into the spinal cord, dye-labelled cells containing both 5-HT and substance P could be observed in the medulla oblongata (Skirboll et al., unpublished). Final evidence for coexistence of substance P and 5-HT in nerve endings has been demonstrated recently by Pelletier et al., (1981) using immunoelectron microscopy (see also Priestley and Cuello, chapter 7).

Numerous neurones in the medullary raphe nuclei and adjacent areas also contain TRH-like peptides (Johansson and Hökfelt, 1980) and a considerable proportion of these TRH-immunoreactive neurones are identical to 5-HT containing ones (Hökfelt et al., 1980a; Johansson et al., 1981). Elution and restaining experiments have demonstrated that, in fact, some neurones contain all three compounds (figure 4.2a-c) (Johansson et al., 1981). Colchicine treatment, transection of the spinal cord as well as neurotoxin treatment causes the same changes with regard to spinal TRH as reported above for substance P and 5-HT, that is, a loss of TRH-immunoreactive nerve endings in the ventral horn after the former types of treatment and accumulation of TRH in dilated axons after colchicine treatment.

We have performed a rough quantitative examination of the proportions of TRH, substance P and 5-HT-immunoreactive neurones in the ventral medulla oblongata (table 4.2). Overall, the substance P and TRH-immunoreactive cell

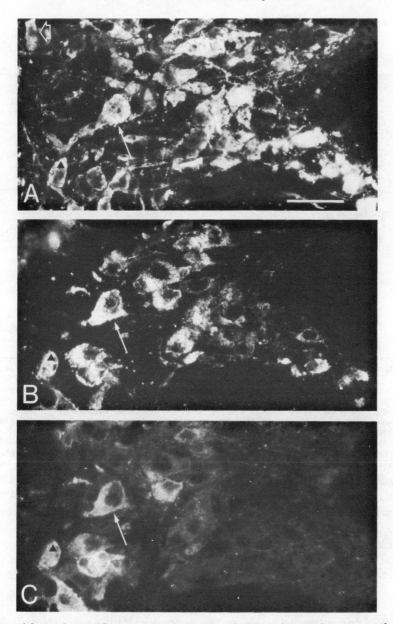

Figure 4.2 *a-c* Immunofluorescence micrographs of the nucleus raphe magnus of col-chicine-treated rat after incubation with antiserum to 5-HT (*a*), TRH (*b*) and substance P (*c*). *a* and *b* are adjacent sections. *b* and *c* show the same section, first incubated with anti-serum to TRH (*b*), then eluted and restained with substance P antiserum (*c*). Arrows and black triangles show two cells which contain all three compounds. Bar indicates 50 μm. Open white arrow in *a* points dorsally. From Johansson *et al.* (1981).

Table 4.2  Quantitative evaluation of 5-HT, TRH and substance P (SP) immunoreactive cell bodies in the rostral (*a*) and caudal (*b*) medulla oblongata of colchicine-treated rat: comparison of the relative distribution within the nuclei

|   | Region | 5-HT (%) | TRH (%) | SP (%) | Number of cells counted (= 100 per cent) |
|---|---|---|---|---|---|
| a | NRM | 53.7 | 24.4 | 21.9 | 1256 |
|   | ARC rm | 76.6 | 21.9 | 1.6 | 192 |
|   | PPP | 56.4 | 17.3 | 26.3 | 1099 |
|   | ARC rl | 78.8 | 18.7 | 2.4 | 860 |
|   | SPP | 62.2 | 18.2 | 19.6 | 1285 |
|   | Others | 63.3 | 18.4 | 18.4 | 109 |
|   | Total (*a*) | 62.2 | 19.9 | 17.9 | 4801 |
| b | NRP | 42.6 | 32.1 | 25.4 | 1525 |
|   | ARC cm | 58.1 | 31.0 | 11.4 | 465 |
|   | NRO | 52.2 | 22.9 | 24.9 | 3016 |
|   | PO | 49.6 | 14.8 | 35.7 | 704 |
|   | ARC cl | 60.4 | 27.5 | 12.2 | 1037 |
|   | Others | 64.4 | 14.4 | 21.3 | 160 |
|   | Total (*b*) | 51.7 | 25.1 | 23.2 | 6907 |
|   | Total (*a* + *b*) | 56.0 | 23.0 | 21.0 | 11,708 |

This table is based on five series of sections used for the quantitative evaluation. The sections have been spaced at different intervals. The total number of cells counted refers to the total number of immunoreactive cells. The borderline between rostral and caudal medulla oblongata has been put at about P 5.5 mm, which approximately represents the caudal ending of nucleus raphe magnus and the rostral beginning of nuclei raphe obscurus and pallidus. The principles for definition of the nuclei have been described. ARC, "Arcuate" region: rm, rostral medial; rl, rostral lateral; cm, caudal medial; cl, caudal lateral. NRM, nucleus raphe magnus; NRO, nucleus raphe obscurus; NRP, nucleus raphe pallidus; PO, "paraolivar" region; PPP, "parapyramidal" region; SPP, "suprapyramidal" region. (From Johansson *et al.*, 1981.)

bodies together equal the number of 5-HT cell bodies, initially suggesting that 5-HT neurones could be subdivided into two subpopulations of about equal size containing substance P and TRH, respectively. Elution and restaining experiments did, however, reveal that at least in some neurones all three compounds were present together and that interesting regional differences in the proportions existed (table 4.2). Thus, nucleus raphe pallidus had comparatively similar proportions of the three compounds indicating the possibility of a high incidence of neurones containing all three compounds, whereas the nucleus arcuatus had low proportions of substance P immunoreactive cells and the interfascicular nucleus (parapyramidal and paraolivar regions) had a low proportion of TRH-immunoreactive cells. Very similar proportions of the three compounds in the nuclei of the ventral medulla were seen in several animals, indicating that they did not reflect chance variations, but rather were characteristic of each region.

Chan-Palay (1979) has reported that cells with low substance P content have a high 5-HT content and that perhaps the levels of the various compounds may fluctuate. As we used cholchicine-treated rats, it is difficult to draw conclusions on these issues from our experiments. Nevertheless, it is an interesting hypothesis, which at present is tested by analysing for example effects of drugs as well as daily rhythms.

In the ventral mesencephalon Dahlström and Fuxe (1964) described several groups of dopamine-containing cells (A8-A10 cell groups) which project in a rostral direction to forebrain areas (Andén *et al.*, 1965; 1966). Subpopulations of these neurones contained a cholecystokinin (CCK)-like peptide (figure 4.3*a* and *b*; 4.4*a*) (Hökfelt *et al.*, 1980*c,d*; Skirboll *et al.*, 1981*a*). Evidence was presented for a clear regional distribution of the CCK-like peptide and dopamine in the mesencephalon. Thus, there were comparatively few CCK-immunoreactive dopamine cells in the zona compacta, and most such cells were observed in the rostral parts of this structure. In the ventral tegmental area (figure 4.3*a* and *b*) (A10) at most half of all dopamine cells seemed to contain CCK-like immuno-reactivity, whereas in the pars lateralis of substantia nigra almost all dopamine cells have the peptide. No CCK-immunoreactive cells have been observed in the pars reticulata, in spite of the fact that at caudal levels numerous dopamine cells are present. Again these proportions were reproducible from animal to animal.

When analysing the forebrain areas known to be innervated by dopamine neurones (see Lindvall and Björklund, 1978), it was found that overlapping CCK-immunoreactive and dopamine terminals were only observed in some of those regions (figure 4.4*b*). Thus high concentrations of CCK-immunoreactive fibres were observed in the caudal ventral-medial nucleus accumbens (figure 4.3*c* and *d*) and the tuberculum olfactorium, in the nucleus interstitialis striae terminalis, in the caudal and the periventricular region of the nucleus caudatus and in the central amygdaloid nucleus, a distribution which suggests primarily limbic projections of the CCK/dopamine neurones. This terminal distribution fits well with the distribution of CCK/dopamine cell bodies in the ventral mesen-cephalon with regard to their known projection areas. The existence of such CCK/dopamine projections from the mesencephalon to the forebrain has been established by combined retrograde tracing experiments, whereby the dye Fast Blue injected into the nucleus accumbens could be visualised in cell bodies in the ventral tegmental area, and these cells also contained both tyrosine hydroxylase and CCK-like immunoreactivity (Hökfelt *et al.*, 1980*c*). There is so far no evidence for the presence of the CCK-like peptide in other dopamine neurones, for example, in the hypothalamus.

Further types of coexistence have been observed in the lower brain stem of the rat brain. Thus, a large proportion of the adrenaline neurones of the C1 (figure 4.5*a-c*) and C2 cell group as well as a population of the noradrenaline neurones of the locus coeruleus (A6 cell group of Dahlström and Fuxe, 1964) contain an avian pancreatic polypeptide (APP)-like peptide (Lundberg *et al.*, 1980*a*; Hunt *et al.*, 1981). APP-immunoreactive nerve fibres were found in several brain stem

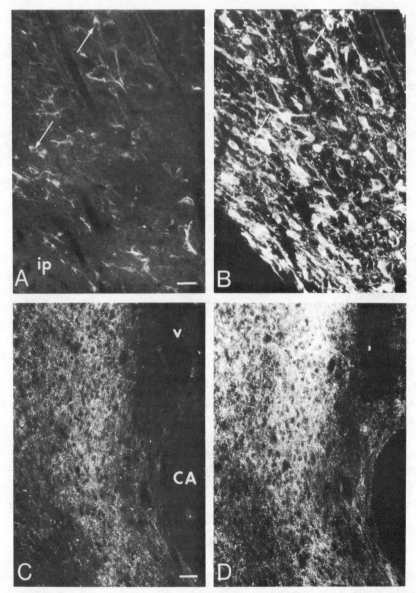

Figure 4.3 *a-d*, Immunofluorescence micrographs of the ventral tegmental area (A10 dopamine cell group (*a* and *b*) and the caudal, medial nucleus accumbens close to the anterior commissure (CA) (*c* and *d*) after incubation with antiserum to gastrin/CCK (*a*) and tyrosine hydroxylase (TH), a marker for dopamine neurones (*b* and *d*). *a* and *b* show the same section, which was first incubated with gastrin/CCK antiserum (*a*) and after photography and elution, restained with TH antiserum (*b*). *c* and *d* show adjacent sections. Note that many cells (arrows) contain both peptide and TH (*a* and *b*). Gastrin/CCK and the TH-immunoreactive nerve endings in the nucleus accumbens have a very similar distribution pattern (*c* and *d*). ip, Interpeduncular nucleus; v, lateral ventricle. Bars indicate 50 μm. From Hökfelt *et al.* (1980*c*).

regions demonstrating a clear overlap with adrenaline containing nerve endings (Hökfelt *et al.*, 1974). There are APP-immunoreactive nerve endings in other brain areas, such as hypothalamus, where an overlap with adrenaline containing nerve endings can be seen in the perifornical region. It is important to emphasize, however, that there are many other APP systems in the hypothalamus and forebrain, for example, in the arcuate nucleus as well as in the cortex (Lorén *et al.*, 1979; see below), which do not coincide with adrenaline or noradrenaline. In the spinal cord APP immunoreactive fibres are present, for example, in the sympathetic lateral column probably being identical to the adrenaline nerve fibres (Lundberg *et al.*, 1980*a*). In addition there are local APP-immunoreactive systems in the spinal cord (Hunt *et al.*, 1981; Hökfelt *et al.*, 1981*a*). Finally, populations of 5-HT neurones in the dorsal and medullary (Skirboll *et al.*, unpublished) raphe nuclei contain enkephalin-like immunoreactivity.

The coexistence situations described so far all involve catecholamines or 5-HT. Recently evidence has been presented that also amino acid transmitters may coexist with a peptide. Thus, Oertel *et al.*, (1981) have demonstrated the GABA-synthesizing enzyme (GAD) and somatostatin in thalamic neurones in the cat.

In conclusion, there is at present evidence for the occurrence of certain peptides in subpopulations of all four types of central monoamine systems so far described, dopamine, noradrenaline, adrenaline and 5-HT and also in GABA neurones. In all cases the peptides seem to be present only in subpopulations of these systems and there are thus many monoamine neurones in the brain which do not seem to contain a peptide. One exception may be adrenaline neurones which to a very high proportion seem to contain the APP-like peptide. It remains to be demonstrated whether the apparent lack of a peptide in a certain part of a monoamine system is real, or whether it is due to low sensitivity of the immunohistochemical technique. One may also envisage the possibility that a family of peptides is present and that all members of this family do not cross react with the antiserum used.

The latter thought brings up the important issue of specificity of the immunoreactions described above. It should be emphasised that in no case has the exact structure of peptides present in the central monoamine neurons been verified. General agreement seems to exist with regard to the uniformity of substance P-like immunoreactivity in the rat brain although minor differences have been reported (Ben-Ari *et al.*, 1978).

With regard to CCK-like immunoreactivity, there exist controversies with regard to identity and different forms have been described, for example, the 33-amino acid CCK, 8-amino acid CCK and 4-amino acid CCK (see Rehfeld, 1978), and according to Dockray *et al.*, (1978) several forms of the octapeptide may exist in the sheep brain.

The identity of the APP-like immunoreactivity is very uncertain. In all probability the peptide is not identical to the recently discovered peptide PYY (Tatemoto and Mutt, 1980; Lundberg *et al.*, 1982*b*). Initially, the use of antisera to bovine PP (BPP) resulted in no immunostaining in the rodent brain (Lorén

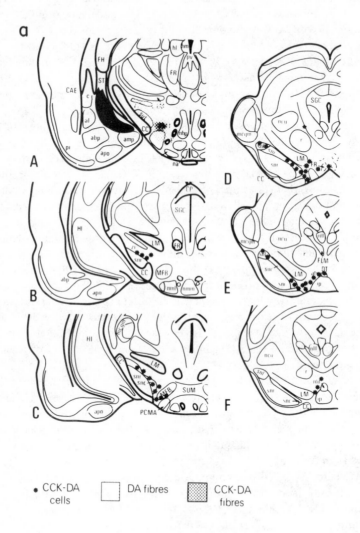

Figure 4.4 Schematic illustration (*a*) of the distribution of dopamine (DA) cell bodies containing a gastrin/CCK-like peptide in the ventral mesencephalon (*a–f* show various frontal levels); and (*b*) of areas with "only" dopamine fibres or with overlapping dopamine

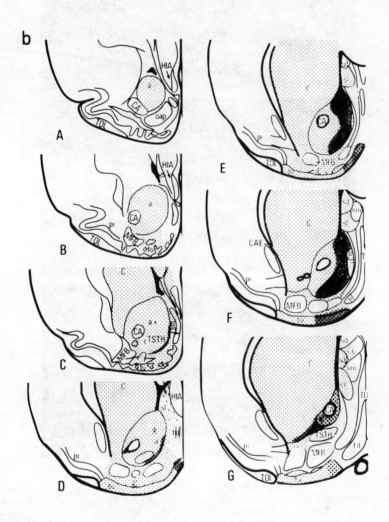

and gastrin/CCK immunoreactive fibres in the rostral telencephalon (*a–g* show various frontal levels mainly of the nucleus caudatus, nucleus accumbens and tuberculum olfactorium). For further details, see Hökfelt *et al.* (1980c), from which these drawings have been taken.

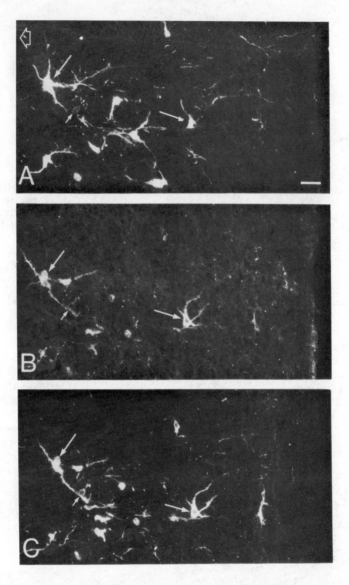

Figure 4.5  Immunofluorescence micrographs of the ventro-lateral, rostral medulla oblongata of colchicine-treated rat after incubation with antiserum to phenylethanolamine *N*-methyl-transferase (PNMT) (*a*), avian pancreatic polypeptide (APP) (*b*) and tyrosine hydroxylase (TH) (*c*). *a* and *b* show adjacent sections. *b* and *c* show the same section, which has been first incubated with APP antiserum (*b*) and, after photography and elution, restained with TH antiserum (*c*). Note that almost all cells (some are indicated by long arrows) contain both PNMT, APP and TH, although APP-like immunoreactivity is much weaker than the immunoreactivity towards the two enzymes. Small arrow points to a cell which is very faintly, if at all, PNMT and APP immunoreactive but shows a fairly strong TH immuno-reaction. Open white arrow in *a* points dorsally. Bar indicates 50 μm.

*et al.*, 1979), but such negative findings must be interpreted with caution as they may be due merely to insufficient "sensitivity" (affinity, avidity) of the antisera. More recently, "staining" with a BPP antiserum in the rat brain and periphery has been reported by Olschowka *et al.*, (1981).

### Functional aspects of central transmitter peptide coexistence

Our understanding of the functional significance of coexistence of a classical transmitter and one or more peptides is at present incomplete. Monoamines, such as the catecholamines and 5-HT, may very well fulfil a transmitter role (see, for example Aghajanian and Wang, 1978; Moore and Bloom, 1978; 1979) and a similar role has also been suggested for several peptides, including substance P, TRH and CCK (Otsuka and Takahashi, 1977; Nicoll *et al.*, 1980; Rehfeld *et al.*, 1980; Dodd and Kelly, 1981). Taken together, these data indicate the possibility of the occurrence of more than one transmitter substance in the same neurone. However, the fact that all these compounds individually have been assigned a role as a transmitter, does of course not enable us to make a statement on their role when they coexist. In fact, it is extremely difficult to design an experiment in the central nervous system that would enable us to study release of several compounds from the same nerve endings with certainty. A problem here is that nerve endings seemingly containing coexisting and non-coexisting compounds are often intermingled. For example, it may very well be that in the nucleus accumbens there are nerve endings containing only dopamine as well as those containing both CCK and dopamine as well as those with only CCK. Whereas the two former ones in all probability originate in the mesencephalon, the CCK nerve endings may do this, but in addition such nerve endings may have a different origin. Thus, any attempt to try to elucidate the possible physiological significance of coexistence of CCK and dopamine in the nucleus accumbens would have to take these possibilities into consideration. In the following we would briefly like to relate some of these findings.

In the spinal cord 5-hydroxytryptophan (5-HTP) the precursor of 5-HT, increases the spontaneous firing of motoneurones (Andén *et al.*, 1964; Myslinski and Anderson, 1977). The work of Otsuka and his collaborators (Konishi and Otsuka, 1974; Otsuka and Takahashi, 1977) has indicated an excitatory action of substance P on spinal motoneurones. Also, TRH produces excitatory effects on motoneurones, although electrophysiologically this has so far only been established in the frog spinal cord (Nicoll, 1977). Several other studies also suggest similar effects of TRH, 5-HT and 5-HTP on spinal reflexes (Shibuya and Anderson, 1968; Cooper and Boyer, 1978; Barbeau and Bedard, 1981). Recently, Barbeau and Bedard (1981) have reported that TRH elicits a strong response in both extensor and flexor muscles of the hind limbs after chronic spinal transection or after injection of the neurotoxin 5, 7-DHT. The effects were identical to those seen after 5-HTP and 5-HT agonists. Interestingly the effects were blocked by cyproheptadine, a 5-HT antagonist, suggesting that TRH acts on

5-HT receptors. TRH may also release 5-HT according to Barbeau and Bedard (1981). The findings suggest interesting interactions of at least two different kinds between TRH and 5-HT, which may reflect a cooperative action of two compounds released from the same nerve endings. Although no similar studies have been carried out for substance P, it may be speculated that also this peptide causes similar effects in view of its demonstrated excitatory action on moto-neurones (Konishi and Otsuka, 1974). It is interesting to note that the effects of TRH were obtained after intravenous administration, indicating that this peptide may pass the blood brain barrier. Whether substance P also does this in a similar experimental situation, remains to be seen.

CCK peptides have been shown to exert effects on various central nervous system functions, both after peripheral and central administration (see for example, Gibbs *et al.*, 1973; Della-Fera and Baile, 1979). Strong excitatory effects on neuronal firing rate of CCK-8 given iontophoretically at very low concentrations suggest that this peptide may act as neurotransmitter or neuromodulator (Dodd and Kelly, 1981). In the ventral tegmental area electrophysiological effects have been recorded after iontopheretic application into the brain tissue as well as after intravenous administration (Skirboll *et al.*, 1981*b*). In both cases dopamine neurones are excited by the peptide. However, there is a characteristic distribution of cells sensitive to CCK (figure 4.6). Thus, these cells are seen in the ventral tegmental area (A10) and in the medial pars compacta of the substantia nigra, but never in the middle portion of pars compacta or in pars reticulata. This distribution fits very well with the distribution of CCK/dopamine cells. The findings indicate that only those dopamine cells which contain CCK are sensitive to the peptide. However, whether these receptors are physiologically activated by a CCK-like peptide released from nerve endings or dendrites in the ventral mesencephalon or if they represent autoreceptors remains to be determined. As there are however, very few CCK immunoreactive nerve endings in this area (Hökfelt *et al.*, 1980*c*), the latter hypotheses may be preferred.

So far, no electrophysiological studies have been carried out on the terminal areas for the CCK/dopamine neurones, which is an essential issue for understanding the physiological role of the dopamine/CCK coexistence. Some indirect evidence has, however, been obtained in studies on dopamine release *in vitro* (Markstein *et al.*, 1981). Thus, the sulphated CCK-7 peptide causes, in low concentrations ($10^{-8}$–$10^{-9}$ M) a dose-dependent increase in electrically induced dopamine release. Whether this effect is direct or indirect is at present uncertain, but the overall effect would agree with the electrophysiological data discussed above showing activation of the dopamine/CCK neurones possibly leading to increased dopamine release. Similar, but less marked effects were also seen in the caudate nucleus, where, in spite of high CCK and dopamine concentrations coexistence of dopamine and CCK seem to occur only to a very limited extent. (Hökfelt *et al.*, 1980*c*). Biochemical studies have demonstrated effects of CCK on dopamine (Fekete *et al.*, 1980; Fuxe *et al.*, 1980; Kovacs *et al.*, 1981). Thus, CCK peptides have been demonstrated to affect dopamine receptor binding,

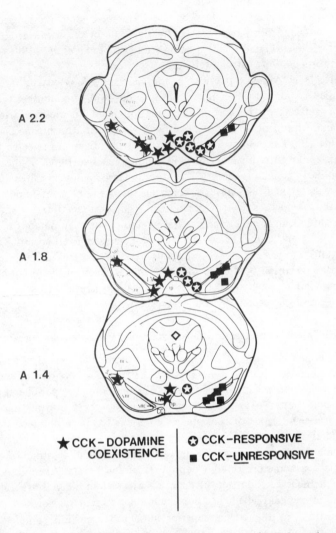

A 2.2

A 1.8

A 1.4

★ CCK – DOPAMINE COEXISTENCE

✪ CCK – RESPONSIVE

■ CCK – UNRESPONSIVE

Figure 4.6  Schematic illustration of the distribution of gastrin/CCK-dopamine cell bodies (left side) compared with the distribution of cells, which respond or do not respond to intravenously or ionotophoretically applied CCK-7 (right side) in the ventral mesencephalon. There is a good correlation between the distribution of cells containing both a gastrin/CCK-like peptide and dopamine with that of cells responsive to the peptide. For further details, see Skirboll *et al.* (1981*b*), from which this drawing has been taken.

resulting in a decrease in the number of binding sites (Fuxe *et al.*, 1981). Such an effect could eventually by way of feedback mechanisms lead to an increased dopamine release as reported above.

The identity of the CCK-like peptides in the brain is at present uncertain as discussed above. A further issue of controversy is the question whether the sulphated or the unsulphated form is active. In most studies discussed above only the sulphated form has proven effective, but in the turnover studies of Kovacs *et al.*, (1981) and in the binding studies of Fuxe *et al.*, (1981) the unsulphated form exhibited strong activity.

The effects of APP-like peptides in the central nervous system have hardly been studied so far. In a preliminary study Fuxe *et al.* (unpublished) reported stimulatory effects on respiration, though not on blood pressure after intraventricular injection of APP, but no effects were seen after bovine pancreatic polypeptide (BPP) injection. This experimental paradigm was selected because of the high concentrations of the APP-immunoreactive fibres in the nucleus tractus solitari, in all probability localized at least mainly in adrenaline neurones. The latter neurones have earlier been reported to be of importance in both central blood pressure and respiratory regulation (see Fuxe *et al.*, 1981).

In conclusion, in several experimental models it has been demonstrated that peptides which are known to coexist with monoamines, exert specific effects in those regions where coexistence situations have been reported. In general, the effect of the co-stored peptide seems to be enhancement of the response caused by the monoamine, suggesting that two coexisting neuroactive substances cooperate in causing a certain physiological response.

## Occurrence in the peripheral nervous system and endocrine and paracrine cells

There are numerous cases of coexistence of a peptide and classical transmitter in the peripheral nervous system. In fact, the first case reported of such a coexistence was observed in the periphery. Furthermore, the peripheral nervous system offers better experimental models and our best information on the physiological significance of coexistence situations has been obtained in studies on peripheral tissues.

In sympathetic ganglia of guinea-pig varying proportions of principal ganglion cells contain a somatostatin-like peptide (figure 4.7a and b) (Hökfelt *et al.*, 1977a). The highest proportion of such cells was seen in the prevertebral ganglia with about 60 per cent labelled cells in the inferior mesenteric ganglion and varying proportions in the coeliac-superior mesenteric ganglion complex (about 50 per cent in the anterior part, 25 per cent in the posterior part). In contrast, in the superior cervical ganglion only a few per cent of the cells contained somatostatin. These somatostatin-immunoreactive cells also contained dopamine β-hydroxylase (DBH) and tyrosine hydroxylase (TH) establishing their noradrenergic nature.

An important issue has been whether the somatostatin-negative noradrenaline cells in these ganglia, in fact, lack this peptide, or if the peptide content is too low to be detected with the present technique, that is, the same problem which was discussed above with regard to central coexistance situations. Recently, a further peptide has been observed in these ganglia in the guinea-pig using an APP antiserum. Both elution and restaining experiments as well as comparison of distribution in adjacent sections, revealed that somatostatin- and APP-immuno-

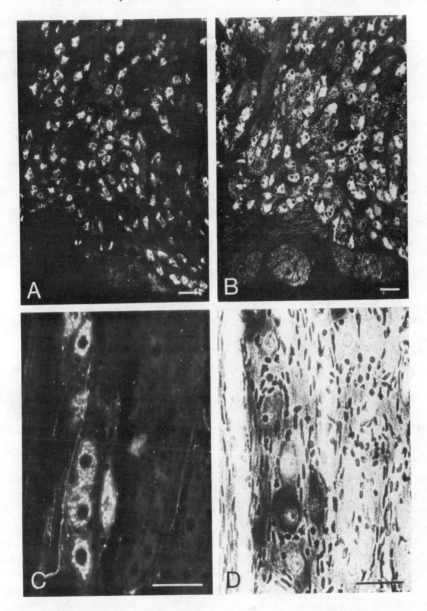

Figure 4.7 Immunofluorescence (a-c) and light (d) micrographs of the inferior mesenteric ganglion of guinea pig (a and b) and the L7 sympathetic ganglion of the cat (c and d) after incubation with antiserum to somatostatin (a), DBH (b), VIP (c) and after staining for AChE (d). a and b: Most of the noradrenergic (DBH-positive) ganglion cell bodies (b) are also somatostatin-immunoreactive (a). c and d: Most of the VIP-immunoreactive ganglion cell bodies (c) are rich in AChE (d). Bars indicate 50 μm. From Hökfelt et al. (1977a) (a and b) and Lundberg et al. (1979) (c and d).

reactive cells were not identical (Lundberg *et al.*, 1982*a*). Thus, peripheral noradrenergic neurones in guinea-pig can be subdivided into at least two populations containing a somatostatin- and APP-like peptide, respectively. Since somatostatin and APP cells do not constitute all ganglion cells, some noradrenaline cells may contain a hitherto unknown peptide, contain no peptide at all, or have too low levels of one or both of the peptides to be detected with the present technique. Finally, small numbers of vasoactive intestinal polypeptide (VIP)-positive cells have been observed in sympathetic ganglia of the guinea-pig (Hökfelt *et al.*, 1977*b*). For example, single cells are seen in the superior cervical ganglion, while in the posterior part of the coeliac-superior mesenteric ganglion complex a somewhat larger proportion of VIP-immunoreactive cells can be seen. In this particular complex APP- and somatostatin-immunoreactive cells are rare. It remains to be established whether these VIP immunoreactive cells represent cholinergic neurones (see below).

In conclusion, in the guinea-pig there seem to exist at least four populations of sympathetic neurones characterized by the presence of detectable amounts of a specific peptide (figure 4.8*a*). In this particular situation no evidence for coexistence of any two of the peptides in the same cells has so far been obtained. It is important to note that considerable species differences seem to exist. Thus, we have not observed somatostatin-like immunoreactivity in sympathetic ganglion cells in the cat, although both APP- and VIP-immunoreactive ganglion cells are present (Lundberg *et al.*, 1980*b*; 1982*a*) (see below).

The analysis of the cat autonomic nervous system has revealed some interesting coexistence situations. In the ganglia of the sympathetic chain, varying proportions of VIP-immunoreactive cells have been observed, with the highest numbers in the L7 ganglion and the stellate ganglion (Lundberg *et al.*, 1979*a*). In these ganglia some 10–15 per cent of all ganglion cells were VIP-immunoreactive. The relative proportions of VIP-immunoreactive cells in these ganglia paralleled the figures calculated for acetylcholinesterase (AChE)-rich cells some 20 years ago by Sjöqvist (1963). It is also consistent with the number of choline acetyltransferase (ChAT)-containing cells in the L7 ganglion as calculated on the basis of microdissection combined with biochemical analysis (Buckley *et al.*, 1967). In fact, a comparative analysis revealed that in most cases VIP-immunoreactive cells corresponded to AChE rich cells (figure 4.7*c* and *d*) (Lundberg *et al.*, 1979), suggesting that the VIP-like peptide is present in cholinergic neurones.

These studies were extended to include also parasympathetic ganglia and similar findings were made in these tissues. In local submandibular ganglia a high proportion of the ganglion cells were VIP-immunoreactive (Lundberg *et al.*, 1980*c*; 1981*a*), and a positive correlation between high AChE activity and VIP immunoreactivity could be established (Lundberg *et al.*, 1980*c*). Since the AChE staining technique is not considered an absolutely specific method for demonstrating cholinergic neurones, the results on the sphenopalatine ganglion offers the hitherto strongest evidence for coexistence of VIP and acetylcholine. This

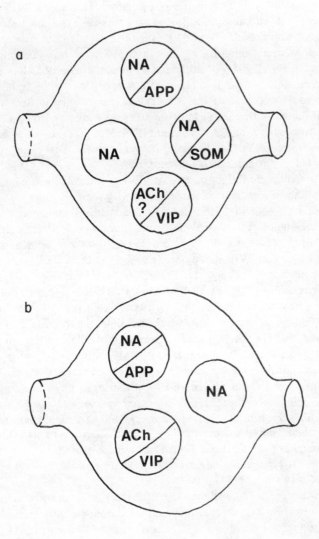

Figure 4.8 Schematic illustration of different types of principal ganglion cell bodies in the inferior mesenteric ganglion of the guinea-pig (*a*) and the L7 ganglion of the sympathetic chain of the cat (*b*). The distinction is based on the possibility to visualise different peptides in sub-populations of the ganglion cells as well as on the possible presence of both adrenergic and cholinergic neurones in these ganglia. So far it seems possible to distinguish four sub-groups in the guinea-pig inferior mesenteric ganglion and three in the cat L7 sympathetic ganglion. No somatostatin-immunoreactive cells have been seen in any cat sympathetic ganglia. It must be emphasised that the presence of cholinergic ganglion cells in the guinea-pig inferior mesenteric ganglion so far only represents a hypothesis. Furthermore, as discussed in the text, it cannot be excluded that the immunohistochemical technique is too insensitive to visualise all peptide stores and that the present subdivision mainly represents differences in peptide levels between different ganglion cells.

ganglion is considered to be a cholinergic ganglion, and in view of the presence
of the peptide in virtually all cells, it is hard to escape the conclusion that, in
fact, VIP and acetylcholine coexist. This is further underlined by experimental
biochemical studies demonstrating that extirpation of this ganglion causes a
parallel loss of ChAT and VIP in the nasal mucosa, a tissue which is innervated
by the sphenopalatine ganglion (Lundberg *et al*., 1981*a*). It will, however, be
important to make combined analyses of these ganglia using antisera to VIP and
ChAT. Antisera to the acetylcholine-synthesising enzyme have in fact been
produced in several laboratories (Eng *et al*., 1974; McGeer *et al*., 1979; Eckenstein
*et al*., 1981), but so far no successful immunohistochemical experiments have
been reported for the autonomic nervous system.

All autonomic ganglia containing AChE-rich and VIP-immunoreactive cell
bodies are known to supply exocrine glands with their cholinergic innervation.
Analysis of such exocrine glands has revealed that VIP-immunoreactive fibres
represent a common feature of these tissues (Bryant *et al*., 1976; Larsson *et al*.,
1978; Uddman, 1980; Lundberg *et al*., 1979*a*; 1980*b*; *c*; 1981*a*, Lundberg,
1981). AChE-rich and VIP-immunoreactive fibres in these glands have a roughly
parallel distribution (Lundberg *et al*., 1979*a*; 1980*b*; *c*; Lundberg, 1981), although
this view has not been held by all groups in the field (see Uddman, 1980). Ultrastructural immunocytochemical analysis has releaved that VIP-like immunoreactivity is present in nerve endings in, for example, the submandibular gland of
the cat, and that the reaction product is mainly confined to large dense cored
vesicles (Johansson and Lundberg, 1981). Parallel routine electron microscopic
analyses has shown that principally only one type of nerve ending can be distinguished on morphological grounds in this gland after sympathectomy, characterised by the presence of large dense cored vesicles and many small empty
vesicles, which confirms earlier findings on the ultrastructural characteristics of
parasympathetic nerve endings in these glands (Garrett, 1974). This type of
nerve ending has generally been assumed to represent cholinergic nerve endings,
in contrast, for example, to adrenergic nerve endings which contain small dense
cored vesicles (Garrett, 1974).

It has therefore been concluded that VIP must reside in nerve endings which
in routine electron microscopic preparations cannot be distinguished from so
called "cholinergic" nerve endings (Johansson and Lundberg, 1981). This is in
contrast to other immunoelectron microscopic studies, which have described
VIP nerve endings as containing a different, larger type of large dense cored
vesicles (Larsson, 1977; Polak and Bloom, 1978). These nerve endings have often
been considered as purinergic nerve endings (see Burnstock, 1972). It may therefore be that VIP-containing nerve endings have a different morphological appearance in different tissues. One explanation could be that cholinergic nerve endings
containing VIP have large dense cored vesicles of about 1000 Å diameter, whereas
other types of VIP nerve endings may contain larger vesicles. Nevertheless, all
immunoelectron microscopic studies suggest that VIP is present mainly in large
dense cored vesicles and no peptide has been reported in the small type vesicles

(diameter 500 Å). Since this may represent a negative artifact, attempts have also been made to analyse the subcellular distribution of VIP and acetylcholine by means of fractionation studies (figure 4.9) (Lundberg *et al.*, 1981*b*). The

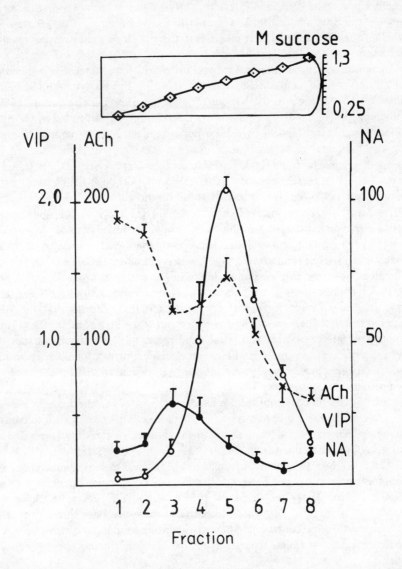

Figure 4.9 Illustration of the distribution of specific activity (pmol/mg protein) for VIP, ACh and NA in whole fractions (sedimentable + soluble portions) of the density gradient of cat submandibular gland. Note that VIP exhibits one distinct peak, which coincides with one of two ACh peaks. The NA peak is distinct from both these peaks. For further details, see Lundberg *et al.* (1981*b*), from which this drawing has been taken.

results indicate that VIP is mainly present in the heavier fractions containing the highest proportions of large dense cored vesicles, whereas only little VIP is present in lighter fractions. In contrast, acetylcholine is found mainly in lighter fractions, although a second smaller peak coincides with the VIP-immuno-reactive one. This could indicate that acetylcholine is mainly stored in small vesicles but that, in addition, a proportion is also stored in larger vesicles. Whether these larger vesicles are identical to the VIP-storing large vesicles remains to be shown.

Sympathetic ganglia in the cat contain many APP-immunoreactive cell bodies, which also are TH- and DBH-immunoreactive and thus produce noradrenaline. They are not identical to the VIP-immunoreactive cells (Lundberg *et al.*, 1980*a*; Lundberg, 1981; Lundberg *et al.*, 1982*a*). Again, there seem to be sympathetic noradrenergic ganglion cells, which do not contain an APP-like peptide, suggesting the existence of at least three principal ganglion cell populations in cat sympathetic ganglia (figure 4.8*b*). APP-immunoreactive nerve fibres are found in many peripheral tissues including exocrine glands. Although their general distribution patterns often are similar to those of the adrenergic ones, interesting differences have been observed. Thus, whereas the DBH- and TH-immunoreactive nerve endings can be found both around blood vessels and close to the secretory elements (acini and ducts), APP-immunoreactive nerve endings are almost exclusively found around blood vessels (Lundberg *et al.*, 1980*a*; 1982*a*). Therefore, it seems as if the population of noradrenaline neurones containing an APP-like peptide preferentially innervates blood vessels. Studies on the nasal mucosa give evidence for a further subspecialisation, namely that the APP-immunoreactive fibres mainly surround arteries (Lundberg *et al.*, 1982*a*). These findings suggest a specialisation and subdivision of the sympathetic nervous system with regard to the type of innervated tissue. Furthermore, it suggests that the coexisting peptide may participate only in certain special functions of the sympathetic nervous system.

Other cases of coexistence have also been reported. In the superior cervical ganglion of the rat a proportion of the ganglion cells has been shown to contain an enkephalin-like peptide after treatment with colchicine locally applied on the ganglion (Schultzberg *et al.*, 1979).

Table 4.1 lists two cases of suspected coexistence including enkephalin and neurotensin in possibly cholinergic preganglionic neurones (Lundberg *et al.*, 1980*b*; 1981*c*; Glazer and Basbaum, 1980). It should, however, be emphasised that no attempts have been made to correlate these neurones with any type of "cholinergic" marker, and that these two peptide-containing systems very well could represent neurones separate from the classical cholinergic preganglionic ones.

In addition to the above mentioned examples of neuronal coexistence, a number of paracrine cells contain both an amine and a peptide. Thus, small intensely fluorescent (SIF) cells in sympathetic ganglia may contain a peptide.

Enkephalin-like immunoreactivity has been reported in such cells in the inferior mesenteric ganglion and in the coeliac-superior mesenteric ganglion complex of guinea-pig (Schultzberg *et al.*, 1979). In the cat coeliac ganglion, SIF cells contain both enkephalin- and somatostatin-like immunoreactivity (Lundberg *et al.*, 1980*b*; 1982*a*) and a substance P-like peptide is also present in these cells in some species (Schultzberg *et al.*, unpublished). In the cat carotid body the type I cells contain enkephalin-like immunoreactivity (Lundberg *et al.*, 1979*b*; Wharton *et al.*, 1980) and a substance P-like peptide has also been reported (Cuello and McQueen, 1980).

Finally, it should be mentioned that peptides have also been observed in the adrenal gland. Thus, a large proportion of the gland cells in the rat (figure 4.10*a*) guinea-pig (figure 4.10*b* and *c*) and cat (figure 4.10*d*) contain enkephalin-like peptides (Schultzberg *et al.*, 1978*a*; *b*). No $\beta$-endorphin-like immunoreactivity was observed in the adrenal gland of any of the species studied. Interestingly, in the normal rat only a small number of enkephalin-immunoreactive gland cells was observed, but after transection of the splanchnic nerve a marked increase in immunoreactivity was seen, resulting in immunofluorescence in most gland cells (figure 4.10*a*) (Schultzberg *et al.*, 1978*b*). Opioid-like material has also been found in the adrenal medulla with biochemical techniques (Viveros *et al.*, 1979; Lewis *et al.*, 1979; Hexum *et al.*, 1980). In a series of elegant papers Udenfriend and his collaborators have demonstrated that the adrenal medulla contains a number of opiate peptides with particularly high concentrations of precursor molecules (Lewis *et al.*, 1979, 1980; Stern *et al.*, 1980). About 25 per cent of the opiate activity is due to the pentapeptides, with high concentration also of the heptapeptide met-enkephalin (Arg$^6$, Phe$^7$) (Stern *et al.*, 1980). The lack of $\beta$-endorphin-like peptides could also be demonstrated biochemically (Viveros *et al.*, 1979; Lewis *et al.*, 1979). The biochemical analysis revealed that the increase in enkephalin-like immunoreactivity, described immunohistochemically after splanchnic nerve sectioning (Schultzberg *et al.*, 1978*b*), is due to increased amount of precursor peptides (Lewis *et al.*, 1981). It is important to note that the adrenal gland in addition contains enkephalin-like material in nerve endings (figure 4.10*b,c*), which disappears after sectioning of the splanchnic nerve (figure 4.10*a*) (Schultzberg *et al.*, 1978*b*).

Also APP immunoreactivity has been observed in some adrenal medullary cells (Lundberg *et al.*, 1980*a*). Finally, neurotensin-like immunoreactivity is present in noradrenaline containing chromaffin cells of the cat adrenal gland (Lundberg *et al.*, 1980*b*; 1981*c*).

Tumours arising from chromaffin cells also contain opioid-like peptides. Thus, both enkephalin- and somatostatin-like immunoreactivities have been demonstrated in pheochromocytoma (Sullivan *et al.*, 1978; Lundberg *et al.*, 1979*c*; Clement-Jones *et al.*, 1980; Giraud *et al.*, 1981; Wilson *et al.*, 1981). For a more detailed account on opioid peptides in adrenal medullary cells and related systems we refer to chapter 5.

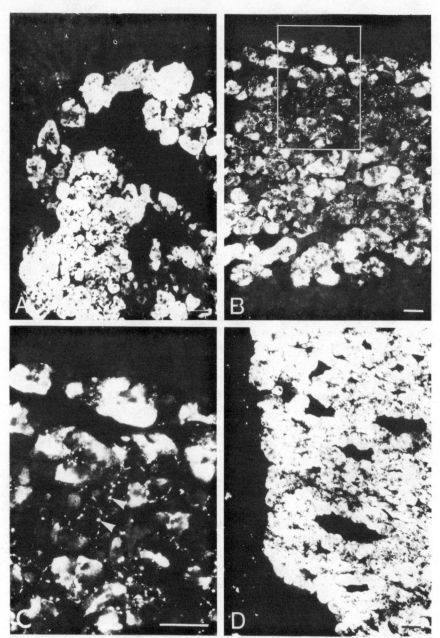

Figure 4.10 Immunofluorescence micrographs of the rat (a), guinea-pig (b and c) and cat (d) adrenal gland after incubation with antiserum to methionine-enkephalin. The rat adrenal gland had been subjected to transection of the splanchnic nerve 24 h before death. Most gland cells in all three species contain enkephalin-like immunoreactivity. Note also the presence of enkephalin-immunoreactive nerve endings in the adrenal medulla of the guinea-pig (b and c). Such nerve endings can also be seen in the rat medulla (not shown), but disappear after section of the splanchnic nerve (a). Bars indicate 50 μm. For further details, see Schultzberg et al. (1978b), from which these micrographs have been taken.

## Functional aspects of peripheral transmitter peptide coexistence

Our best knowledge so far with regard to functional significance of coexisting classical transmitters and peptides is based on studies on the peripheral nervous system, more precisely the submandibular salivary gland of cat. This gland has been used as an *in vivo* model due to its accessability for experimental work. It is, however, likely that, at least in the cat, similar mechansims operate in most exocrine glands. In fact, preliminary studies on, for example, sweat glands and nasal mucosa suggest the existence of similar mechanisms for the control of secretion and vasodilation.

It has long been known that parasympathetic nerve stimulation at a high frequency causes salivary secretion and a marked increase in blood flow through the gland (Bernard, 1858). Whereas salivation can be completely blocked by atropine, this drug has little effect on vasodilation as noted already by Heidenhain (1872) (figure 4.11c). The background for these experimental findings has been a subject of controversy for many years, and explanations have included occurrence of special noncholinergic vasodilatory nerves as well as nervous release of an enzyme, kallikrein, which causes production of vasodilating peptides, for example, bradykinin (see Hilton and Lewis, 1955a; b). It may be noted that sweat glands represent a special case, as the cholinergic fibres innervating them have their cell bodies in ganglia of the sympathetic chain. In agreement with the concept of a cholinergic control of exocrine glands, these tissues can be demonstrated to contain numerous AChE-rich nerves. As discussed above, these glands also have more or less overlapping networks of VIP-immunoreactive fibres and there is evidence that VIP is present in the cholinergic neurones, suggesting the possibility of a concomitant release of these two compounds from the same nerve endings.

This hypothesis has been extensively tested by Lundberg and collaborators. It has been demonstrated that parasympathetic stimulation of the submandibular gland causes, together with secretion and increase in blood flow, a marked release of immunoreactive VIP (figure 4.11) (Lundberg *et al.*, 1980c; Bloom and Edwards, 1980). VIP release is dependent on stimulation frequency and is particularly large at high frequencies with an about ten fold increase in VIP output at 15 Hz as compared to 6 Hz (figure 4.11b and c) (Lundberg *et al.*, 1981d). Preliminary studies have also demonstrated a concomitant release of acetylcholine and VIP during nerve stimulation (Lundberg *et al.*, unpublished). Whereas atropine totally abolished submandibular secretion at all frequencies, it reduced only the initial and maintained vasodilatory response at lower frequencies (figure 4.11a-c). Interestingly, at higher frequencies atropine caused a marked increase in overflow of VIP, accompanied by an increased duration of the vasodilatory response (figure 4.11) (Lundberg *et al.*, 1981a;e; Lundberg, 1981).

It has therefore been speculated that release of VIP is controlled by inhibitory muscarinic autoreceptors. Thus, the increased levels of VIP after atropine treatment could be due to a blockade of these presynaptic inhibitory receptors (figure

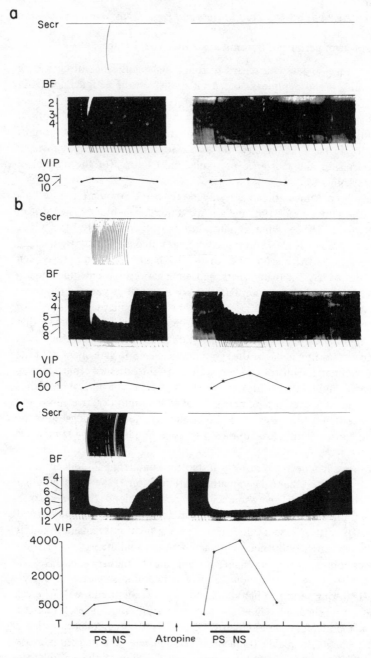

Figure 4.11 Effects of parasympathetic nerve stimulation at (a) 2 Hz, (b) 6 Hz and (c) 15 Hz on cat submandibular blood flow (BF, ml/min), salivary secretion (Secr, drops) and VIP release (VIP), expressed as VIP output (fmol $min^{-1}$ $g^{-1}$). Each tenth drop of saliva and blood is separately marked. Systemic arterial blood pressure was between 110 and 120 mm Hg in all cases. Time scale (T) between thick bars = 1 min. Atropine 0.5 mg/kg intravenously was given before the second stimulation. Note the different scales for VIP output. (From Lundberg, 1978.)

4.15). These findings suggest an interesting possibility of interaction between two coexisting transmitter-like compounds. In conclusion the effects of atropine suggest that, whereas acetylcholine is responsible for secretion, both acetylcholine and VIP seem to be of importance for vasodilation. However, in the latter response acetylcholine seems to be mainly involved in the initial phase and at low frequency stimulation. The contribution of VIP in the vasodilatory response increases with time and frequency.

The lack of pharmacological agents interfering with peptide mechanisms at synapses is a general problem in attempts to elucidate the functional role of peptides. Lundberg and collaborators (1980c; 1981e), using VIP antiserum or IgG isolated from VIP antiserum, have demonstrated that infusion of such antiserum or IgG reduced both vasodilation and salivary secretion at 2 Hz (figure 4.12). These findings may indicate that VIP is released also at a low frequency stimulation and is of importance also for the initial vasodilatory phase.

The importance of VIP for vasodilation can also be ascertained by infusion

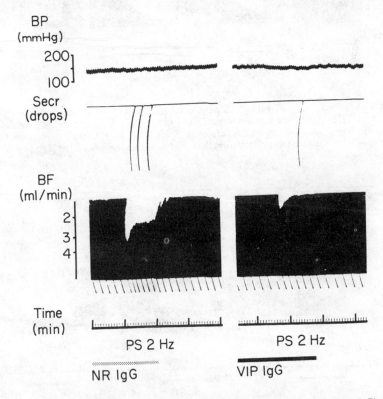

Figure 4.12 Effects of local intra-arterial infusion of normal rabbit IgG (NR IgG) or IgG isolated from VIP antiserum (VIP IgG) on vasodilation (BF) and salivary secretion (Secr) from the cat submandibular gland induced by parasympathetic nerve stimulation (PS 2 Hz). BP, Blood pressure. Recordings are as in figure 8.11. (From Lundberg *et al.*, 1981e.)

of the peptide, but even at a very high dose no salivary secretion can be observed (figure 4.13) (Shimizu and Taira, 1979; Bloom and Edwards, 1980; Lundberg *et al.*, 1980*c*; 1981*f*). VIP-induced vasodilation could not be blocked by atropine. Infusion of acetylcholine alone caused both vasodilation and salivary secretion (figure 4.14). To obtain maximal vasodilation, about 100 times higher doses of acetylcholine than VIP had to be infused. When acetylcholine and VIP were infused together, an enhancement of vasodilation and secretory response was

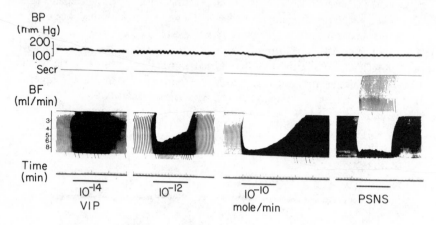

Figure 4.13  Effects of local intra-arterial infusion of VIP and parasympathetic nerve stimulation at 15 Hz (PSNS) on submandibular gland blood flow (BF) and salivary secretion (secr.). BP, Blood pressure. Recordings are as in figure 4.11. Note the marked vasodilatory response of VIP infusions but no salivation is seen. (From Lundberg *et al.*, 1981*f*.)

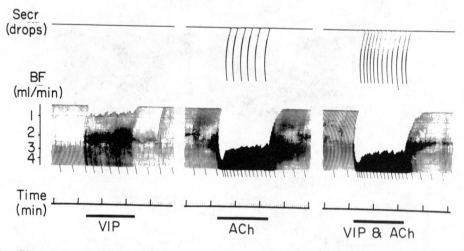

Figure 4.14  Effects of local intra-arterial infusions of VIP, ACh, and VIP combined with ACh on submandibular gland blood flow (BF) and salivary secretion (secr.). Doses were VIP 0.1 pmol/min and ACh 50 pmol/min. (From Lundberg, 1981.)

observed with an additive effect on vasodilation with lower doses of acetylcholine and VIP. The salivary secretion induced by acetylcholine could be potentiated by VIP (figure 4.14). Acetylcholine-induced salivation could be potentiated even with low doses of VIP, which did not cause major additional changes in blood flow (figure 4.14). Furthermore, increase in blood flow induced by isoprenaline was much less potent in potentiating acetylcholine-induced salivation. These findings suggest that the effects of VIP are not only related to effects on blood flow (Lundberg *et al.*, 1981*f*; Lundberg, 1981).

The exact mechanisms of action of VIP and acetylcholine in inducing vasodilation and salivary secretion in the submandibular gland have not been elucidated. Lundberg (1981) has discussed this question extensively and pointed out that VIP, probably by way of specific receptors, activates adenylate cyclase with subsequent intracellular cyclic AMP formation, whereas acetylcholine by way of action on muscarinic receptors may, *inter alia*, lead to an increase in $Ca^{2+}$ permeability and formation of cyclic GMP by way of activation of guanylate cyclase (figure 4.15). It is also of interest to draw parallels to *in vitro* experiments on the guinea-pig exocrine pancreas by Gardner and his associates (Gardner and Jackson, 1977; Gardner, 1979). These authors have concluded that agents which simultaneously activate cyclic AMP and cyclic GMP mechanisms interact in "some presently unknown way", causing a potentiation of the functional response, which in their case is enzyme secretion. Other types of interactions can, however, also occur, and it has, in fact, been demonstrated by Lundberg and his associates that VIP can increase binding of acetylcholine to muscarinic receptors in the cat submandibular gland (Lundberg *et al.*, 1982). Furthermore, VIP and acetylcholine seem to interact at the second messenger level, that is, cyclic AMP formation (Fredholm and Lundberg, 1981). Again, the interaction of the two coexisting compounds is to increase the physiological responses and this interaction may occur at different levels (figure 4.15), as was discussed also for coexisting compounds in the central nervous system (see above).

A comparison of acetylcholine and VIP as compounds stored and released from the same nerve endings, reveals striking differences at many levels (figure 4.15). Whereas acetylcholine can be synthesised within the nerve endings due to the presence of the synthesising enzyme (ChAT), VIP as a peptide is in all probability only produced in the cell bodies on ribosomes, and each molecule released at the nerve ending will therefore have to be transported along the axon to the release site. Thus, the replacement of released acetylcholine can occur rapidly by way of uptake of choline and immediate synthesis and storage of acetylcholine, whereas VIP has to be replaced by axonal transport, which then suggests a slow turnover (see Lundberg *et al.*, 1981*h*). Another issue, which could be addressed on the basis of these findings, is whether the two compounds could be considered as neurotransmitters or neuromodulators. For discussion on the definition of this issue see, for example, Burnstock *et al.*, (1979). Also this issue has been discussed by Lundberg (1981): briefly acetylcholine can be considered as a transmitter with regard to its action on secretion and possibly on vasodilation, but it

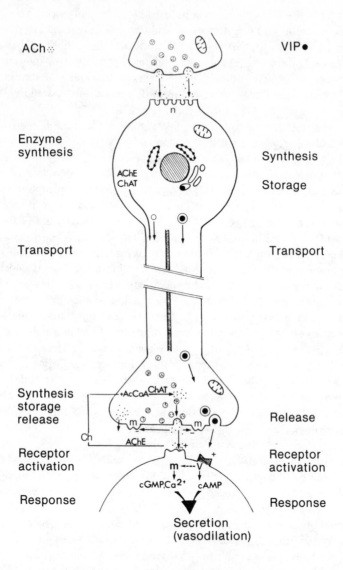

ACh                                                    VIP●

Enzyme
synthesis
                                                       Synthesis

                                                       Storage

Transport                                              Transport

Synthesis
storage
release
                                                       Release

Receptor
activation
                                                       Receptor
                                                       activation

Response                                               Response

Secretion
(vasodilation)

Figure 4.15 Schematic illustrations of major characteristics of synthesis, transmitter release, and so on, for a postganglionic ACh/VIP containing neurone in the cat submandibular gland. The preganglionic cholinergic nerve ending (top), exocrine or smooth muscle effector cell (bottom), and organelles like small clear vesicles, large dense cored vesicles, mitochondria, RER, Golgi and axonal microtubuli have been briefly outlined. ACh is indicated by small dots; n, nicotinic receptors; AChE, acetylcholine esterase; ChAT, choline acetyltransferase; Ch, choline; AcCoA, acetyl coenzyme A; m, muscarinic receptor; inhibition of release; +, stimulation of receptor; VIP, filled circle; V, VIP receptor. For details see text. (From Lundberg, 1981.)

acts as a modulator on the hypothetical presynaptic muscarinic receptors controlling VIP release (figure 4.15). VIP, on the other hand, could be considered as a transmitter with regard to its action on vasodilation, whereas its presumed effects on secretion seem to be of modulatory nature.

Of interest also is the possible interaction of acetylcholine/VIP neurones with the sympathetic nervous system. As described above, the nasal mucosa and the submandibular gland (and other exocrine glands) contain in addition to acetylcholine/VIP neurones, sympathetic nerve terminals, some of which seem to contain an APP-immunoreactive substance and noradrenaline, and some which may only contain noradrenaline. Whereas the latter innervate exocrine elements, the APP/noradrenaline neurones have been found preferentially around arterial vessels (Lundberg *et al.*, 1982*a*). This offers a morphological basis for interaction in the control of blood flow. Lundberg and collaborators (Lundberg *et al.*, 1980*d*; Lundberg, 1981) have shown that infusion of APP can inhibit both the vasodilation induced by parasympathetic nerve stimulation as well as the concomitant salivary secretion (figure 4.16).

APP did not inhibit VIP release to any major extent which suggests that the APP in some way reduces the effector cell response to the mediator substances which are released during nerve stimulation (Lundberg, 1981). This is also indicated by the finding that local infusion of APP can also inhibit VIP-induced vasodilation (figure 4.17). It is interesting that in the sympathetic nerves APP cooperates with the classical transmitter, noradrenaline, in the functional response, just as there is a cooperative effect between VIP and acetylcholine. It must be emphasised that the interpretation of these findings is preliminary. As discussed above, the nature of the APP-like immunoreactivity has not been elucidated. In fact, it seems unlikely that the peptide present in the tissue is genuine APP. In line with this, BPP has also been tested. In fact, both this peptide and APP in higher doses seem to have direct vasoconstrictory effects suggesting an interaction with noradrenaline of similar type as has been reported for VIP and acetylcholine (Lundberg, unpublished).

## PEPTIDE/PEPTIDE COEXISTENCE

During the past decade numerous peptides have been mapped in the central and peripheral nervous system with immunohistochemical techniques. It was often found that certain areas in the brain such as hypothalamus, the amygdaloid complex, and several areas in the lower brain stem, such as the nucleus tractus solitari contained many, if not all, peptides investigated. However, analysis of the distribution patterns of the cell bodies containing different immunoreactivities suggested that, at large, peptides were present in separate systems. The areas rich in peptides were often rich in classical transmitters, for example, catecholamines and indolamines and, as described above, the subsequent detailed analyses revealed interesting situations, where a classical transmitter and a peptide coexisted. Similarly, the detailed comparison of distribution patterns of peptide

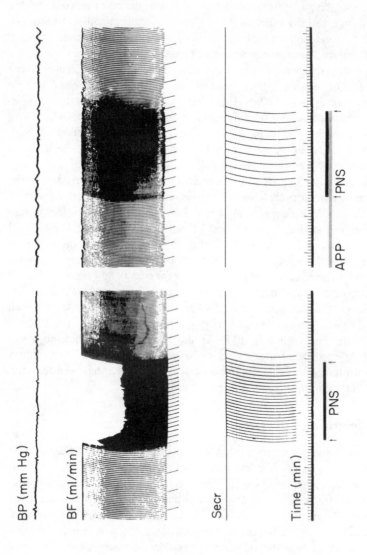

Figure 4.16  Effects of local intra-arterial infusion of APP on the response to parasympathetic nerve stimulation in the cat submandibular gland. BF, Blood flow; BP, blood pressure, S, secretion. Note that APP infusion inhibits both the vasodilatory and salivation response without having any effect per se on those parameters. (From Lundberg *et al.*, 1980*d*.)

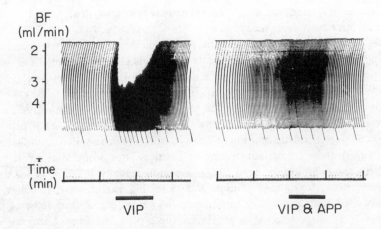

Figure 4.17  Effects of local intra-arterial infusion of APP (2 pmol/min) on submandibular vasodilation (BF) induced by VIP (20 pmol/min). (From Lundberg, 1981.)

containing neurones have revealed that certain situations occur, where two or more peptides are found in the same neurone. (table 4.3).

The first example of such a coexistence was the so called proopiocortin system. These neurones are located in the hypothalamus and they contain, *inter alia* ACH and β-endorphin (Bloch *et al.*, 1978; Watson *et al.*, 1978; Nilaver *et al.*, 1979). These neurones are, however, not identical to any of the numerous enkephalin systems in the brain (Bloom *et al.*, 1978). This multiple peptide coexistence could be explained by the fact that all these peptides have a common precursor (Mains *et al.*, 1977; Roberts and Herbert, 1977; Nakanishi *et al.*, 1979). Interestingly, in spite of the fact that the pentapeptide enkephalin is present in this molecule (within the β-endorphin part), most antisera do not indicate enkephalin in these cells. The work of Udenfriend and his collaborators (see Lewis *et al.*, 1980) have now demonstrated that the enkephalins have completely different precursors than β-endorphin. In the following we would, however, not like to deal with these systems, but concentrate on some other peptide/peptide

Table 4.3   Coexistence of peptides*

| Peptide I | Peptide II | |
|-----------|------------|---|
| ACTH | β-endorphin | CNS (hypothalamus) |
| Enkephalin | Somatostatin | CNS (hypothalamus) |
| Enkephalin | Neurophysin | CNS (hypothalamus) |
| Enkephalin | APP | CNS (spinal cord) |
| Substance P | TRH | CNS (medulla) |
| Substance P | CCK | CNS (periaquaductal grey) |
| Somatostatin | APP | CNS (forebrain) |
| Somatostatin | CCK/gastrin | PNS (submucous plexus of large intestine) |

*For references see text. See also footnotes to table 4.1.

coexistence situations, for which no apparent explanation with regard to precursor identity is available today.

The gastro-intestinal tract contains numerous peptide neurones, including immunoreactive substance P, somatostatin, enkephalin, bombesin, CCK, and many others (for summaries on such studies, see Furness and Costa, 1980; Jessen *et al.*, 1980; Schultzberg *et al.*, 1980; and Leander *et al.*, 1981). These peptides are distributed in cell bodies present in the two ganglionic layers and in nerve terminals in all layers of the intestinal wall. Although each peptide exhibits characteristic distribution patterns (Costa and Furness, 1980; Schultzberg *et al.*, 1980), there are certain striking similarities. Thus, somatostatin, VIP and gastrin/CCK-immunoreactive cell bodies are preferentially localised in the submucous plexus. In detailed elution and restaining experiments, it could be demonstrated that in the large intestine of the guinea pig, at least some of the somatostatin cells contained a gastrin/CCK-like peptide (figure 4.18*a* and *c*), whereas VIP was present in a different population of cells (figure 4.18*b*) (Schultzberg *et al.*, 1980). These findings illustrate that coexistence of peptides may occur in subpopulations of neurones and that differences in the gross distribution patterns cannot be taken as a guarantee for the existence of completely separate systems. In fact, coexistence both with regard to peptide/classical transmitter and peptide/peptide always seems to occur in subpopulations of neurones.

In the central nervous system enkephalin-somatostatin coexistence has been described in the median eminence (Tramu and Leonardelli, 1979), enkephalin and neurophysin in the posterior pituitary (Coulter *et al.*, 1981), and somatostatin and an APP-like peptide in nerve cell bodies in, for example, nucleus caudatus, cerebral cortex, nucleus accumbens and the hippocampus (figure 4.18*d* and *e*) (Vincent *et al.*, 1982). In the rostral mesencephalic periaqueductal central grey a population of neurones contains both a substance P and a CCK-like peptide (figure 4.18*f* and *g*) (Skirboll *et al.*, 1981) and these neurones seem to project to the spinal cord (Skirboll *et al.*, unpublished). In the lower medulla oblongata cell bodies in the raphe nuclei (raphe pallidus, raphe obscurus and raphe magnus) and adjacent areas contain both a substance P- and TRH-like peptide (figure 4.2*b* and *c*) (Johansson *et al.*, 1981). These neurones also project to the spinal cord. In the spinal cord, Hunt *et al.*, (1981) have observed a population of neurones at the lumbar and sacral levels, which contains both an enkephalin- and an APP-like peptide. Whether the enkephalin immunoreactive neurones in the rat superior cervical ganglion (Schultzberg *et al.*, 1979) also contain an APP-like peptide remains to be demonstrated.

Again, this coexistence seems to be confined to small populations of all neurones containing the respective peptide. As discussed above, the crucial question is whether or not peptides, in fact, are limited to the neurone populations where they can be observed with immunohistochemistry. It is well known that the technique is often not sufficiently sensitive to demonstrate peptides (and other compounds) in all systems where they occur. Thus negative results should be interpreted with great caution. Perhaps, therefore, better and

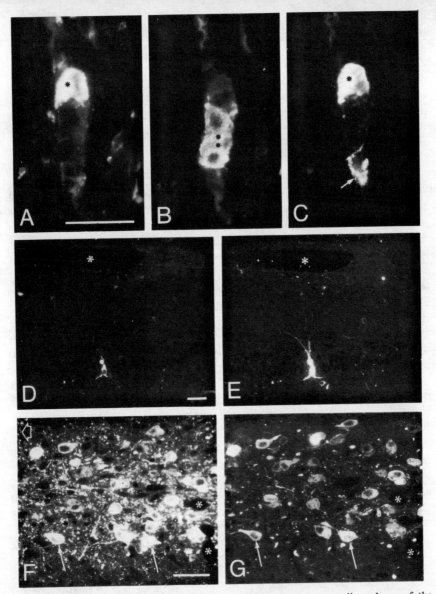

Figure 4.18 Immunofluorescence micrographs of the submucous ganglion plexus of the proximal colon of vinblastine-treated (local treatment) guinea-pig (*a-c*), of the hippocampus (*d* and *e*) and periaqueductal central grey (*f* and *g*) of colchicine-treated rat after incubation with antiserum to gastrin/CCK (*a* and *g*), VIP (*b*), somatostatin (*c* and *e*), APP (*d*) and substance P (*f*). *a-c* represent the same section, which has been first incubated with gastrin/CCK antiserum (*a*), then eluted and restained with VIP antiserum (*b*) and finally eluted again and restained with somatostatin antiserum (*c*). Gastrin/CCK (one asterisk in *a*) and somatostatin (one asterisk in *c*), but not VIP (two asterisks in *b*) immunoreactivities are present in the same cells. Note that somatostatin in addition is present in a further cell (arrow in *c*). *d* and *e* represent the same section which was first stained with APP antiserum (*d*), then eluted and restained for somatostatin (*e*). Somatostatin- and APP-like immunoreactivities are seen in the same cell in the CA-1 region of the dorsal hippocampus. Asterisks denote the same blood vessel. *f* and *g* represent adjacent sections. Many nerve cells in the ventral PAG (arrows indicate some) contain both substance P- and gastrin/CCK-like immunoreactivities. Bars indicate 50 μm. *a-c* are from Schultzberg *et al.* (1980); *d* and *e* from Vincent *et al.* (1982); and *f* and *g* from Skirboll *et al.* (1982).

more sensitive antisera as well as more sensitive techniques will reveal more numerous and more extensively distributed coexistence situations both with regard to classical transmitter and peptide as well as to peptide/peptide coexistence.

## CONCLUSIONS

We have summarised morphological evidence for the coexistence of peptides and classical transmitters in neurones. Although direct evidence for coexistence is mainly given for cell somata, indirect evidence exists also for coexistence in nerve endings, that is the sites from which transmitters and neuromodulators are released. Very recently, direct ultrastructural evidence has been presented that two compounds in fact are present in the same nerve endings and even in the same storage vesicles. With regard to functional significance, results have recently been obtained, particularly in studies on the peripheral nervous system, suggesting interesting possibilities of interaction between, for example, acetylcholine and VIP in exocrine glands. In this model the two compounds seem to cooperate in causing a full functional response, and principally similar types of cooperation may occur in other coexistence situations in other tissues.

It will be an important task to elucidate whether the coexistence situations described here are permanent and represent expressions of genetic regulation, or whether they represent functional fluctuation as suggested by Chan-Palay (1979). It has been shown that substance P levels in *inter alia*, the substantia nigra markedly fluctuate in a diurnal cycle (Kerdelhue *et al.*, 1979), perhaps depending on, for example, a functional state. Studies are now under way to see if coexistence occurs with similar distribution patterns in other species, in different ages and in different experimental situations. It may be speculated that in certain physiological conditions a neurone will only express one of the peptides. This will allow the neurone to change and increase its capability to convey information and transmit differentiated messages across the synapses. Whether these messages always are of transmitter or neuromodulatory nature, or whether peptides are involved in other functions, such as recognition and regulation of trophic function, remains to be shown. Finally, it may be interesting to analyse whether or not disturbances in the balance between two or more neuroactive substances released from a neurone may be of importance for certain pathophysiological conditions such as mental illness or disorders of the autonomic nervous system.

## ACKNOWLEDGEMENTS

This study was supported by grants from the Swedish Medical Research Council (04X-2887; 04X-04495; 17X-5438), Knut och Alice Wallenbergs Stiftelse, Magnus Bergvalls Stiftelse, Sven och Ebba-Kristina Hagbergs Stiftelse, Olli och Elof Erikssons Stiftelse and Svenska Tobaksbolaget. The article was in part prepared during a stay of Tomas Hökfelt at the National Institutes of Health as a

Fogarty Fellow. The Fellowship is gratefully acknowledged. The support of Dr M. Brownstein (NIMH) is gratefully acknowledged. We thank Miss Annika Edin, Mrs Waldtraut Hiort, and Miss Anne Peters for skilful technical assistance.

# REFERENCES

Aghajanian, G. R., and Wang, R. Y. (1978). Physiology and pharmacology of central serotonergic neurons. *Psychychopharmacology: A Generation of Progress* (ed. M. A. Lipton, A. Dimascio and K. F. Killam), Raven Press, New York, pp. 171–183

Andén, N-E., Dahlström, A., Fuxe, K., and Larsson, K. (1965). Further evidence for the presence of nigro-neostriatal dopamine neurones in the rat. *Am. J. Anat.*, **116**, 329–334

Andén, N-E., Dahlström, A., Fuxe, K., Larsson, K., Olson, L. and Ungerstedt, U. (1966). Ascending monoamine neurons to the telencephalon and diencephalon. *Acta Physiol. Scand.*, **67**, 313–326

Andén, N-E., Jukes, M. and Lundberg, A. (1964). Spinal reflexes and monoamine liberation. *Nature London*, **202**, 1222–1223

Avrameas, S. (1969). Coupling of enzymes to proteins with glutaldehyde. Use of the conjugates for the detection of antigens and antibodies. *Immunochemistry* **6**, 43–47

Barbeau, H. and Bedard, P. (1981). Similar motor effects of 5-HT and TRH in rats following chronic spinal transection and 5, 7-dihydroxytryptamine injection. *Neuropharmacology*, **20**, 477–481

Baumgarten, H. G., Björklund, A., Lachenmayer, L. and Nobin, A. (1973). Evaluation of the effects of 5, 7-dihydroxytryptamine on serotonin and catecholamine neurons in the rat CNS. *Acta Physiol. Scand.*, suppl., **391**, 1–19

Baumgarten, H. G., Björklund, A., Lachenmayer, L., Nobin, A. and Stenevi, V. (1971). Long lasting selective depletion of brain serotonin by 5, 6-di-hydroxytryptamine. *Acta Physiol. Scand.*, suppl., **373**, 1–15

Ben-Ari, Y., Pradelles, P., Gros, C., and Dray, F. (1979). Identification of authentic substance P in striatonigral and amygdaloid nuclei using combined high performance liquid chromatography and radioimmunoassay. *Brain Res.*, **173**, 360–363

Bernard, C. (1858). De l'influence de deux ordres de nerfs qui déterminent les variations di couleur du sang veineux dans les organes glandulaires. *C.r. Acad. Sci. Paris*, **47**, 245–253

Björklund, A., Emson, P. C., Gilbert, R. T. F., and Skagerberg, G. (1979). Further evidence for the possible coexistence of 5-hydroxytryptamine and substance P in medullary raphe neurons of rat brain. *Br. J. Pharmac.*, **66**, 112–113

Bloch, B., Bugnon, C., Fellman, D. and Lenys, D. (1978). Immunocytochemical evidence that the same neurons in the human infundibular nucleus are stained with anti-endorphins and antisera of other related peptides. *Neurosci. Lett.*, **10**, 147–152

Bloom, F. E., Battenberg, E., Rossier, J., Ling, N. and Guillemin, R. (1978). Neurons containing β-endorphin in rat brain exist separately from those containing enkephalin: immunocytochemical studies. *Proc. natn. Acad. Sci., U.S.A.*, **75**, 1591–1595

Bloom, S. R. and Edwards, T. (1980). Vasoactive intestinal peptide in relation to atropine resistant vasodilatation in the submaxillary gland of the cat. *J. Physiol. Lond.* **129**, 253–271

Brownstein, M. J., Saavedra, J. M., Axelrod, J., Zeman, G. H. and Carpenter, D. O. (1974). Coexistence of several putative neurotransmitters in single identified neurons of *Aplysia*. *Proc. natn. Acad. Sci. U.S.A.*, **7**, 4662–4665

Bryant, M. G., Polak, J. M., Modlin, J., Bloom, S. R., Albuquerque, R. J. and Pearse, A. G. E. (1976). Possible dual role of vasoactive intestinal polypeptide as gastrointestinal hormone and neurotransmitter candidate. *Lancet*, **i**, 991–993

Buckley, G., Consolo, S., Giacobini, E. and Sjöqvist, F. (1967). Cholineacetylase in innervated and denervated sympathetic ganglia and ganglion cells of the cat. *Acta Physiol. Scand.*, **71**, 348–356

Burn, J. H. and Rand, M. J. (1965). Acetylcholine in adrenergic transmission. *A. Rev. Pharmac.*, **5**, 163–182

Burnstock, G. (1972). Purinergic nerves. *Pharmac. Rev.*, **24**, 509–581

Burnstock, G. (1976). Do some cells release more than one transmitter? *Neuroscience*, **1**, 239–248

Burnstock, G., Hökfelt, T., Gershon, M. D., Iversen, L. L., Kosterlitz, H. W., Szurszewski, J. H. (1979). Non-adrenergic, non-cholinergic autonomic neurotransmission mechanisms. *Neurosci. Res. Progr. Bull.*, **17**, 377–519

Chan-Palay, V. (1979). Combined immunocytochemistry and autoradiography after in vivo Injections of monoclonal antibody to substance P and $^3$H serotonin: coexistence of two putative transmitters in single raphe cells and fiber plexuses. *Anat. Embryol.*, **156**, 241–254

Chan-Palay, V. Jonsson, G. and Palay, S. L., (1978). Serotonin and substance P coexist in neurons of the rat's central nervous system. *Proc. natn. Acad. Sci. U.S.A.*, **75**, 1582–1586

Clement-Jones, V., Corder, R. and Lowry, P. J. (1980). Isolation of human met-enkephalin and two groups of putative precursors (2K-pro-met-enkephalin) from an adrenal medullary tumour. *Biochem. biophys. Res. Commun.*, **95**, 665–673

Coons, A. H. (1958). Fluorescent antibody methods. In *General Cytochemical Methods* (ed. J. F. Danielli), Academic Press, New York, pp. 399–422

Cooper, B. R. and Boyer, C. E. (1978). Stimulant action of thyrotropin-releasing hormone on cat spinal cord. *Neuropharmacology*, **17**, 153–156

Cottrell, G. A. (1976). Does the giant cerebral neurone of *Helix* release two transmitters, acetylcholine and serotonin. *J. Physiol. Lond.*, **259**, 44–45P

Coulter, D., Elde, R. P., and Unveizagt, S. L. (1981). Co-localization of neurophysin- and enkephalin-like immunoreactivity in cat pituitary. *Peptides*, suppl., **1**, 51–55

Cuello, A. C. and McQueen, D. S. (1980). Substance P: a carotid body peptide. *Neurosci. Lett.*, **17**, 215–219

Dahlström, A. (1971). Effects of vinblastine and colchicine on monoamine containing neurons of the rat with special regard to the axoplasmic transport of amine granules. *Acta Neuropatol. Berlin*, suppl., **5**, 226–237

Dahlström, A. and Fuxe, K. (1964). Evidence of the existence of monoamine-containing neurons in the central nervous system. I. Demonstration of monoamines in the cell bodies of brain stem neurons. *Acta Physiol. Scand.*, **62**, suppl., **232**, 1–55

Daly, J., Fuxe, K. and Jonsson, G. (1973). Effects of intracerebral injections of 5, 6-dihydroxytryptamine on central monoamine neurons: Evidence for selective degeneration of central 5-hydroxytryptamine neurons. *Brain Res.*, **49**, 476–482

Daly, J., Fuxe, K. and Jonsson, G. (1974). 5, 7-dihydroxytryptamine as a tool for the morphological and functional analysis of central 5-hydroxytryptamine neurons. *Res. Commun. chem. Path. Pharmac.*, **7**, 175–187

Della-Fera, M. and Baile, C. A. (1979). Cholecystokinin octapeptide: continuous picomole injections into the cerebral ventricles of sheep supress feeding. *Science*, **206**, 471–473

Dockray, G. J., Gregory, R. A., Hutchinson, J. B., Harris, J. J. and Runswick, M. J. (1978). Isolation, structure and biological activity of two cholecystokinin octapeptides from sheep brain. *Nature London*, **274**, 711–713

Dodd, J. and Kelly, J. S. (1981). The actions of cholecystokinin and related peptides on pyramidal neurones of the mammalian hippocampus. *Brain Res.*, **205**, 337–350

Eckstein, F., Barde, Y. A., Thoenen, H. (1971). Production of specific antibodies to choline acetyltransferase purified from pig brain. *Neuroscience*, **6**, 993–1000

Eng, L., Uyeda, C. T., Chao, L. P. and Wolfgram, F. (1974). Antibody to bovine choline acetyltransferase and immunofluorescent localization of the enzyme in neurons. *Nature London*, **250**, 243–245

Falck, B. (1962). Observations on the possibilities of the cellular localization of monoamines by a fluorescence method. *Acta Physiol. Scand.*, suppl. **56**, 197

Falck, B., Hillarp, N. A., Thieme, G., and Torp, A. (1962). Fluorescence of catecholamines and related compounds condensed with formaldehyde. *J. Histochem. Cytochem.*, **10**, 348–354

Fekete, M., Varszegi, M., Penke, B., Kovacs, K. and Telegdy, G. (1980). Effects of intracerebroventricular administration of cholecystokinin octapeptide sulfate ester on dopamine, norepinephrine and serotonin contents of different brain structures. *Neuroendocrinol. Lett.*, **2**, 67–72

Fuxe, K., Agnati, L. F., Ganten, D., Goldstein, M., Yukimura, T., Jonsson, G., Bolme, P.,

Hökfelt, T., Andersson, K., Härfstrand, A., Unger, T. and Rascher, W. (1981). The role of noradrenaline and adrenaline neuron systems and substance P in the control of central cardiovascular functions. In *Central Nervous System Mechanisms in Hypertension* (ed. J. P. Buckley and C. M. Ferrario), Raven Press. New York, pp. 89–113

Fuxe, K., Agnati, L. F., Köhler, C., Kuonen, D., Ögren, S-O., Andersson, K. and Hökfelt, T. (1981). Characterization of normal and supersensitive dopamine receptors: effects of ergot drugs and neuropeptides. *J. Neural Transmission*, 51, 3–37

Fuxe, K., Andersson, K., Locatelli, V., Agnati, L. F., Hökfelt, T., Skirboll, L. and Mutt, V. (1980). Cholecystokinin peptides produce marked reduction of dopamine turnover in discrete areas in the rat brain following intraventricular injection. *Eur. J. Pharmac.*, 67, 329–332

Fredholm, B. and Lundberg, J. M. (1981). VIP-induced cyclic AMP formation in the cat submandibular gland. Potentiation by carbacholine. *Acta Physiol. Scand.* (in press)

Furness, J. and Costa, M. (1980). Types of nerve in the enteric nervous system. *Neuroscience*, 5, 1–20

Gardner, J. (1979). Regulations of pancreatic exocrine functions in vitro: Initial steps in the actions of secretogogues. *A. Rev. Physiol.*, 41, 55–66

Gardner, J. and Jackson, M. (1977). Regulations of amylase release from dispersed pancreatic acinar cells. *J. Physiol. Lond.* 270, 439–454

Garrett, J. R. (1974). Innervation of salvary glands, morphological considerations. In *Secretory Mechanisms of Exocrine Glands* (ed. N. A. Thorn and O. H. Petersen), Munksgaard, Copenhagen, pp. 17–27

Gibbs, J., Young, R. and Smith, G. P. (1973). Cholecystokinin elicits satiety in rats with open gastric fistulas. *Nature London*, 245, 323–325

Gilbert, R. F. T., Emson, P. C., Hunt, S. P., Bennett, G. W., Marsden, C. A., Sandberg, B. E. B., Steinbusch, H. and Verfiofstad, A. A. J. (1982). The effects of monoamine neurotoxins on peptides in the rat spinal cord. *Neuroscience*, 7, 69–88

Giraud, P., Eiden, L. E., Audiopei, Y., Gillioz, P., Conte-Devolx, B., Boudouresque, F., Eskay, R. and Oliver, C. (1981). Enkephalins, ACTH, α-MSH and β-endorphin in human pheochromocytomas. *Neuropeptides*, 1, 237–252

Glazer, E. J., and Basbaum, A. I. (1980). Leucine enkephalin: localization in and ceroplasmic transport by sacral parasympathetic preganglionic neurons. *Science*, 208, 1479–1481

Hanley, M. R. and Cottrell, G. A. (1974). Acetylcholine activity in an identified 5-hydroxytryptamine-containing neurone. *J. Pharm. Pharmac.*, 26, 980

Hanley, M. R., Cottrell, G. A., Emson, P. C., and Fonnum, F. (1974). Enzymatic synthesis of acetylcholine by a serotonin-containing neurone from *Helix. Nature New Biol.*, 251, 631, 633

Heidenhain, R. (1872). Ueber die Wirkung einiger Gifte auf die Nerven der glandula submaxillaris. *Pflügers Archs*, 5, 309–318

Hexum, T. D., Yang, H. Y. T., and Costa, E. (1980). Biochemical characterization of enkephalin-like immunoreactive peptides of adrenal glands. *Life Sci.*, 27, 1211–1216

Hilton, S. M. and Lewis, G. P. (1955a). The cause of the vasodilatation accompanying activity in the submandibular salivary gland. *J. Physiol. Lond.*, 128, 235–248

Hilton, S. M. and Lewis, G. S. (1955b). The mechanisms of the functional hyperaemia in the submandibular salivary gland. *J. Physiol. Lond.*, 129, 253–271

Hökfelt, T., Fuxe, K., Goldstein, M. and Joh, T. H. (1973). Immunohistochemical localization of three catecholamine synthesizing enzymes: Aspects of methodology. *Histochemistry*, 33, 231–254

Hökfelt, T., Fuxe, K., Goldstein, M. and Johansson, O. (1974). Immunohistochemical evidence for the existence of adrenaline neurons in the rat brain. *Brain Res.* 66, 235–251

Hökfelt, T., Fuxe, K. and Joh, T. H. (1975). Applications of immunohistochemistry to studies on monoamine cell systems with special reference to nerve tissues. *Ann. N.Y. Acad. Sci.* 254, 407–432

Hökfelt, T., Elfvin, L. G., Elde, R., Schultzberg, M., Goldstein, M. and Luft, R. (1977a) Occurrence of somatostatin-like immunoreactivity in some peripheral sympathetic noradrenergic neurons. *Proc. natn. Acad. Sci. U.S.A.*, 74, 3587–3591

Hökfelt, T., Elfvin, L-G., Schultzberg, M., Fuxe, K., Said, S. I., Mutt, V. and Goldstein, M. (1977b). Immunohistochemical evidence of vasoactive intestinal polypeptide-containing neurons and nerve fibers in sympathetic ganglia. *Neuroscience*, 2, 885–896

Hökfelt, T., Ljungdahl, A., Steinbusch, H., Verhofstad, A., Nilsson, G., Brodin, E., Pernow, B., and Goldstein, M. (1978). Immunohistochemical evidence of substance P-like immunoreactivity in some 5-hydroxytryptomine-containing neurons in the rat central nervous system. *Neuroscience*, 3, 517–538

Hökfelt, T., Lundberg, J. M., Schultzberg, M., Johansson, O., Ljungdahl, A. and Rehfeld, J. (1980a). Coexistence of peptides and putative transmitters in neurons. In *Neural Peptides and Neuronal Communication* (ed. E. Costa and M. Trabucchi), Raven Press, New York, pp. 1–23

Hökfelt, T., Johansson, O., Ljungdahl, A., Lundberg, J. M. and Schultzberg, M. (1980b). Peptidergic neurons. *Nature London*, 284, 515–521

Hökfelt, T., Skirboll, L., Rehfeld, J. F., Goldstein, M., Markey, K. and Dann, O. (1980c). A subpopulation of mesencephalic dopamine neurons projecting to limbic areas contains a cholecystokinin-like peptide: Evidence from immunohistochemistry combined with retrograde tracing. *Neuroscience*, 5, 2093–2124

Hökfelt, T., Rehfeld, J. F., Skirboll, L., Ivemark, B., Goldstein, M. and Markey, K. (1980d). Evidence for coexistence of dopamine and CCK in mesolimbic neurones. *Nature London*, 285, 476–478

Hökfelt, T., Johansson, O., Fuxe, K., and Goldstein, M. (1982). Catecholamine neurons – distribution and cellular localization as revealed by immunohistochemistry. In *Catecholamines II* (ed. N. Weiner and U. Trendelenburg), Springer, Berlin, in press

Hunt, S. P., and Emson, P. C., Gilbert, R., Goldstein, M. and Kimmel, J. R., (1981). Presence of avian pancreatic polypeptide-like immunoreactivity in catecholamine and methionine enkephalin containing neurons within the central nervous system. *Neurosci. Lett.* 21, 125–130

Jaim-Etcheverry, G. and Zieher, L. M. (1971). Ultrastructural cytochemistry and pharmacology of 5-hydroxytryptamine in adrenergic nerve endings. III. Selective increase of norepinephrine in the rat pineal gland consecutive to depletion of neuronal 5-hydroxytryptamine. *J. Pharmac. exp. Ther.*, 178, 42–48

Jessen, K. R., Saffrey, M. J., van Noorden, S., Bloom, S. R., Polak, J. M. and Burnstock, G. (1980). Immunohistochemical studies of the enteric nervous system in tissue culture and *in situ*: Localization of vasoactive intestinal polypeptide (VIP), substance-P and enkephalin immunoreactive nerves in the guinea-pig gut. *Neuroscience*, 5, 1717–1735

Johansson, O. and Hökfelt, T. (1980). Thyrotropin releasing hormone, somatostatin, and enkephalin: distribution studies using immunohistochemical techniques. *J. Histochem. Cytochem.*, 28, 364–366

Johansson, O. and Lundberg, J. M. (1981). Ultrastructural localization of VIP-like immunoreactivity in large dense cored vesicles of "cholinergic type" nerve terminals in cat exocrine glands. *Neuroscience*, 5, 847–862

Johansson, O., Hökfelt, T., Pernow, B., Jeffcoate, S. L., White, N., Steinbusch, H. W. M. Verhofstad, A. A. J., Emson, P. C. and Spindel, E. (1981). Immunohistochemical support for three putative transmitters in one neuron: Coexistence of 5-hydroxytryptamine-, substance P-, and thyrotropin releasing hormone-like immunoreactivity in medullary neurons projecting to the spinal cord. *Neuroscience*, 6, 1857–1881

Jonsson, G. (1981). Lesion methods in neurobiology. In *Techniques in Neuroanatomical Research* (ed. Ch. Heym and W-G. Forssman), Springer-Verlag, Berlin, pp. 71–99

Kerdelhue, B., Palkovits, M., Karteszi, M. and Reinberg, A. (1981). Circadian variations in substance P, luliberin (LH-RH) and thyroliberin (TRH) contents in hypothalamic and extrahypothalamic brain nuclei of adult male rats. *Brain Res.*, 206, 405–413

Kerkut, G. A., Sedden, C. B. and Walker, R. J. (1967). Uptake of DOPA and 5-hydroxytryptamine by monoamine-forming neurons in the brain of Helix aspersa. *Comp. Biochem. Physiol.*, 23, 159–162

Konishi, S. and Otsuka, M. (1974). Excitatory action of hypothalamic substance P on spinal motoneurones of newborn rats. *Nature London*, 252, 734–735

Kovacs, G., Szabo, G., Penke, B. and Telegdy, G. (1981). Effects of cholecystokinin octapeptide on striatal dopamine metabolism and on apomorphine-induced stereotyped cage-climbing in mice. *Eur. J. Pharmac.*, 69, 313–319

Larsson, L. I. (1977). Ultrastructural localization of a new neuronal peptide (VIP). *Histochemistry*, 54, 153–176

Larsson, L-I., Sundler, F. and Håkanson, R. (1975). Fluorescence histochemistry of poly-peptide hormone-secreting cells in the gastro-intestinal mucosa. In *Progress in Gastro-intestinal Endocrinology* (ed. J. C. Thompson), University of Texas Press, Austin, pp. 169-195

Larsson, L-I., Fahrenkrug, J., Holst, J. J. and Schaffalitzky de Muckadell, O.B. (1978). Innervation of the pancreas by vasoactive intestinal polypeptide (VIP) immunoreactive nerves. *Life Sci.*, 22, 773-780

Leander, S., Håkanson, R. and Sundler, F. (1981). Nerves containing substance P, vasoactive intestinal polypeptide, enkephalin, or somatostatin in the guinea-pig taenia coli: Distri-bution, ultrastructure and possible functions. *Cell Tissue Res.*, 215, 21-39

Lewis, R. V., Stein, A. S., Rossier, J., Stein, S. and Udenfriend, S. (1979). Putative enke-phalin precursors in bovine adrenal medulla. *Biochem. biophys. Res. Commun.*, 89, 822-829

Lewis, R. V., Stein, A. S., Kimura, S., Rossier, J., Stein, S. and Udenfriend, S. (1980). An about 50 000-dalton protein in adrenal medulla: a common precursor of met- and leu-enkephalin. *Science*, 208, 1459-1461

Lewis, R., Stein, A. S., Kilpatrick, D., Gerber, L., Rossier, J. J., Stein, S. and Udenfriend, S. (1981). Marked increases in large enkephalin containing polypeptides in the rat adrenal gland following denervation. *Neuroscience*, 1, 80-82

Lindvall, O. and Björklund, A. (1978). Organization of catecholamine neurons in the rat central nervous system. In *Handbook of Psychopharmacology*, 9: *Chemical Pathways in the Brain* (ed. L. L. Iversen, S. D. Iversen and S. H. Snyder), Plenum Press, New York, pp. 139-231

Ljungdahl, Å., Hökfelt, T. and Nilsson, G. (1978). Distribution of substance P like immuno-reactivity in the central nervous system of the rat. I. Cell bodies and nerve terminals. *Neuroscience*, 3, 861-943

Lorén, I., Alumets, J., Håkanson, R. and Sundler, F. (1979). Immunoreactive pancreatic polypeptide (PP) occurs in the central and peripheral nervous system: Preliminary immunocytochemical observations. *Cell Tissue Res.*, 200, 179-186

Lundberg, J. M. (1981). Evidence for coexistence of vasoactive intestinal polypeptide (VIP) and acetylcholine in neurons of cat exocrine glands. *Acta Physiol. Scand.*, suppl., 112, 1-57

Lundberg, J. M., Hökfelt, T., Schultzberg, M., Uvnäs-Wallensten, K., Köhler, C. and Said, S. J. (1979a). Occurrence of vasoactive intestinal polypeptide (VIP)-like immunoreactivity in certain cholinergic neurons of the cat. Evidence from combined immunohistochemistry and acetylcholinesterase staining. *Neuroscience*, 4, 1539-1559

Lundberg, J. M., Hökfelt, T., Fahrenkrug, J., Nilsson, G. and Terenius, L. (1979b). Peptides in the cat carotid body (glomus caroticum): VIP-, enkephalin- and substance P-like immunoreactivity. *Acta Physiol. Scand.*, 107, 279-281

Lundberg, J. M., Hamberger, B., Schultzberg, M., Hökfelt, T., Granberg, P. O., Efendic, S., Terenius, L., Goldstein, M. and Luft, R. (1979c). Enkephalin- and somatostatin-like immunoreactivities in human adrenal medulla and pheochromocytoma. *Proc. natn. Acad. Sci. U.S.A.*, 76, 4079-4083

Lundberg, J. M., Hökfelt, T., Änggård, A., Kimmel, J., Goldstein, M. and Markey, K. (1980a). Coexistence of an avian pancreatic polypeptide (APP) immunoreactive substance and catecholamines in some peripheral and central neurons. *Acta Physiol. Scand.*, 110, 107-109

Lundberg, J. M., Hökfelt, T., Änggård, A., Uvnäs-Wallensten, K., Brimijoin, S., Brodin, E. and Fahrenkrug, J. (1980b). Peripheral peptide neurons: Distribution, axonal transport and some aspects on possible functions. In *Adv. Biochem. Psychopharmac.*, 22, Raven Press, New York, pp. 25-36

Lundberg, J. M., Änggård, A., Fahrenkrug, J., Hökfelt, T. and Mutt, V. (1980c). Vasoactive intestinal polypeptide in cholinergic neurons of exocrine glands: functional significance of coexisting transmitters for vasodilation and secretion. *Proc. natn. Acad. Sci. U.S.A.*, 77, 1651-1655

Lundberg, J. M., Änggård, A., Hökfelt, T. and Kimmel, J. (1980d). Avian pancreatic poly-peptide (APP) inhibits atropine resistant vasodilation in cat submandibular salivary gland and nasal mucosa: Possible interaction with VIP. *Acta Physiol. Scand.*, 110, 199-201

Lundberg, J. M., Ånggård, A., Emson, P., Fahrenkrug, J. and Hökfelt, T. (1981a). VIP-ergic and cholinergic mechanisms in the cat nasal mucosa: Studies on choline acetyltransferase and VIP release. *Proc. natn. Acad. Sci. U.S.A.*, 78, 5255–5259

Lundberg, J. M., Fried, G., Fahrenkrug, J., Holmstedt, B., Hökfelt, T., Lagercrantz, H. Lundgren, G. and Ånggård (1981b). Subcellular fractionation of cat submandibular gland: Comparative studies on the distribution of acetylcholine and vasoactive intestinal polypeptide (VIP). *Neuroscience*, 6, 1101–1010

Lundberg, J. M., Rökaeus, A., Hökfelt, T., Rosell, S., Brown, M. and Goldstein, M. (1981c). Neurotensin-like immunoreactivity in the preganglionic sympathetic nerves and in the adrenal medulla of the cat. *Acta Physiol. Scand.*, in press

Lundberg, J. M., Ånggård and Fahrenkrug, J. (1981d). Complementary role of vasoactive intestinal polypeptide (VIP) and acetylcholine for cat submandibular gland blood flow and secretion. I. VIP release. *Acta Physiol. Scand.*, 113, 317–327

Lundberg, J. M., Ånggård, A. and Fahrenkrug, J. (1981e). Complementary role of vaso-active intestinal polypeptide (VIP) and acetylcholine for cat submandibular gland blood flow and secretion. II. Effects of cholinergic antagonists and VIP antiserum. *Acta Physiol. Scand.*, 113, 329–336

Lundberg, J. M., Ånggård, A. and Fahrenkrug, J. (1981f). Complementary role of vasoactive intestinal polypeptide (VIP) and acetylcholine for cat submandicular gland blood flow and secretion. III. Effects of local infusions. *Acta Physiol. Scand.*, in press

Lundberg, J. M., Hedlund, B. and Bartfai, T. (1981g). Vasoactive intestinal polypeptide (VIP) enhances muscarinic ligand binding in the cat submandibular salivary gland. *Nature London*, 295, 147–149

Lundberg, J. M., Brimijoin, S. and Fahrenkrug, J. (1981h). Characteristics of the axonal transport of vasoactive intestinal polypeptide (VIP) in nerves of the cat. *Acta Physiol. Scand.*, 112, 427–436

Lundberg, J. M., Hökfelt, T., Ånggård, A., Terenius, L., Elde, R., Kimmel, J., Goldstein, M. and Markey, K. (1982a). Organization principles in the peripheral sympathetic nervous system: Subdivision by coexisting peptides (somatostatin-, avian pancreatic polypeptide-and vasoactive intestinal polypeptide-like immunoreactivity materials). *Proc. natn. Acad. Sci. U.S.A.*, in press

Lundberg, J. M., Tatemoto, K., Terenius, L., Hellström, P. M., Mutt, V., Hökfelt, T. and Hamberger, B. (1982b). Localization of the polypeptide (PYY) in gut endocrine cells and effects on intestinal blood flow and motility. *Proc. natl. Acad. Sci. U.S.A.*, in press

Mains, R. E., Eipper, B. A. and Ling, N. (1977). Common precursor to corticotropins and endorphins. *Proc. natn. Acad. Sci. U.S.A.*, 74, 3014–3018

Markstein, R., Skirboll, L. and Hökfelt, T. (1981). The effect of cholecystokinin-like peptides on dopamine release *in vitro*. *Eur. J. Pharmac.*, in press

McGeer, E. G., McGeer, P. L., Hattori, T. and Singh, V. K. (1979). Immunohistochemistry of choline acetyltransferase. *Progr. Brain Res.*, 49, 59–70

Moore, R. Y. and Bloom, F. E. (1978). Central catecholamine neuron systems: Anatomy and physiology of the dopamine system. *A. Rev. Neurosci.*, 7, 129–169

Moore, R. Y. and Bloom, F. E. (1979). Central catecholamine neuron systems: Anatomy and physiology of the norepinephrine and epinephrine systems. *A. Rev. Neurosci.*, 2, 113–168

Myslinski, N. R. and Anderson, E. G. (1977). The effect of serotonin precursors on moto-neuron activity. *J. Pharmac. exp. Ther.*, 204, 19–26

Nakane, P. N. and Pierce, G. B. (1967). Enzyme-labeled antibodies for the light and electron microscopic localization of tissue antigens and antibodies. *J. Cell Biol.*, 33, 307–311

Nakanishi, S., Inogue, A., Kita, T., Nakamura, M., Change, A. C. Y., Cohen, S. N. and Numa, S. (1979). Nucleotide sequence of cloned cDNA for bovine corticotropin-β-lipotropin precursor. *Nature London*, 278, 423–427

Nicoll, R. A. (1977). Excitatory action of TRH on spinal motoneurones. *Nature London*, 265, 242–243

Nicoll, R. A., Alger, B. E. and Jahr, C. E. (1980). Peptides as putative excitatory neuro-transmitters: Carnosine, enkephalin, substance P and TRH. *Proc. R. Soc. Lond.*, B210, 133–149

Nilaver, G., Zimmerman, E. A., Defendin, R., Liotta, A. S., Krieger, D. T. and Brownstein, M. J. (1979). Adrenocorticotropin and β-lipotropin in the hypothalamus; localization in the same arcuate neurons by sequential immunocytochemical procedures. *J. Cell Biol.*, 81, 50–58

Oertel, W., Graybiel, A., Mugnaini, E., Elde, R., Schmechel, D. and Kopin, I. (1981). Coexistence of glutamate decarboxylase immunoreactivity and somatostatin-like immunoreactivity in neurons of nucleus reticularis thalami of the cat. *Abstr. Soc. Neurosci.*, 7, 223

Olschowka, J. A., O'Donohue, T. L. and Jacobowitz, D. M. (1981). The distribution of bovine pancreatic polypeptide-like immunoreactivity in the rat central nervous system. *Abstr. Soc. Neurosci.*, 7, 914

Osborne, N. N. (1977). Do snail neurones contain more than one transmitter? *Nature*, 270, 622–623

Osborne, N. N. (1979). Is Dale's principle valid? *Trends in Neurosci.*, 2, 73–75

Otsuka, M. and Takahashi, T. (1977). Putative peptide neurotransmitters. *A. Rev. Pharmac. Toxicol.*, 17, 425–439

Owman, Ch. (1964). Sympathetic nerves probably storing two types of monoamines in the rat pineal gland. *Int. J. Neuropharmac.*, 2, 97–127

Owman, Ch., Håkanson, R. and Sundler, F. (1973). Occurrence and function of amines in polypeptide hormone producing cells. *Fedn Proc. Fedn Am. Soc. exp. Biol.*, 32, 1785–1791

Patterson, P. H. (1978). Environmental determination of autonomic neurotransmitter functions. *A. Rev. Neurosci.*, 1, 1–18

Pearse, A. G. E. (1969). The cytochemistry and ultrastructure of polypeptide hormone producing cells of the APUD series and the embryologic physiologic and pathologic implications of the concept. *J. Histochem. Cytochem.*, 17, 303–313

Pearse, A. G. E. and Polak, J. M. (1975). Bifunctional reagents as vapour- and liquid-phase fixatives for immunohistochemistry. *Histochem. J.*, 7, 179–186

Pearse, A. G. E. and Takor, T. (1979). Neuroendocrine embryology and the APUD concept. *Clin. Endocrinol.*, suppl., 5, 2295–2345

Pelletier, G., Steinbusch, H. W. and Verhofstad, A. (1981). Immunoreactive substance P and serotonin present in the same dense core vesicles. *Nature London*, 293, 71–72

Polak, J. M. and Bloom, S. R. (1978). Peptidergic nerves of the gastrointestinal tract. *Invest. Cell Pathol.*, 1, 301–326

Potter, D. D., Landis, S. C. and Furshpan, E. J. (1981). Adrenergic-cholinergic dual function in cultured sympathetic neurons of the rat. In *Development of the Autonomic Nervous System*, Ciba Foundation Symposium, 83, pp. 123–138

Rehfeld, J. F. (1978). Immunochemical studies on cholecystokinin. II. Distribution and molecular heterogenecity in the central nervous system and small intestine of man and dog. *J. biol. Chem.*, 253, 4022–4030

Rehfeld, J. F., Goltermann, N., Larsson, L-I., Emson, P. M. and Lee, C. M. (1979). Gastrin and cholecystokinin in central and peripheral neurons. *Fedn Proc.*, 38, 2325–2329

Roberts, J. L. and Herbert, E. (1977). Characterization of a common precursor to corticotropins and β-lipotropin peptides and their arrangement relative to corticotropin in the precursor synthesized in a cell free system. *Proc. natn. Acad. Sci. U.S.A.*, 74, 5300–5304

Schultzberg, M., Hökfelt, T., Lundberg, J. M., Terenius, L., Elfvin, L-G. and Elde, R. (1978a). Enkephalin-like immunoreactivity in nerve terminals in sympathetic ganglia and adrenal medulla and in adrenal medullary gland cells. *Acta Physiol. Scand.*, 103, 475–477

Schultzberg, M., Lundberg, J. M., Hökfelt, T., Terenius, L., Brandt, J., Elde, R. and Goldstein, (1978b). Enkephalin-like immunoreactivity in gland cells and nerve terminals of the adrenal medulla. *Neuroscience*, 3, 1169–1186

Schultzberg, M., Hökfelt, T., Terenius, L., Elfvin, L-G., Lundberg, J. M., Brandt, J., Elde, R. P. and Goldstein, M. (1979). Enkephalin immunoreactive nerve fibres and cell bodies in sympathetic ganglia of the guinea pig and rat. *Neuroscience*, 4, 249–270

Schultzberg, M., Hökfelt, T., Nilsson, G., Terenius, L., Rehfeld, J. F., Brown, M., Elde, R., Goldstein, M. and Said, S. J. (1980). Distribution of peptide- and catecholamine-containing neurons in the gastro intestinal tract of the rat and guinea-pig: Immunohisto-chemical studies with antisera to substance P, vasoactive intestinal polypeptide, enkephalins, somatostatin, gastrin/CCK, neurotensin and dopamine-β-hydroxylase. *Neuroscience*, 5, 689–744

Shibuya, T. and Anderson, E. G. (1968). The influence of chronic cord transection on the effects of 5-hydroxytrytophan, L-tryptophan and paragyline on spinal neural activity. *J. Pharmac. exp. Ther.*, 164, 185–190

Shimizu, T. and Taira, N. (1979). Assessment of the effects of vasoactive intestinal peptide (VIP) on blood flow through the salivation of the dog salivary gland in comparison with those of secretin, glucagon and acetylcholine. *Br. J. Pharmac.*, 65, 683–687

Singer, E., Sperk, G., Placheta, P. and Leeman, S. E. (1979). Reduction of substance P levels in the ventral cervical spinal cord of the rat after intracisternal 5,7-dihydroxytryptamine injections. *Brain Res.*, 174, 362–365

Sjöqvist, F. (1963). Pharmacological analysis of acetylcholinesterase-rich ganglion cells in the lumbosacral sympathetic system of the cat. *Acta. Physiol. Scand.*, 57, 352–362

Skirboll, L., Hökfelt, T., Grace, A. A., Hommer, D. W., Rehfeld, J., Markey, K., Goldstein, M. and Bunney, B. S. (1981a). The coexistence of dopamine and a CCK-like peptide in a subpopulation of midbrain neurons: Immunocytochemical and electrophysiological studies. In *Apomorphine and other Dopaminomimetics*, 1: *Basic Pharmacology* (ed. G. L. Gessa and G. V. Corsini), Raven Press, New York, pp. 65–77

Skirboll, L., Grace, A. A., Hommer, D. W., Rehfeld, J., Goldstein, M., Hökfelt, T. and Bunney, B. S. (1981b). Peptide-monoamine coexistence: studies of the actions of cholecystokinin-like peptide on the electrical activity of midbrain dopamine neurons. *Neuroscience*, 6, 2111–2124

Skirboll, L., Hökfelt, T., Rehfeld, J., Cuello, C. and Dockray, G. (1981). Coexistence of substance P- and cholecystokinin-like immunoreactivity in neurons of the mesencephalic periaqueductal central gray. *Neurosci. Lett.*, in press

Solcia, E., Capella, C., Vassallo, G. and Buffa, R. (1975). Endocrine cells of the gastric mucosa. *Int. Rev. Cytol.*, 42, 283–286

Stein, A. S., Lewis, R. V., Kimura, J., Rossier, J., Stein, S. and Undenfriend, S. (1980). Opioid hexapeptides and heptapeptides in adrenal medulla and brain; possible impli-cations on the biosynthesis of enkephalins. *Arch. biochem. Biophys.*, 205, 606–613

Sternberger, L. A. (1979). *Immunocytochemistry*, second edition, Wiley, New York

Sternberger, L. A., Hardy, P. H. Jr., Cuentis, J. J. and Meyer, H. G. (1970). The unlabeled antibody enzyme method of immunohistochemistry. Preparations and properties of soluble antigen-antibody complex (horseradish peroxidase-antihorseradish peroxidase) and its use in identifications of spirochetes. *J. Histochem. Cytochem.*, 18, 315–324

Sullivan, S. N., Bloom, S. R. and Polak, J. M. (1978). Enkephalin in peripheral neuro-endocrine tumours. *Lancet*, 3, 986–987

Tatemoto, K. and Mutt, V. (1980). Isolation of two novel candidate hormones using a chemical method for finding naturally occurring polypeptides. *Nature London*, 285, 417–418

Tramu, G. and Leonardelli, J. (1979). Immunohistochemical localization of enkephalins in median eminence and adenohypophysis. *Brain Res.*, 168, 457–471

Tramu, G., Pillez, A. and Leonardelli, J. (1978). An efficient method of antibody elution for the successive or simultaneous localization of two antigens by immunocytochemistry. *J. Histochem. Cytochem.*, 26, 322–324

Uddman, R. (1980). Vasoactive intestinal polypeptide. Distribution and possible role in the upper respiratory and digestive region. MD Thesis, University of Lund, Lund.

Vandesande, F. and Dierickx, K. (1975). Identification of the vasopressin producing neurons in the hypothalamic magnocellular neurosecretory system of the rat. *Cell Tiss. Res.*, 164, 153–162

Vincent, S. R., Skirboll, L., Hökfelt, T., Johansson, O., Lundberg, J. M., Elde, R. P., Terenius, L. and Kimmel, J. (1982). Coexistence of somatostatin- and avian pancreatic polypep-tide (APP)-like immunoreactivity in some forebrain neurons. *Neuroscience*, 7, 439–446

Viveros, O. H., Diliberto, E. J., Hazum, E. and Chang, K-J. (1979). Opiate materials in the adrenal medulla: Evidence for storage and secretion with catecholamines. *Molec. Pharmac.*, 16, 1101–1108

Watson, S., Akil, H., Richard III, C. W. and Barchas, J. D. (1978). Evidence for two separate opiate peptide neuronal systems. *Nature London*, 275, 226–228

Wharton, J., Polak, J. M., Pearse, A. G. E., McGregor, G. P., Bryant, M. G., Bloom, S. R., Emson, P. C., Bisgard, G. E. and Will, J. A. (1980). Enkephalin-, VIP- and substance P-like immunoreactivity in the carotid body. *Nature London*, 28, 269–271

Wilson, S. P., Cubeddu, L. X., Chang, K-J. and Viveros, O. H. (1981). Met-enkephalin, leu-enkephalin and other opiate-like peptides in human pheochromocytoma tumours. *Neuropeptides*, 1, 273–281

# 5

# The adrenal medulla: a model for studying synthesis, co-storage and co-secretion of peptides and catecholamines

O. Humberto Viveros and Steven P. Wilson (Department of Medicinal Biochemistry, Wellcome Research Laboratories, Research Triangle Park, North Carolina 27709, USA)

## INTRODUCTION

The possibility of simultaneous storage and release of multiple chemical messengers from secretory cells has become the centre of increasing interest during recent years (Pearse, 1969; Burnstock, 1976; Hökfelt et al., 1980; Larsson, 1980). A multimessenger system requires that a single secretory cell synthesise, store and release two or more molecules, each in quantities capable of generating a change in the biological activity of an effector cell through interaction with specific receptors. Storage of multiple messengers in the same secretory vesicle is central to studies of the cotransmission hypothesis since most, if not all, neurones and endocrine cells belong to the general class of merocrine cells where the secretory products are segregated in, and released from storage/secretory vesicles.

For those who wonder why the adrenal medulla is included in a symposium dealing with synapses that operate with more than one neurotransmitter, it should suffice to say that although adrenal chromaffin cells are not true neurones *in situ*, they share a common ancestry with postganglionic sympathetic neurones (Coupland, 1965) and can extend axonal projections and form synapses when transplanted to the anterior chamber of the eye (Olson et al., 1980; Unsicker et al., 1980) or when cultured under special conditions (Unsicker et al., 1980; Livett and Dean, 1980). A second reason to believe that findings in the adrenal medulla may be applicable to true neurones is historical. The adrenal medulla has repeatedly proven useful as a model for studying peripheral and central catecholaminergic systems. A number of important discoveries were first made using the adrenal medulla, to cite only a few: the isolation and chemical characterisation of adrenaline as the first catecholamine messenger (Oliver and Schafer, 1895; Takamine, 1901), the identification of the enzymes for catecholamine biosynthesis (Nagatsu *et al.*, 1964, Levin *et al.*, 1960; Kirshner and Goodall, 1957), the first isolation and characterisation of a neurohormone storage vesicle (Blaschko and Welch, 1953; Hillarp *et al.*, 1953), the morphological and biochemical demonstration of exocytosis as the mechanism for neurotransmitter secretion, (De Robertis and Vaz Ferreira, 1957; Douglas, 1968; Viveros, 1975), and the first evidence for long-term regulation of transmitter synthesis by induction of catecholamine synthesis enzymes (Mueller *et al.*, 1969; Viveros *et al.*, 1969*a*). The latest addition to this list, and the subject of this report, is the synthesis, storage and secretion of enkephalins and enkephalin-related peptides by adrenomedullary chromaffin cells (Schultzberg *et al.*, 1978; Viveros *et al.*, 1979*a*, 1980*a*; Wilson *et al.*, 1980*a*; Hexum *et al.*, 1980; Lewis *et al.*, 1979).

From the first isolation of adrenomedullary chromaffin vesicles (Blaschko and Welch, 1953; Hillarp *et al.*, 1953) it became obvious that these organelles were more than just membrane-enclosed bags filled with catecholamines waiting for the stimulus to trigger their release. These vesicles were found to contain, in addition to catecholamines, large amounts of heterogeneous soluble proteins and peptides, high concentrations of ATP and substantial amounts of calcium and magnesium (Blaschko and Welch, 1953; Hillarp *et al.*, 1953; Hillarp, 1958; Smith, 1968; Roda and Hogue-Angeletti, 1979). All of these vesicular components are released as a quantal package during exocytotic secretion (Viveros, 1975; Viveros *et al.*, 1969*b*). These diverse molecules, which are stored in and secreted from chromaffin vesicles, are then possible comessengers of the adrenal catecholamines; the only other qualification needed to fulfill the role of cohormones is the ability to modify the functional state of a target cell.

The adrenal medulla is part of the general psychoneuroendocrine system that maintains homeostasis and responds to situations of stress and coping (Lewis, 1975; Frankenhaeuser, 1979). Many of the stressful stimuli that activate adrenomedullary secretion also induce significant analgesia, which can be, at least in part, blocked by opiate antagonists (Bodner *et al.*, 1978; Lewis *et al.*, 1980*a*). Thus we first explored the possibility that some of the non-catecholamine components in the chromaffin vesicle might have opiate activity.

## OPIOID PEPTIDES IN ADRENOMEDULLARY CHROMAFFIN CELLS

### Presence and chemical characterisation

In preliminary experiments, we found that a water lysate prepared from chromaffin vesicles of bovine adrenal medulla was highly cross-reactive with Leu-enkephalin and Met-enkephalin antibodies and competed with $[^{125}I]$-(D-Ala$^2$,

D-Leu[5]) enkephalin for binding to rat brain membrane opiate receptors (Viveros *et al.*, 1979*b*). Similar results were obtained with acidic extracts of adrenal medullae from different species (Viveros *et al.*, 1979*a*; Viveros *et al.*, 1980*a*; Saria *et al.*, 1980) (table 5.1). All opiate activity was lost on incubation of the extracts with pronase, indicating the peptidergic nature of the adrenomedullary opioids (Viveros *et al.*, 1979*a*; Viveros *et al.*, 1980*a*). While this work was in progress, two other groups independently determined the presence of opioid peptides in the adrenal medulla (Schultzberg, 1978; Hexum *et al.*, 1980). The presence of these peptides and their initial chemical characterisation have been the subject of recent reviews (Viveros *et al.*, 1980*a*; Viveros and Wilson, 1982). We will briefly summarise only that information necessary for the understanding of the more recent work included in this report.

Table 5.1  Opioid peptide content in the adrenal medulla of several species

| Species | n | Opioid peptides | Catecholamines | CA / OP |
|---|---|---|---|---|
| | | (nmol/g wet wt) | ($\mu$mol/g wet wt) | (X 10$^{-3}$) |
| Rat | (6) | 0.29 ± 0.03 | – | – |
| Hamster | (5 pooled) | 0.50 | – | – |
| Rabbit | (6) | 0.85 ± 0.15 | – | – |
| Guinea Pig | (12) | 1.2  ± 0.15 | 7.7 ±  0.7 | 7.02 ± 0.63 |
| Cat | (5) | 3.2  ± 0.7 | 31.7 ±  2.9 | 9.91 ± 0.62 |
| Ox | (8) | 6.8  ± 0.7 | 58.6 ±  2.1 | 8.62 ± 0.57 |
| Dog | (6) | 21.2  ± 1.1 | 23.7 ±  2.7 | 1.12 ± 0.09 |
| Human | | | | |
| Internal disease or sudden death | (7) | 1.99 ± 0.32 | 12.1 ±  1.5 | 7.03 ± 1.42 |
| Cranial trauma or internal haemorrhage | (8) | 0.26 ± 0.06 | 6.4 ±  1.6 | 31.83 ± 9.19 |
| Phaeochromocytoma | (10) | 0.3 – 173 | 5.5 – 66.6 | – |

Adrenal medullae were rapidly dissected from the cortex in the cold and homogenized in 1 M acetic acid. Values represent mean ± s.e. mean of duplicate determination on medulla extracts except for human phaeochromocytoma where the range of values is included. Opioid peptide values are expressed as Met-enkephalin equivalents. (Data modified from Viveros *et al.*, 1979*a*; 1980*a*; Saria *et al.*, 1980; Wilson *et al.*, 1981*c*.)

The opiate activity of adrenal medullary extracts is enhanced several fold when the extracts are treated with trypsin and even more when limited carboxypeptidase B digestion follows trypsin treatment (Lewis *et al.*, 1979; Lewis *et al.*, 1980*b*). Molecular sieve chromatography of the extracts reveals a large heterogeneity of peptides with native and with cryptic opiate activity; the approximate molecular weights range from 500 to 30 kilodaltons. Of the total opiate activity that can be measured with a radioreceptor assay in the adrenal extracts, approximately one-fourth is contributed by the pentapeptides Met-enkephalin and Leu-enkephalin; the next most abundant peptide in this group is the heptapeptide

Met-enkephalin (Arg[6], Phe[7]) (Stern *et al.*, 1980). No significant amounts of $\beta$-endorphin or dynorphin have been found in normal adrenal medulla (Schultzberg, 1978; Viveros *et al.*, 1979*a*; Lewis *et al.*, 1979; Watson *et al.*, 1981). The enhanced opiate activity after trypsin and carboxypeptidase B treatment results from the release of large numbers of Met-enkephalin and Leu-enkephalin sequences present in the larger molecular weight peptides that have no or only slight activity on the radioreceptor assay when tested in their native form (Lewis *et al.*, 1980*b*). Figure 5.1 shows the elution profile from a P-100 chromatography

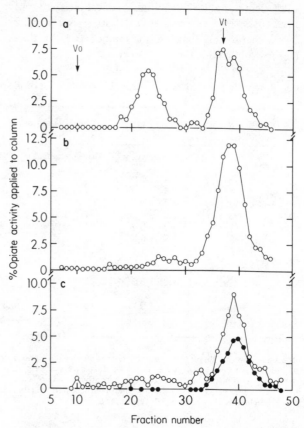

Figure 5.1 Biogel P-100 gel filtration chromatography of opioid peptides from various tissues. Acetic acid (1.0 M) extracts of cultured bovine adrenal chromaffin cells (*a*), partially purified human pheochromocytoma chromaffin vesicles (*b*), or highly purified bovine splenic nerve large dense-core vesicles (*c*) were neutralised and applied (250–500 $\mu$l) to a 0.9 × 30 cm column of Biogel P-100. The elution buffer was 50 mM Tris · HCL, pH 8.1 at 4°C. The buffer flow rate was 5 ml/h and fractions of 520 $\mu$l were collected. Aliquots of the collected fractions were assayed for opiate activity following sequential digestion with trypsin and carboxypeptidase B (○) or without enzyme treatment (●). The data are shown as the percentage of the opiate activity, after enzyme treatment, of the unfractionated material applied to the column. Recoveries of opiate activity were 75, 91, and 70 per cent in panels *a*, *b*, and *c*, respectively; recovery of the sample without enzyme treatment (panel *c*) was 78 per cent.

column of total opioid peptide activity (native and cryptic) of an acid extract of bovine adrenal chromaffin cells after 4 d in primary culture. The opioid material eluting at the total column volume corresponds to peptides of molecular weight below 5 kilodaltons and includes Met-enkephalin, Leu-enkephalin and other small opioid peptides. The broad peak eluting between fractions 18 and 28 corresponds to molecular weights from 10 to 20 kilodaltons. No opiate activity is found in this larger molecular weight region unless the fractions are treated with trypsin and carboxypeptidase B before the assay.

## Synthesis of opioid peptides

A decrease in adrenal catecholamines *in vivo* resulting from exocytotic secretion or selective amine depletion by reserpine treatment (table 5.2) produces an increase in the opioid peptide content of the adrenal medulla (Viveros *et al.*,

Table 5.2 Effect of insulin hypoglycemia and reserpine on adrenomedullary opioid peptides and catecholamine stores in the cat

|  | $n$ | Catecholamines ($\mu$mol/ g wet wt) | Opioid peptides (nmol/ g wet wt) | $\dfrac{CA}{OP}$ |
|---|---|---|---|---|
| Control | 4 | 31.72 ± 2.85 | 3.08 ± 1.08 | 14,407 ± 4,008 |
| Insulin (6 h) | 3 | 4.43 ± 0.65** | 0.50 ± 0.11* | 13,500 ± 7,000 |
| Reserpine (24 h) | 4 | 5.65 ± 0.98** | 3.20 ± 0.66 | 2,437 ± 725* |
| Reserpine (7 d) | 3 | 8.37 ± 2.90** | 9.50 ± 3.61*,† | 1,171 ± 663** |

Insulin 40 IU/kg was given intravenously and reserpine 2 mg/kg daily was given intraperitoneally on 2 successive days. Animals were killed 6 h, 24 h or 7 d after the last drug administration. Data are expressed as mean ± s.e. mean.
Statistical differences: *$P < 0.01$; **$P < 0.001$ compared with control; †$P < 0.05$ compared with reserpine 24 h.

1980) and of bovine chromaffin cells in culture (Wilson *et al.*, 1980*a*; Viveros *et al.*, 1980*b*; Wilson *et al.*, 1981*a*; Wilson *et al.*, 1981*b*) in spite of the inability of these cells and storage vesicles to take up opioid peptides from the medium (Viveros *et al.*, 1980*a*). The content of peptides with cryptic opiate activity is also enhanced by reserpine treatment (Wilson *et al.*, 1981*b*). These increases, which are blocked by inhibitors of protein synthesis (Viveros *et al.*, 1980*a*; Wilson *et al.*, 1981*a*), are similar to the induction of tyrosine hydroxylase and dopamine $\beta$-hydroxylase that follows catecholamine depletion or increased neurogenic stimulation of the adrenal gland (Mueller, 1969; Viveros *et al.*,

1969*a*), suggesting a coordinated regulation of the synthesis of these different cellular proteins.

Cultured cells incubated simultaneously with radiolabelled methionine and tyrosine incorporate both amino acids into Met-enkephalin and only tyrosine into Leu-enkephalin (Wilson *et al.*, 1980, 1981*b*) (table 5.3). This experiment demonstrates the *de novo* synthesis of enkephalins by chromaffin cells and an increase in the rate of enkephalin synthesis induced by reserpine treatment.

Table 5.3   Reserpine increases the content and synthesis of enkephalins in chromaffin cells in culture

| Treatment | Met-enkephalin | | | | Leu-enkephalin | | |
|---|---|---|---|---|---|---|---|
| | Total content (pmol) | New synthesis | | | Total content (pmol) | New synthesis | |
| | | From [$^3$H]-Tyr (pmol) | From [$^{35}$S]Met (pmol) | Fraction labelled | | From [$^3$H]-Tyr (pmol) | Fraction labelled |
| None | 13.8 | 1.7 | 2.1 | 0.14 | 21.4 | 2.1 | 0.10 |
| Reserpine (100 nM) | 53.4 | 12.8 | 10.5 | 0.22 | 35.9 | 6.5 | 0.18 |

Data correspond to amounts extracted from $7.7 \times 10^6$ bovine chromaffin cells for each treatment. Cells in culture were incubated for 3 d with [$^3$H]-tyrosine (572 d.p.m./pmol) and [$^{35}$S]-methionine (715 d.p.m./pmol). Enkephalins were purified by Amberlite XAD-2 and HPLC. (Data and methodological details from Wilson *et al.*, 1980*a*.)

Furthermore, the preferential increase in total Met-enkephalin over Leu-enke-phalin levels and the greater labelling of Met-enkephalin provides evidence for differential control of the synthesis and storage of the two enkephalins. If both enkephalins originate from the same macromolecular precursor as has been pro-posed (Lewis *et al.*, 1980*b*), these experiments suggest differential processing of the common precursor.

## Storage of opioid peptides in catecholamine-containing chromaffin vesicles

Immunocytochemical studies have shown enkephalin-like immunoreactivity in adrenomedullary cells and in a few nerve fibres in the adrenal medulla and adrenal cortex (Schultzberg *et al.*, 1978; Linnoila *et al.*, 1980). Less than three per cent of the opioid peptide in the dog adrenal gland is found in the isolated cortex, and all of it can be accounted for by medullary contamination (Viveros *et al.*, 1979*a*). While the adrenal medullae of all vertebrates examined contain opioid peptides (table 5.1), there is almost a 100-fold difference in concentra-tion between various species. The number of enkephalin-like immunoreactive cells also varies with the species and, in general, is proportional to the opioid peptide content as measured by radioreceptor assay. For example, the rat, the species with the lowest content of opioid peptides in the adrenal, has only a few enkephalin-like immunoreactive chromaffin cells. By contrast, in the dog every chromaffin cell immunostains with antibodies specific for Met-enkephalin and Leu-enkephalin (figure 5.2), indicating that in this species both adrenaline and noradrenaline-containing cells contain both pentapeptides (Linnoila, Diliberto, Wilson and Viveros, unpublished).

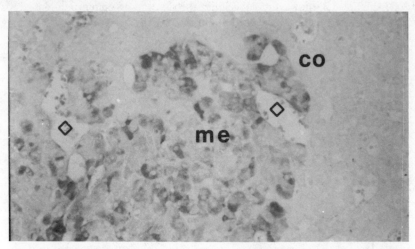

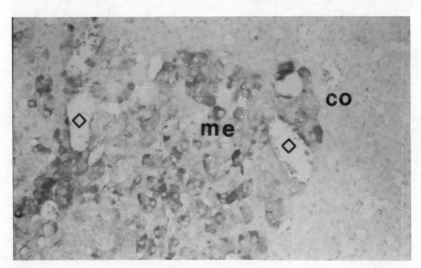

Figure 5.2 Enkephalin-like immunoreactivity in the dog adrenal gland as revealed by the peroxidase-antiperoxidase staining technique. (*a*) Section through the adrenal medulla and cortex following incubation with anti-serum to Met-enkephalin. (*b*) An immediately adjacent section following incubation with antiserum to Leu-enkephalin. Note the dark immunostaining of all the medullary cells and no staining of the adrenal cortex in the upper left corner of the photomicrographs. For technical details see Linnoila *et al.*, 1980. (Courtesy of Dr R. I. Linnoila.)

The catecholamine-containing chromaffin vesicles are easily isolated with high purity and yield by differential and sucrose gradient centrifugation (Viveros *et al.*, 1969). The separation of these vesicles can be readily followed by the catecholamine content and by the presence of other specific markers such as dopamine β-hydroxylase, an enzyme that is in part soluble inside the vesicle and in part an integral protein of the vesicle membrane (Viveros *et al.*, 1969*b*; Duch *et al.*, 1968). Figure 5.3 shows the subcellular distribution of opioid peptides, dopamine β-hydroxylase and catecholamines in the dog adrenal medullar homogenate.

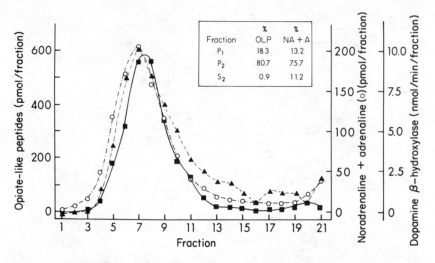

Figure 5.3 Distribution of opioid peptides (■), catecholamines and dopamine β-hydroxylase (▲) on sucrose density centrifugation of a dog adrenal medullary large granular fraction. The insert shows the distribution of opioid peptides (OLP) and catecholamines on differential centrifugation. The resulting P₂ sediment was resuspended and layered over a linear gradient between 61.6 per cent (fraction 1) and 19.2 per cent w/w (fraction 20) sucrose in water and centrifuged to equilibrium. (Modified from Viveros *et al.*, 1979*a*.)

Eighty per cent of the opioid peptides sediment at $26,000g$ for 20 min ($P_2$ fraction). When the $P_2$ fraction is further resolved by isopynic centrifugation through a linear sucrose gradient, the opioid peptide-containing particles equilibrate at the same density as particles containing the catecholamines and dopamine β-hydroxylase, indicating the storage of all three components in the same secretory vesicle (Viveros *et al.*, 1979*a*). This co-storage of opioid peptides and catecholamines has been confirmed in bovine adrenal glands (Viveros *et al.*, 1980*a*) and in bovine chromaffin cells in primary culture (Wilson *et al.*, 1981*b*).

## Co-secretion of opioid peptides and catecholamines

Secretion from the adrenal medulla is a quantal, all-or-none, exocytotic release of the chromaffin vesicle content (Viveros, 1975; Viveros *et al.*, 1969*b*). As dopamine β-hydroxylase, the largest soluble component of the vesicle, is secreted with cate-cholamines (Viveros *et al.*, 1968), it follows that all the other vesicular compon-ents will be secreted. As predicted, opioid peptides and catecholamines are secreted in a molar ratio identical to the ratio within the cell (Viveros *et al.*, 1979*a*, 1980*a*, 1980*b*; Wilson *et al.*, 1981*b*, 1981*d*). This secretion of opioid peptides is illustrated in figure 5.4. As the catecholamine secretion varies with the different experimental conditions there is a perfect proportionality in the

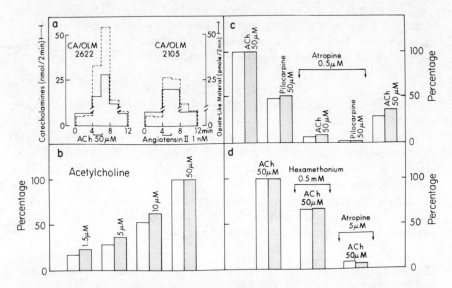

Figure 5.4 Effect of secretagogues and antagonists on the secretion of opioid peptides and catecholamines from perfused dog adrenals. The effluent from the perfused glands was col-lected every two minutes and assayed for catecholamines and opioid peptides. Each period of stimulation lasted 2 min. Bars in panels *b*, *c*, and *d* correspond to the cumulative secretion of catecholamines (open bars) and opioid peptides (stippled bars) during the two minutes of stimulation and the 6 min washout period; 100 per cent is the effect of 50 μM acetylcholine. (Data from Viveros *et al.*, 1980*a*.)

amount of peptide secreted. Adrenal medulla opioid peptides and catecholamines are also co-secreted *in vivo* (Viveros *et al.*, 1980*a*). Because of the variety in structure and origin of the endogenous opiates present in blood, the rapid degradation of enkephalins in plasma, the possibility of diffusion barriers, and the clearance of the secreted peptides through the adrenal lymphatics, we have preferred to estimate *in vivo* secretion by the difference in opioid peptide con-tent before and after splanchnic stimulation rather than trying to measure pep-tide levels in the adrenal vein. This approach has been successfully used in previous studies on the secretion of dopamine β-hydroxylase (Viveros *et al.*, 1980*a*, 1969*b*).

Table 5.2 shows the proportional decrease in opioid peptide content and cate-cholamines in the adrenal glands of cats where splanchnic nerve discharge had been increased reflexly by insulin-induced hypoglycemia. The administration of a moderate dose of reserpine, that acts by selectively depleting vesicular catecholamines, leaving the other vesicular components unaltered, shows that the decrease in opioid peptide content is not a consequence of the decrease in catecholamine levels resulting from the insulin treatment. As will be discussed later, reserpine treatment triggers the induction of opioid peptide synthesis such that the content is markedly increased 7 d after drug treatment. The opioid peptides present in human adrenals may also be secreted (table 5.1): there is a marked decrease in catecholamine and peptide content in the glands of subjects who died in shock as a consequence of traumatic injury when compared with individuals who were autopsied after sudden death or who died after prolonged disease.

To avoid some of the uncontrollable factors involved in studies of opioid peptide secretion *in vivo* or in the perfused glands, we have developed a chemically defined medium where chromaffin cells in primary culture maintain the morphology and many of the biochemical characteristics of differentiated adrenomedullary cells for long periods of time (Wilson and Viveros, 1981). Table 5.4 shows the proportional secretion of opioid peptides and catecholamines from bovine adrenal medullary cells in culture when stimulated by a number of secretagogues that induce exocytotic release by a variety of mechanisms. The bovine chromaffin cells secrete in response to the activation of nicotinic acetylcholine receptors; this effect is completely abolished by the nico-

Table 5.4   Co-secretion of catecholamines and opioid peptides from chromaffin cell cultures

| Secretagogue | Percentage cell content secreted* | |
| --- | --- | --- |
| | Catecholamines | Opioid peptides |
| Acetylcholine 50 $\mu$M | 25.1 ± 2.0 | 27.6 ± 2.5 |
| Nicotine 10 $\mu$M | 24.2 ± 0.6 | 27.1 ± 2.6 |
| Nicotine 10 $\mu$M + (d)-tubocurarine 10 $\mu$M | 0 | 0 |
| Nicotine 10 $\mu$M, no calcium | 0 | 0 |
| BaCl$_2$ 2 mM, no calcium | 42.4 ± 1.7 | 44.7 ± 1.7 |
| Veratridine 200 $\mu$M | 19.3 ± 1.4 | 18.8 ± 1.5 |
| KCl 50 mM | 21.0 ± 2.1 | 18.3 ± 1.8 |
| Ionomycin 20 $\mu$M | 35.6 ± 1.4 | 32.5 ± 4.9 |

*Mean ± s.e. mean ($n$ = 3). Basal secretion was substracted from all values.

tinic antagonist (*d*)-tubocurarine or by omission of calcium ions from the incubation medium. Barium, which induces catecholamine secretion in the absence of calcium, also induces a proportional release of opioid peptides. Veratridine (an activator of voltage-dependent sodium channels), potassium depolarisation and the calcium ionophore Ionomycin stimulate the coordinated secretion of amines and peptides. A detailed study of the effect of calcium concentration on the proportional secretion of amines and peptides by chomaffin cells in culture can be found in figure 5.6.

*Are peptides with cryptic opiate activity secreted?*
Most of our studies have dealt with the peptides that are active in the opiate-receptor assay without enzymatic activation. The culture system seemed especially suited to test whether the peptides with cryptic opiate activity and the natively active peptides were in common or separate secretory pools. Table 5.5 shows that stimulation of the cells with nicotine produces an identical secretion of both types of peptides. Similar results were obtained when the cells were

Table 5.5   Secretion of peptides with cryptic opiate activity from chromaffin cells

|  | Cell content (pmol/culture) | Secreted (pmol/culture) | Percentage content secreted |
|---|---|---|---|
| Native opioid peptides | 33 ± 2 | 9 ± 1 | 27 ± 3 |
| Total opioid peptides | 158 ± 9 | 43 ± 5 | 27 ± 3 |
| Cryptic opioid peptides | 125 ± 7 | 34 ± 4 | 28 ± 4 |

Chromaffin cells were incubated with or without nicotine 10 $\mu$M for 20 min. At the end of the incubation, cells were extracted and aliquots assayed for opiate activity prior (native) and after digestion with trypsin and carboxypeptidase B (total opioid peptides). Data are shown as mean ± s.e. mean (*n* = 3).

stimulated with barium or Ionomycin. Secretion of the larger peptides containing enkephalin sequences has also been observed by analysing the effluent of perfused bovine adrenal glands (Kilpatrick *et al.*, 1980*b*) and from bovine chromaffin cells that had adopted neuronal characteristics in culture (Rossier *et al.*, 1981).

*Adrenaline or noradrenaline cells as the source of opioid peptide secretion*
The dog adrenal has a marked predominance of adrenaline over noradrenaline and, as shown in figure 5.2, all chromaffin cells contain enkephalin-like immunoreactivity; thus, the dog is not a convenient species to study which of the catecholamine-containing cell types stores and secretes opioid peptides. Recently, it has been stated that enkephalins are stored only in the adrenaline-containing cells in the bovine adrenal medulla (Livett *et al.*, 1981). The initial ratio of

adrenaline to noradrenaline (three to two) in bovine chromaffin cells is retained with little or no change during three weeks in culture (Wilson and Viveros, 1981). These cells also maintain the morphological differences characteristic of adrenaline and noradrenaline-containing cells (Wilson and Viveros, 1981).

When the secretion of adrenaline and that of noradrenaline were determined individually, we found that several different secretagogues (nicotine, potassium ions, veratridine) were more potent at inducing noradrenaline than adrenaline secretion (Wilson and Viveros, unpublished). This difference in the sensitivity of noradrenaline and adrenaline cells was large enough to study the correlation between opioid peptide secretion and the secretion of each amine. Figure 5.5 shows that the noradrenaline response to nicotine stimulation was displaced to

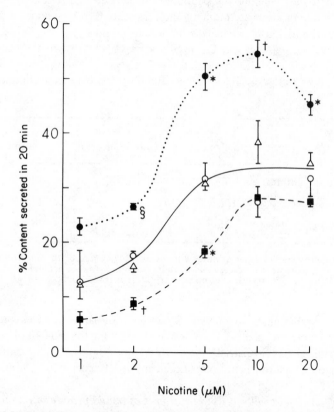

Figure 5.5 Correlation of opioid peptide secretion with total catecholamine secretion. The secretion of adrenaline (■), noradrenaline (●), total catecholamines (△) and opioid peptides (○) induced by exposing bovine chromaffin cells in culture to different concentrations of nicotine for 20 min was determined. Cultures had been plated 4 d before; on the day of the experiment the proportion of adrenaline was $64 \pm 1$ per cent ($n = 24$) of total catecholamines. The data are shown as mean $\pm$ s.e. mean ($n = 3$). Statistically significant differences of catecholamine secretion when compared with opioid peptide secretion: $*P < 0.025$; $\dagger P < 0.005$; $\S P < 0.001$.

the left of the adrenaline response. The dose-response curve for opioid peptide secretion is significantly different from the dose-response relationship of adrenaline and noradrenaline secretion but it is superimposable on the dose-response curve for total catecholamine release. These results indicate that the opioid peptides are being secreted from both types of cells and in the same proportion as each of the amines is being released.

### The mechanism of catecholamine-peptide secretion

We have already mentioned some of the morphological and biochemical evidence which suggests that exocytosis is the mechanism of secretion from adrenal chromaffin cells. This hypothesis is further supported by the proportionality in the release of catecholamines and opioid peptides reported above. Recently, Uvnäs and Aborg (1973, 1980) have offered an alternative hypothesis for quantal catecholamine secretion by an ion-exchange mechanism. The activation of the chromaffin cell, or of a nerve terminal, increases sodium conductance across the plasma membrane; the increase in ion conductance that occurs in the area of contact of plasma and storage vesicle membrane would lead to exchange of sodium for catecholamines at ionic binding sites in the vesicular storage complex, thus releasing catecholamines. The release of the other vesicular components is considered to be a rather infrequent disposal of worn out vesicles (Uvnäs and Aborg, 1980).

One fundamental prediction of the ion-exchange hypothesis is that the amount of catecholamines released does not depend on the quantity of transmitter stored in each vesicle, but rather on the factors that determine the ion conductrance of the area of fused vesicle-cell membrane (Uvnäs, 1973). The quantal hypothesis of transmitter secretion as originally proposed by Del Castillo and Katz (1954) and later extended to the adrenal medulla (Viveros, 1975; Viveros *et al.*, 1979*b*) predicts that the amount of transmitter, or hormone, secreted by a fixed stimulus is a direct function of vesicle number and content. As mentioned above, agents which inhibit catecholamine uptake into chromaffin vesicles produce an increase in the opioid peptide content of adrenal chromaffin cells *in vivo* (Viveros *et al.*, 1979*a*) and in culture (Wilson *et al.*, 1980*a*; Viveros *et al.*, 1980*b*; Wilson *et al.*, 1981*a*, 1981*c*). These observations provided a system to subject either hypothesis to experimental testing.

Table 5.6 clearly shows that the secretion of either opioid peptides or catecholamines is strictly proportional to the corresponding increase in opioid peptide content and decrease in catecholamine levels. The increase in opioid peptide content could be distributed among pre-existing vesicles or represent an increase in the number of chromaffin vesicles per cell. Whether the decreased catecholamine content remains only in the initial vesicles or is also distributed to newly synthesised vesicles, the decrease in catecholamine secretion strongly supports the quantal all-or-none exocytic secretion from chromaffin cells and contradicts the ion-exchange hypothesis.

Table 5.6 Proportional secretion of catecholamines and opioid peptides from chromaffin cells treated with reserpine or tetrabenazine

| Experiment | Addition to culture medium | Catecholamines/Culture | | Opioid peptides/Culture | |
|---|---|---|---|---|---|
| | | Cell content (nmol) | Nicotine-evoked secretion (nmol) | Cell Content (pmol) | Nicotine-evoked secretion (pmol) |
| 1 | None | 55.3 ± 1.4 | 12.8 ± 0.8 | 24.2 ± 1.2 | 6.9 ± 0.3 |
| | Reserpine | 9.4 ± 0.2 | 1.8 ± 0.1 | 48.2 ± 1.7 | 14.6 ± 0.6 |
| | Ratio | 0.17 | 0.14 | 1.99 | 2.12 |
| 2 | None | 112.0 ± 1.2 | 26.4 ± 1.9 | 27.7 ± 1.9 | 7.7 ± 0.9 |
| | Tetrabenazine | 20.5 ± 0.9 | 4.7 ± 0.4 | 72.5 ± 2.1 | 19.6 ± 1.9 |
| | Ratio | 0.18 | 0.18 | 2.62 | 2.55 |

Chromaffin cells were used 3 d after indicated additions of reserpine 100 nM or tetra-benazine 100 $\mu$M to the culture medium. Cells were stimulated with nicotine 20 $\mu$M for 10 min (experiment 1) or nicotine 10 $\mu$M for 20 min (experiment 2). Cell contents represent the amounts of catecholamines and opioid peptides present in unstimulated cells after the incubation period. Nicotine-evoked secretion values are the losses in cell content evoked by exposure to nicotine. The data are expressed as mean ± s.e. mean ($n$ = 3 for experiment 1 and $n$ = 6 for experiment 2). Ratio indicates the quotient of the drug-treated value over the untreated value.

## OPIOID PEPTIDES IN HUMAN PHAEOCHROMOCYTOMA AND IN POSTGANGLIONIC SYMPATHETIC NERVES

We have recently attempted to extend the new knowledge on opioid peptides from the adrenal medulla to other ontogenically related cells like the sympathetic postganglionic neurone and phaeochromocytoma tumour cells. Although opioid peptides have been found in these cells, there are interesting differences and similarities when compared to the adrenomedullary chromaffin cell.

### Human phaeochromocytoma

Opioid peptides including Met-enkepahlin, Leu-enkephalin and Met-enkephalin-[Arg[6], Phe[7]] and peptides with cryptic opiate activity (figure 5.1) have been identified in human pheochromocytoma (Sullivan *et al.*, 1978; Lundberg *et al.*, 1979; Clement-Jones *et al.*, 1980; Giraud *et al.*, 1981; Wilson *et al.*, 1981c). The opioid peptide content varies widely between and within tumours (table 5.1). Since the catecholamine content of different regions of a phaeochromocytoma varies independently from the concentration of opioid peptides, the ratio of these two substances may differ as much as four-fold between areas of the same tumour (Wilson, Cubeddu, Chang and Viveros, unpublished). Some tumour cells may preferentially synthesise and store enkephalins with no, or only small amounts of, catecholamines, and vice versa. This possibility is supported by the visualisation of enkephalin-like immunoreactivity in human phaeochromocytoma cells which lack dopamine β-hydroxylase immunoreactivity, a situation never observed in human adrenal glands (Linnoila *et al.*, 1980; Lundberg *et al.*, 1979).

Similar to the adrenal medulla, most of the opioid peptides sediment with the catecholamine-containing particles (Wilson *et al.*, 1981*c*) and opioid peptide levels of phaeochromocytoma cells in culture can be induced by reserpine or nicotine treatment (Wilson *et al.*, 1981*b*). As expected, a number of stimuli activate secretion of opioid peptides from phaeochromocytes in culture (Wilson *et al.*, 1918*d*). Despite the similarities, the secretion of opioid peptides, catecholamines and preloaded [$^3$H]-noradrenaline differs in several significant respects from the secretion of these molecules from normal chromaffin cells (compare figure 5.6*a* and *c*). Adrenal medulla cells, in all conditions examined, secrete opioid peptides and catecholamines in the same proportion, and the ratio of amines to peptides secreted is the same as the corresponding ratio within the cell (figure 5.6*c* and *d* and above).

In contrast, in phaeochromocytoma all secretagogues tested are more potent in inducing secretion of opioid peptides than catecholamines (Wilson *et al.*, 1981*d*). Whereas in normal chromaffin cells secretion of [$^3$H]-catecholamines is identical to the secretion of endogenous monoamines (Kilpatrick *et al.*, 1980*a*), in phaeochromocytoma cells the secretion of [$^3$H]-noradrenaline is consistently greater than the secretion of endogenous amines, and in maximal conditions of stimulation it becomes the same as the secretion of opioid peptides. The calcium dependence of the secretory response to nicotine is identical for catecholamines and opioid peptides in normal cells (figure 5.6), whereas in phaeochromocytoma cells nicotine stimulates secretion of opioid peptides at much lower concentrations of extracellular calcium than are required to elicit endogenous catecholamine secretion. These results suggest heterogeneous storage pools of opioid peptides and catecholamines in phaeochromocytoma cells and even heterogeneity in the sites for recently stored [$^3$H]-noradrenaline as compared to endogenous catecholamines.

This can be seen more clearly in figure 5.6*b*, which shows that there is a good correlation between [$^3$H]-noradrenaline and catecholamine secretion, although the positive Y intercept indicates that the fraction of the stored label can be secreted in the absence of endogenous catecholamine secretion. No significant correlation is found between the secretion of opioid peptides and amines. Although other interpretations are possible, if we consider these results in light of the variable ratios of catecholamines to opioid peptides in different regions of the same tumour and the immunocytochemical observations on opioid peptides and dopamine β-hydroxylase distribution (Lundberg *et al.*, 1979) discussed above, it seems likely that there is a spectrum from highly responsive phaeochromo-

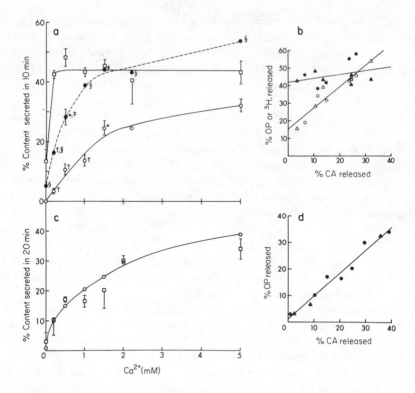

Figure 5.6   Dependency of opioid peptide, endogenous catecholamine and [³H]-noradren-
aline secretion induced by nicotine on the external concentration of calcium ions. *a* and *b*,
Human phaeochromocytoma cells; *c* and *d*, bovine chromaffin cells in primary culture. The
nicotine concentration was $10 \mu$M for both cell types. In panels *a* and *c*, bars representing
s.e. mean are shown only when the value is larger than the symbol used for the mean. Endogenous catecholamines (○), preloaded [³H]-noradrenaline (●) and opioid peptide (□)
secretion are shown. *$P < 0.05$ compared with opioid peptide secretion; †$P < 0.01$ compared with opioid peptide secretion; ‡$P < 0.05$ compared with catecholamine secretion;
§$P < 0.01$ compared with catecholamine secretion. Panels *b* and *d* show the correlation
between secretion of opioid peptides and endogenous catecholamines (●, ▲) and between
secretion of [³H]-catecholamines and endogenous catecholamines (○, △). Regression coef-
ficients: chromaffin cells opioid peptide compared with catecholamines, $r = 0.98$; phaeochromocytoma cells label compared with catecholamines, $r = 0.94$; phaeochromocytoma
cells opioid peptides compared with catecholamines, $r = 0.11$.

cytoma cells that contain only or mainly opioid peptides, to less responsive cells
that preferentially synthesise and store catecholamines. [³H]-noradrenaline may
be taken up preferentially, but not exclusively, into the storage vesicles of the
catecholamine-containing cells.

The very high concentration of opioid peptides in some phaeochromocytomas,
the large size these tumours can reach compared with the adrenal medulla, and
the low secretory threshold of the tumour cells, may result in massive releases
of opioid peptides into the circulation. Part of the clinical pleomorphism of this

disease may be attributed to the opioid peptides released from the tumours (Wilson *et al.*, 1981*c*). Phaeochromocytoma patients may be under hypertensive therapy for prolonged periods of time. Because catecholamine-depleting agents as well as other autonomic-acting drugs induce the synthesis of opioid peptides, the treatment needed to control blood pressure may concurrently exacerbate the symptoms derived from the excessive production of opioid peptides.

### Postganglionic sympathetic nerves

Enkephalin-like immunoreactivity has been visualised in a small number of adrenergic perikarya in rat sympathetic ganglia (Schultzberg *et al.*, 1979), but it is difficult to assess to what extent the initial biochemical characterisation done in extracts of whole sympathetic ganglia (Hughes *et al.*, 1977; DiGiulio *et al.*, 1978) reflects the biochemistry of the postganglionic sympathetic neurone or that of the small intensely fluorescent cells and the nerve terminal network which also contain opioid peptides (Schultzberg *et al.*, 1979).

The bovine splenic nerve was selected to study the subcellular distribution and chemical composition of sympathetic neurone opioid peptides because 98 per cent of the axons are sympathetic C-fibres and nerve vesicles can be prepared with high purity and yield (Klein *et al.*, 1979). As in the adrenal medulla, 85 per cent of the nerve opioid peptides sediment with catecholamines in a particulate fraction (Wilson *et al.*, 1980*b*). When resolved by sucrose density centrifugation, 90 per cent of this material is in the noradrenergic, large dense-cored vesicles, giving a high molar ratio of opioid peptides to catecholamines (1 in 60). There is no evidence for processing of the peptides during axonal transport. Of the total opioid peptides in the noradrenergic vesicles, at least 50 per cent could be accounted for by Met-enkephalin and Leu-enkephalin in a ratio of between one and two to one, only a small amount of material (10 per cent after correction for recovery and relative potency) eluted from a high performance liquid chromatography column at the position of Met-enkephalin [$Arg^6$, $Phe^7$] (Wilson *et al.*, 1980*b*).

The sucrose-$D_2O$ density gradient previously used for particle separation concentrates the noradrenergic, large dense-cored vesicles too close to the bottom of the gradient (Wilson *et al.*, 1980*b*). In an attempt to separate opioid peptide-containing vesicles from noradrenaline-containing particles the two fractions that contain the highest concentration of opioid peptides and noradrenaline were pooled, diluted and recentrifuged in two other gradients with a different density profile. Figure 5.7 shows that in both gradients, there was a good correspondence of opioid peptides and norepinephrine distribution. The slight displacement of dopamine $\beta$-hydroxylase towards lower densities is indicative of a few partially empty vesicles. Trypsin/carboxypeptidase B digestion of acid extracts of the purified vesicles produced only a two-fold increase in opiate activity (figure 5.1), against a five- to ten-fold increase typically seen with extracts of the bovine adrenal medulla or chromaffin cells in culture. Most of the receptor-

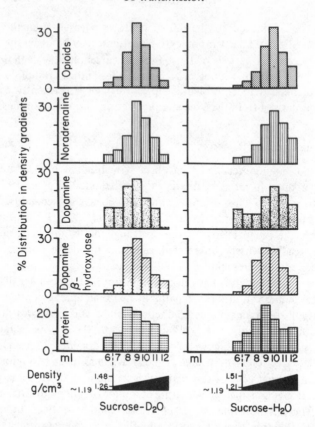

Figure 5.7 Distribution of opioid peptides, noradrenaline, dopamine, dopamine β-hydroxy-lase and protein on density gradient centrifugation of a purified large dense-cored vesicle fraction from bovine splenic nerves. Purified noradrenergic nerve vesicles were prepared as described by Wilson *et al.* (1980*b*) through a sucrose-D$_2$O gradient of densities 1.10 to 1.27 g/cm$^3$. Purified vesicles were recovered from the two bottom fractions of the first gradient, diluted and layered on top of the sucrose-D$_2$O or the sucrose-H$_2$O gradients of higher density. After centrifugation to equilibrium, 1-ml fractions were collected and analysed as previously described (Klein *et al.*, 1979; Wilson *et al.*, 1980*b*). Note the co-sedimentation of opioid peptides, catecholamines and dopamine β-hydroxylase.

active peptides eluted at the total volume of the Biogel P-100 column (apparent molecular weight below 5 kilodaltons), even after enzymatic digestion of the eluates.

These experiments confirm the previous data on the storage of opioid peptides with norepinephrine in the same particle and further support the notion that the different peptides with cryptic opiate activity found in the noradrenergic, large dense-cored vesicles are final secretory products and that processing is probably done at an early stage at the neuronal perikaryon. As not all principal neurones in sympathetic ganglia show enkephalin-like immunoreactivity (Hughes *et al.*, 1977), it is possible that the opioid peptides may be stored in only a fraction of the total noradrenergic large dense-cored vesicle population. These findings suggest the exocytotic co-secretion of noradrenaline and opioid peptides from those nerve terminals that contain both substances.

## CONCLUSIONS: PHYSIOLOGICAL IMPLICATIONS OF MULTIMESSENGER SYSTEMS IN THE PERIPHERAL ADRENERGIC SYSTEM

The presence of adrenomedullary opioid peptides in the circulation, the large variety of actions of these peptides outside the central nervous system, and the possible physiological roles for the opioid peptides secreted with the catecholamines have recently been discussed elsewhere (Viveros and Wilson, 1982). We will restrict our discussion to only two aspects of the possible role of multimessenger communication originating at the peripheral adrenergic system.

### Adrenomedullary secretion and opioid-mediated stress-induced analgesia

Evidence for participation of endogenous opioids in analgesia induced by stress factors that markedly stimulate secretion of the adrenal medulla led us to examine the presence of opioids in the adrenal medulla. Recent studies, though still preliminary, support such a role and will be summarised here. Lewis *et al.* (1980*a*, 1981*a*) have recently characterised, in the rat, two forms of analgesia induced by inescapable foot shock. A short exposure to continuous foot shock produces a non-opioid-mediated analgesia whereas intermittent shock for 30 min causes profound analgesia that is antagonised by naloxone (Lewis *et al.*, 1980*a*) and shows cross-tolerance to morphine (Lewis *et al.*, 1981*a*). Adrenalectomy, adrenal demedullation and adrenal medullary denervation antagonized the opioid but not the non-opioid analgesia induced by stress. Testing for analgesia after reserpine, given on a treatment schedule that should have depleted catecholamines and increased opioid peptide content, significantly enhanced the naloxone-sensitive analgesia (Lewis *et al.*, 1981*b*). These findings strongly suggest that the opioid peptides secreted from the adrenal medulla are critically involved in certain forms of stress-induced analgesia.

### Mono-, dual- or multi-messenger chemical communication in the peripheral adrenergic system

From the biochemical data provided in this report and from cytochemical information provided by others (Schultzberg *et al.*, 1978; 1979; Linnoila *et al.*, 1980; Lundberg *et al.*, 1979), it is obvious that there is a large variability in the amount of opioid peptides present in the adrenal medulla, sympathetic nerves and phaeochromocytoma tumors in different species. This variability is also present within the same individual: not every sympathetic ganglion or every cell in the ganglia or the adrenal medulla contains equal amounts of enkephalin-like immunoreactivity (Schultzberg *et al.*, 1978; Lundberg *et al.*, 1979). In fact, some adrenomedullary cells seem to contain only Met-enkephalin or only Leu-enkephalin

(Linnoila *et al.*, 1980) and the content can change depending on the cell's functional state (Schultzberg *et al.*, 1978; Viveros *et al.*, 1980*b*; Wilson *et al.*, 1980*a*; 1981*a*). Furthermore, other non-opioid biologically active peptides have been found in significant amounts in peripheral noradrenergic sympathetic neurones, which may or may not simultaneously contain enkephalins (Hökfelt *et al.*, 1980; Schultzberg *et al.*, 1979). We prefer to believe that this large variability in the association of catecholamines and neuropeptides represents specialised functions for the particular combination of messengers rather than an accidental or vestigial presence of these peptides.

In contrast to the variability in the presence of neuropeptides, all noradrenergic and adrenergic vesicles also contain high concentrations of ATP and soluble dopamine β-hydroxylase. Little has been done to identify specific functions for these other vesicular components after they are secreted from nerve terminals or from the adrenal medulla. Recent evidence has suggested that the non-cholinergic, non-adrenergic residual contraction of the cat nictating membrane, induced by sympathetic nerve stimulation, is due to the secretion of ATP from the sympathetic nerve terminals (Langer and Pinto, 1976). Thomas *et al.* (1980, 1981) have found that dopamine β-hydroxylase modulates the β-receptor sensitivity of pinealocytes and circulating lymphocytes, suggesting that this protein may have important functions as a co-messenger in addition to its well known role in catecholamine biosynthesis. Opioid peptides, ATP and ATP metabolites, and dopamine β-hydroxylase may not only exert effects at very short-range (synaptic) or long-range (hormonal) targets but may have paracrine actions influencing the adrenal microcirculation, neighbouring adrenocortical cells or the blood elements traversing the adrenal gland.

The release of all the many soluble components, in addition to the classical messenger, that have been found to be present in hormone, neurohormone and neurotransmitter storage vesicles may not be just a futile secretion but may contain a wealth of significant information for the pre- and post-synaptic cellular elements, thus contributing to the integrated, holistic response of the neuroeffector (or hormone-target) physiological unit. An excellent example of such a structured synaptic message has already been unravelled by the work of Hökfelt and his associates in the integrated response of exocrine glands to the co-secretion of acetycholine and vasoactive intestinal peptide (Hökfelt *et al.*, 1980; Lundberg *et al.*, 1980). Although one can trace the origins of the idea of co-storage and co-secretion of neurotransmitters for at least 25 years (Abrahams *et al.*, 1957), the multimessenger concept of neural and hormonal transmission is finally coming of age and may well drastically modify our understanding of integrative physiology.

## REFERENCES

Abrahams, V. C., Koelle, G. B. and Smart, P. (1957). Histochemical demonstration of cholinesterases in the hypothalamus of the dog. *J. Physiol. Lond.*, **139**, 137–44
Blaschko, H. and Welch, A. D. (1953). Localization of adrenaline in cytoplasmic particles of the bovine adrenal medulla. *Arch. exp. Path. Pharmac.*, **219**, 17–22

Bodner, R. J., Kelly, D. D., Spiaggia, A., Ehrenberg, C. and Glusman, M. (1978). Dose-dependent reduction by naloxone of analgesia induced by cold-water stress. *Pharmac. Biochem. Behav.*, 8, 667–72

Burnstock, J. (1976). Do some nerve cells release more than one transmitter. *Neuroscience*, 1, 239–48

Clement-Jones, V., Corder, R. and Lowry, P. J. (1980). Isolation of human Met-enkephalin and two groups of putative precursors (2K-pro-met-enkephalin) from an adrenal medullary tumour. *Biochem. biophys. Res. Commun.*, 95, 665–73

Coupland, R. E. (1965). *The Natural History of the Chromaffin Cell*. Longman, London

Del Castillo, J. and Katz, B. (1954). Quantal components of the end plate potential. *J. Physiol. Lond.*, 124, 560–73

DiGiulio, A. M., Yang, H.-Y. T., Lutold, B., Fratta, W., Hong, J. and Costa, E. (1978). Characterization of enkephalin-like material extracted from sympathetic ganglia. *Neuropharmacology*, 17, 989–92

Douglas, W. W. (1968). Simulus-secretion coupling: the concept and clues from chromaffin and other cells. *Br. J. Pharmac.*, 34, 451–74

Duch, D. S., Viveros, O. H. and Kirshner, N. (1968). Endogenous inhibitors in adrenal medulla of dopamine β-hydroxylase. *Biochem. Pharmac.*, 17, 255–64

Frankenhaeuser, M. (1979). Psychoneuroendocrine approaches to the study of emotion as related to stress and coping. In *Nebraska Symposium on Motivation*, (ed. H. E. Howe and R. A. Dienstbier), University of Nebraska Press, Nebraska, pp. 123–61

Giraud, P., Eiden, L. E., Audigier, Y., Gillioz, P., Conte-Devolx, B., Boudouresque, F., Eskay, R. and Oliver, C. (1981). Enkephalins, ACTH, α-MSH and β-endorphin in human pheochromocytomas. *Neuropeptides*, 1, 237–52

Hexum, T. D., Yang, H.-Y. T. and Costa, E. (1980). Biochemical characterization of enkephalin-like immunoreactive peptides of adrenal glands. *Life Sci.*, 27, 1211–6

Hillarp, N.-Å. (1958). Isolation and some biochemical properties of the catecholamine granules in the cow adrenal medulla. *Acta Physiol. Scand.*, 43, 82–96

Hillarp, N.-Å., Lagerstedt, S. and Nilson, B. (1953). The isolation of a granule fraction from the suprarenal medulla, containing the sympathomimetic catecholamines. *Acta Physiol. Scand.*, 29, 251–63

Hökfelt, T., Lundberg, J. M., Schultzberg, M., Johansson, O., Ljungdahl, Å and Rehfeld, J. (1980). Coexistence of peptides and putative transmitters in neurons. In *Neuronal Peptides and Neuronal Communciation*, (ed. E. Costa and M. Trabucchi), Raven Press, New York, pp. 1–23

Hughes, J., Kosterlitz, H. W. and Smith, T. W. (1977). The distribution of methionine-enkephalin and leucine-enkephalin in the brain and peripheral tissues. *Br. J. Pharmac.*, 61, 639–47

Kilpatrick, D. L., Ledbetter, F. H., Carson, K. A., Kirshner, A. G., Slepetis, R. and Kirshner, N. (1980a). Stability of bovine adrenal medulla cells in culture. *J. Neurochem.*, 35, 679–92

Kilpatrick, D. L., Lewis, R. V., Stein, S. and Udenfriend, S. (1980b). Release of enkephalins and enkephalin-containing polypeptides from perfused beef adrenal glands. *Proc. natn. Acad. Sci. U.S.A.*, 77, 7473–5

Kirshner, N. and Goodall, McC. (1957). The formation of adrenaline from noradrenaline. *Biochem. biophys. Acta*, 24, 658–9

Klein, R. L., Thureson-Klein, A. K., Yen, S.-H. C., Baggett, J. McC., Gasparis, M. S. and Kirksay, D. F. (1979). Dopamine β-hydroxylase distribution in density gradients: physiological and artefactual implications. *J. Neurobiol.*, 10, 291–307

Langer, S. Z. and Pinto, J. E. B. (1976). Possible involvement of a transmitter different from norepinephrine in the residual responses to nerve stimulation of the cat nictitating membrane after pretreatment with reserpine. *J. Pharmac. exp. Therap.*, 196, 697–713

Larsson, L. I. (1980). On the possible existence of multiple endocrine, paracrine and neurocrine messengers in secretory cell systems. *Invest. Cell Path.*, 3, 73–85

Levin, E. Y., Levenberg, B. and Kaufman, S. (1960). The enzymatic conversion of 3,4-dihydroxyphenylethylamine to norepinephrine. *J. biol. Chem.*, 235, 2080–6

Lewis, J. P. (1975). Physiological mechanisms controlling secretory activity of adrenal medulla. In *Handbook of Physiology*, Section 7: *Endocrinology*, VI: *Adrenal Gland* (ed.

H. Blaschko, G. Sayers and A. D. Smith), American Physiological Society, Washington, D.C., pp. 309–19

Lewis, R. V., Stern, A. S., Kimura, S., Rossier, J., Stein, S. and Udenfriend, S. (1980b). An about 50,000-dalton protein in adrenal medulla: a common precursor of [met-] and [leu-] enkephalin. *Science*, 208, 1459–61

Lewis, R. V., Stern, A. S., Rossier, J., Stein, S. and Udenfriend, S. (1979). Putative enkephalin precursors in bovine adrenal medulla. *Biochem. biophys. Res. Commun.*, 89, 822–9

Lewis, J. W., Cannon, J. T. and Liebeskind, J. C. (1980a). Opioid and non-opioid mechanisms of stress analgesia. *Science*, 208, 623–5

Lewis, J. W., Sherman, J. E. and Liebeskind, J. C. (1981a). Opioid and nonopioid stress analgesia: assessment of tolerance and cross-tolerance with morphine. *J. Neurosci.*, 1, 358–363

Lewis, J. W., Tordoff, M. G., Sherman, J. E. and Liebeskind, J. C. (1981). Role of the adrenal medulla in opioid stress analgesia. *Sco. Neurosci. Abstra.*, 7, 735

Linnoila, R. I., Diaugustine, R. P., Hervonen, A. and Miller, R. J. (1980). Distribution of [met$^5$]- and [leu$^5$]-enkephalin-, vasoactive intestinal polypeptide- and substance p-like immunoreactivities in human adrenal glands. *Neuroscience*, 5, 2247–59

Livett, B. G. and Dean, D. M. (1980). Distribution of immunoreactive enkephalins in adrenal paraneurons: preferential localization in varicose processes and terminals. *Neuropeptides*, 1, 358–63

Livett, B. G., Dean, D. M., Whelan, L. G., Udenfriend, S. and Rossier, J. (1981). Co-release of enkephalin and catecholamines from cultured chromaffin cells. *Nature*, 289, 317–9

Lundberg, J. M., Änggård, A., Fahrenkrug, J., Hökfelt, T. and Mutt, V. (1980). Vasoactive intestinal polypeptide in cholinergic neurons of exocrine glands. Functional significance of coexisting transmitters for vasodilation and secretion. *Proc. natn. Acad. Sci. U.S.A.*, 77, 1651–5

Lundberg, J. M., Hamberger, B., Schultzberg, M., Hökfelt, T., Grandberg, P. Efendić, S., Terenius, L., Goldstein, M. and Luft, R. (1979). Enkephalin- and somatostatin-like immunoreactivities in human adrenal medulla and pheochromocytoma. *Proc. natn. Acad. Sci. U.S.A.*, 76, 4079–83

Mueller, R. A., Thoenen, H. and Axelrod, J. (1969). Increase in tyrosine hydroxylase activity after reserpine administration. *J. Pharmac. exp. Ther.*, 169, 74–9

Nagatsu, T., Levitt, M. and Udenfriend, S. (1964). Tyrosine hydroxylase – the initial step in norepinephrine biosynthesis. *J. biol. Chem.*, 239, 2910–7

Oliver, J. and Schafer, E. A. (1895). Phsyiological effect of extracts of the suprarenal capsules. *J. Physiol. Lond.*, 18, 230–79

Olson, L., Seiger, A., Freedman, R. and Hoffer, B. (1980). Chromaffin cells can innervate brains tissue: evidence from intraocular double grafts. *Exp. Neurol.*, 70, 414–26

Pearse, A. G. E. (1969). The cytochemistry and ultrastructure of polypeptide hormone-producing cells of the APUD series and the embryologic, physiologic and pathologic implications of the concept. *J. Histochem. Cytochem.*, 17, 303–13

De Robertis, E. D. P. and Vaz Ferreira, A. (1957). Electron microscope study of the excretion of catechol-containing droplets in the adrenal medulla. *Expl. Cell Res.*, 12, 568–74

Roda, L. G. and Hogue-Angeletti, R. A. (1979). Peptides in the adrenal medulla chromaffin granule. *FEBS Lett.*, 107, 393–7

Rossier, J., Dean, D. M., Livett, B. G. and Udenfriend, S. (1981). Enkephalin congeners and precursors are synthesized and released by primary cultures of adrenal chromaffin cells. *Life Sci.*, 28, 781–9

Saria, A., Wilson, S. P., Molnar, A., Viveros, O. H. and Lembeck, F. (1980). Substance P and opiate-like peptides in human medulla. *Neurosci. Lett.*, 20, 195–200

Schultzberg, M., Hökfelt, T., Terenius, L., Elfvin, L.-G., Lundberg, J. M., Brandt, J., Elde, R. P. and Goldstein, M. (1979). Enkephalin immunoreactive nerve fibres and cell bodies in sympathetic ganglia of the guinea pig and rat. *Neuroscience*, 4, 249–70

Schultzberg, M., Lundberg, J. M., Hökfelt, T., Terenius, L., Brandt, J., Elde, R. P. and Goldstein, M. (1978). Enkephalin-like immunoreactivity in gland cells and nerve terminals of the adrenal medulla. *Neuroscience*, 3, 1169–86

Smith, A. D. (1968). Biochemistry of adrenal chromaffin granules. In *The Interaction of Drugs and Subcellular Components in Animals Cells*, (ed. P. N. Campbell), Churchill, London, pp. 239–92

Stern, A. S., Lewis, R. V., Kimura, S., Rossier, J., Stein, S. and Udenfriend, S. (1980). Opioid hexapeptides and heptapeptides in adrenal medulla and brain; possible implications on the biosynthesis of enkephalins. *Arch. Biochem. Biophys.*, **205**, 606–13

Sullivan, S. N., Bloom, S. R. and Polak, J. M. (1978). Enkephalin in peripheral neuroendocrine tumors. *The Lancet*, i, 986–7

Takamine, J. (1901). Adrenaline, the active principle of the suprarenal glands and its mode of preparation. *Am. J. Pharm.*, **73**, 523–31

Thomas, J. A., Sakai, K. K., Holck, M. I. and Marks, B. H. (1980). Dopamine β-hydroxylase: a modulator of beta adrenergic receptor activity. *Res. Comm. chem. Path. Pharmac.*, **29**, 3–13

Thomas, J. A. Unverferth, D. V. and Marks, B. H. (1981). Lymphocyte beta-adrenoreceptor function in congestive heart failure: modulation by dopamine-beta-hydroxylase. In *Catecholamines in the Heart*, (ed. P. Gerlach), Springer Verlag, Heidelberg, in press

Unsicker, K., Griesser, J-H., Lindmar, R., Löffelhoz, K. and Wolf, U. (1980). Establishment, characterization and fibre outgrowth of isolated bovine adrenal medullary cells in long-term culture. *Neuroscience*, **5**, 1445–60

Uvnäs, B. (1973). An attempt to explain nervous transmitter release as due to nerve impulse-induced cation exchange. *Acta Physiol. Scand.*, **87**, 168–75

Uvnäs, B. and Aborg, C.-H. (1980). Possible role of nerve impulse induced sodium ion flux in a proposed multivesicular fractional release of adrenaline and noradrenaline from the chromaffin cell. *Acta. Physiol. Scand.*, **109**, 363–8

Viveros, O. H. (1975). Mechanism of secretion of catecholamines from adrenal medulla. In *Handbook of Physiology*, Section 7: *Endocrinology*, VI: *Adrenal Gland*, (ed. H. Blaschko, J. Sayers and A. D. Smith), American Physiological Society, Washington, D.C., pp. 389–426

Viveros, O. H., Arqueros, L. and Kirshner, N. (1968). Release of catecholamines and dopamine-β-oxidase from the adrenal medulla. *Life Sci.*, **7**, 609–18

Viveros, O. H., Arqueros, L., Connett, R. J. and Kirshner, N. (1969*a*). Mechanism of secretion from the adrenal medulla: IV. The fate of the storage vesicles following insulin and reserpine administration. *Molec. Pharmac.*, **5**, 69–82

Viveros, O. H., Arqueros, L. and Kirshner, N. (1969*b*). Quantal secretion from adrenal medulla: all-or-none release of storage vesicle content. *Science*, **165**, 911–3

Viveros, O. H., Diliberto, E. J. Jr., Hazum, E. and Chang, K.-J. (1979*a*). Opiate-like materials in the adrenal medulla: evidence for storage and secretion with catecholamines. *Molec. Pharmac.*, **16**, 1101–8

Viveros, O. H., Hazum, E., Diliberto, E. J. Jr, Cuatrecasas, P. and Chang, K.-J. (1979*b*). Concomitant storage and secretion of opioid-like peptides with catecholamines from the storage vesicles of the adrenal medulla in different species. *Abstr. Seventh Int. Meetg ISN*, Jerusalem, Israel, p. 636

Viveros, O. H., Diliberto, E. J. Jr., Hazum, E. and Chang, K.-J. (1980*a*). Enkephalins as possible adrenomedullary hormones: storage, secretion, and regulation of synthesis. In *Neural Peptides and Neuronal Communication*, (ed. E. Costa and M. Trabucchi), Raven Press, New York, pp. 191–204

Viveros, O. H. and Wilson, S. P. (1982). Opioid peptides in the peripheral sympathetic system and in pheochromocytoma. In *Norepinephrine: Clinical Aspects*, (ed. M. J. Ziegler and C. R. Lake), William and Wilkins, Baltimore, in press

Viveros, O. H., Wilson, S. P., Diliberto, E. J., Jr, Hazum, E. and Chang, K.-J. (1980*b*). Enkephalins in adrenomedullary chromaffin cells and sympathetic nerves. In *Advances in Physiological Sciences*, **14**: *Endocrinology, Neuroendocrinology, Neuropeptides*, **II**, (ed. E. Stark, E. B. Makara, B. Halász and Gy Rappay), Pergamon Press, New York, pp. 349–53

Watson, S. J., Akil, H., Ghazarossian, V. E. and Goldstein, A. (1981). Dynorphin immunocytochemical localization in brain and peripheral nervous system: preliminary studies. *Proc. natn. Acad. Sci. U.S.A.*, **78**, 1260–3

Wilson, S. P., Abou-Donia, M. M., Chang, K.-J. and Viveros, O. H. (1981*a*). Reserpine increase opiate-like peptide content and tyrosine hydroxylase activity in adrenal medullary chromaffin cells in culture. *Neuroscience*, 6, 71–9

Wilson, S. P., Chang, K.-J. and Viveros, O. H. (1980*a*). Synthesis of enkephalins by adrenal medullary chromaffin cells: reserpine increases incorporation of radiolabeled amino acids. *Proc. natn. Acad. Sci. U.S.A.*, 77, 4364–7

Wilson, S. P., Chang, K.-J. and Viveros, O. H. (1981*b*). Opioid peptide synthesis in bovine and human adrenal chromaffin cells. *Peptides*, suppl. 1, 2, 83–8

Wilson, S. P., Cubeddu, L. X., Chang, K.-J. and Viveros, O. H. (1981*c*). Met-enkephalin, leu-enkephalin and other opiate-like peptides in human pheochromocytoma tumors. *Neuropeptides*, 1, 273–81

Wilson, S. P., Klein, R. L., Chang, K.-J., Gasparis, M. S., Viveros, O. H. and Yang, W.-H. (1980*b*). Are opioid peptides co-transmitters in noradrenergic vesicles of sympathetic nerves? *Nature*, 288, 707–9

Wilson, S. P., Slepetis, R., Chang, K.-J., Kirshner, N. and Viveros, O. H. (1981*d*). Secretagogues that act by different mechanisms induce secretion of opioid peptides and catecholamines from chromaffin and pheochromocytoma cells. *Soc. Neurosci. Abstr.*, 7, 203

Wilson, S. P. and Viveros. O. H. (1981). Primary culture of adrenal medullary chromaffin cells in a chemically defined medium. *Expl. Cell Res.*, 133, 159–69

# 6

# The co-transmitter hypothesis, with special reference to the storage and release of ATP with noradrenaline and acetylcholine

G. Burnstock (Department of Anatomy and Embryology, and Centre for Neuroscience, University College, Gower Street, London WC1E 6BT, UK)

## INTRODUCTION

For many years most of us have accepted the idea that one nerve fibre makes and releases only one transmitter. This has become known as 'Dale's principle', although this nomenclature is not strictly correct and the history behind it is curious (see Eccles, 1976). In the Northnagel Lecture in 1934, Dale speculated in relation to the "axon reflex", that different endings of a sensory neurone (one a central synapse, the other concerned with antidromic vasodilatation of skin vessels) probably released the same transmitter. In the mid-1950s, it was Eccles who coined the words Dale's principle (apparently not entirely with the agreement of Dale), and defined it as "at all the axonal branches of a neurone, there is liberation of the same transmitter substance or substances". Ironically, this definition does not exclude the possibility of "co-transmitters".

Largely on the basis of our studies of the evolution of the autonomic nervous system (see Burnstock, 1969) and some evidence for coexistence of transmitters in certain invertebrate nerves (for example, Brownstein *et al.*, 1974; Cottrell, 1976; see also Osborne, chapter 9), I questioned whether Dale's principle was as universal as generally thought in a commentary in *Neuroscience* entitled "Do some nerve cells release more than one transmitter?" (Burnstock, 1976). This suggestion for the existence of co-transmitters was received with some resistance at the time, so it is gratifying to see the high level of current interest in the topic.

The first consideration of the coexistence of transmitters concerned the hypothesis that acetylcholine (ACh) and noradrenaline (NA) coexisted in sympathetic neurones (Burn and Rand, 1965). This possibility has been supported in recent years for developing sympathetic neurones both *in vitro* (see Patterson, 1978; Bunge *et al.*, 1978; Le Douarin, 1981; Potter *et al.*, 1981), and *in vivo* (Hendry *et al.*, 1981; Black *et al.*, 1981). Most sympathetic neurones are "programmed" to become either adrenergic or cholinergic soon after birth, but the question that remains is whether some sympathetic neurones of some species retain the ability to store and release both ACh and NA in the adult (see Burnstock, 1978*a*). The current focus of interest regarding coexistence of transmitters concerns established transmitters such as ACh, NA or 5-hydroxytryptamine (5-HT) with a variety of biologically active polypeptides that have been localised by immunocytochemistry (see Chan-Palay *et al.*, 1978; Hökfelt *et al.*, 1980; and Gilbert *et al.*, Chan-Palay; Hökfelt *et al.* and Priestley and Cuello, chapter 7).

The hypothesis that a purine nucleotide, probably ATP, is the transmitter in non-adrenergic, non-cholinergic autonomic nerves supplying the smooth muscle of the gastrointestinal tract and bladder was first proposed in 1972 (Burnstock, 1972). Since that time considerable evidence has accumulated in favour of this hypothesis (see Burnstock, 1979; 1981*a*), although it is not yet universally accepted.

In this article, the focus of attention will be on the evidence that ATP is stored and released together with the established transmitters in some adrenergic and cholinergic nerves. The various roles of ATP released from adrenergic and cholinergic nerves will also be discussed, including its actions: as a cotransmitter on postjunctional $P_2$-purinoceptors; as a prejunctional modulator of the release of the principal transmitter by way of $P_1$-purinoceptors on the nerve terminals; and as a modulator of the extent and/or duration of the postjunctional actions of the principal transmitter.

## ACETYLCHOLINE AND ATP

### Storage of ATP and its release from cholinergic nerves

*Electric organ of fish*
Cholinergic vesicles isolated from the electric organ of various elasmobranch fish contain ATP in addition to the principal transmitter ACh: *Torpedo marmorata* (Dowdall *et al.*, 1974; Israel *et al.*, 1979; Zimmerman and Bokor, 1979; Zimmerman *et al.*, 1979); *Narcine brasiliensis* (Boyne, 1976); and *Electrophorus electricus* (Zimmerman and Denston, 1976). The ACh:ATP molar ratio in all three species is 4–10:1. The major nucleotide in these vesicles is ATP (83 per cent of the total), with ADP (15 per cent) and traces of AMP also being present (Dowdall *et al.*, 1974; Zimmerman, 1978; (see also Zimmerman, chapter 12).

Studies of the turnover of adenine nucleotides in cholinergic synaptic vesicles have shown that ATP and ACh are depleted to the same extent (about 50 per cent) during nerve stimulation, that adenosine is an effective precursor of vesicular adenine nucleotides and that the new population of vesicles that appear following nerve stimulation has a high turnover rate for both ATP and ACh (Zimmerman and Denston, 1977; Zimmerman, 1978; 1979). Furthermore, a saturable uptake system for adenosine into nerve terminals isolated from the *Torpedo* electric organ with a $K_m$ value of 1 $\mu$M has been reported, which is comparable with that of the high affinity choline uptake system (Dowdall, 1978). Evidence for axonal flow of ATP, as for ACh, in organelles other than mitochondria has also been reported (Davies, 1978).

Israel and his co-workers have presented evidence to suggest that ATP is also released from postsynaptic sites as a result of the depolarisation produced by ACh (Meunier *et al.*, 1975; Israel *et al.*, 1976). They showed that depolarisation of postsynaptic membranes by $K^+$ also led to ATP release, but some experiments by this group have shown that ATP can also be released by $K^+$ depolarisation from nerve terminals isolated from electric tissue (Meunier, 1978).

### Rat diaphragm

Considerable quantities of ATP (up to 0.1 mM) have been reported to be released from the endings of phrenic nerves in the rat diaphragm during stimulation (Silinsky and Hubbard, 1973; Silinsky, 1975). This compares well with the levels of ATP released on stimulation of some regions of the cortex (Pull and McIlwain, 1972; Heller and McIlwain, 1973; Wu and Phillis, 1978).

### Stomach and bladder

Stimulation of the cholinergic nerves in the cervical sympathetic nerve trunk before it joined the vago-sympathetic trunk to the stomach of the toad failed to lead to increase in release of purine compounds into the venous effluent (Burnstock *et al.*, 1970). However, botulinum neurotoxin virtually abolished the atropine-resistant response of the guinea-pig bladder to field stimulation, suggesting that ATP, which is a strong contender for the non-cholinergic transmitter to this preparation (Burnstock *et al.*, 1978), is being released as a co-transmitter with ACh (MacKenzie *et al.*, 1982). Hoyes *et al.* (1975) presented ultrastructural evidence which supports this view.

### Brain

Release of [$^3$H] -adenine derivatives has been shown to occur in the cholinergic septal system, which were considered as possible cotransmitters with ACh (Rose and Schubert, 1977).

## Actions of purine nucleotides and nucleosides on cholinergic transmission

### Presynaptic actions

ATP and adenosine have been shown to act on presynaptic purinergic receptors leading to modulation of the release of ACh from cholinergic motor nerves in skeletal muscle of rat diaphragm (Ginsborg and Hirst, 1971; 1972; Ribeiro and Walker, 1975; Ribeiro and Dominguez, 1978), frog sartorius (Ribeiro and Walker, 1975; Ribeiro and Dominguez, 1978; Brănisteanu *et al.*, 1979), fish electric organ (Israel *et al.*, 1977), brain (Kluge *et al.*, 1977) and intestine (Kosterlitz and Lees, 1972; Takagi and Takayanagi, 1972; Mori *et al.*, 1973; Gintzler and Musacchio, 1975; Sawynok and Jhamandas, 1976; Vizi and Knoll, 1976; Leighton and Parmeter, 1977; Starke, 1977; Gustafsson *et al.*, 1978; Hayashi *et al.*, 1978; Moritoki *et al.*, 1978; Okwuasaba and Cook, 1980). These responses are blocked by methylxanthines (Ginsborg and Hirst, 1971; Sawynok and Jhamandas, 1976; Vizi and Knoll, 1976; Ribeiro and Dominguez, 1978), indicating that they are mediated by $P_1$-purinoceptors (Burnstock, 1978*b*). ATP does not act by way of $P_2$-purinoceptors, but is rapidly broken down to AMP and adenosine which occupy the $P_1$-purinoceptors on the cholinergic nerve terminals (Moody and Burnstock, 1982). It has been suggested that occupation of the presynaptic $P_1$-purinoceptors leads to decrease in the entry of $Ca^{2+}$, with consequent reduction in release of transmitter (Ribeiro, 1979; Dowdle and Maske, 1980; Israel *et al.*, 1980; Hayashi *et al.*, 1981).

Evidence that the actions of adenosine (and ATP) are presynaptic at the motor endplates in both rat diaphragm and frog sartorius is that, while the frequency of miniature endplate potentials (m.e.p.p.s.), representing spontaneous release of ACh, is reduced and the amplitude of the nerve-evoked endplate potentials is reduced, the mean amplitude of the mepps is not reduced (Ginsborg and Hirst, 1972; Ribeiro and Walker, 1975). Neither adenosine nor ATP modifies the action potential in frog sciatic nerve (Okamoto *et al.*, 1964; Ribeiro and Dominguez, 1978). Furthermore, ATP in concentrations sufficient to produce modulatory effects (0.01–0.2 mM), which are comparable to the amounts collected during nerve stimulation (see above), had no postsynaptic action (Ribeiro, 1977), although at high concentrations, ATP potentiated the post-junctional action of ACh (see below). Reduction of evoked excitatory post-synaptic potentials (e.p.s.p.s.) in brain to half control values by way of pre-synaptic receptors to low concentrations of adenosine (or ATP) have also been reported (Kuroda *et al.*, 1976; Scholfield, 1978). Silinsky (1980) has suggested that two types of adenosine receptor may be present at cholinergic endings, one mediating depression and the other enhancing of ACh release.

*Postsynaptic actions*

Apart from the direct action of ATP on $P_2$-purinoceptors on postjunctional cells (see Burnstock, 1981*a*; Stone, 1981), ATP can act as a postjunctional modulator of the action of ACh.

Increase of ACh receptor sensitivity by ATP has also been demonstrated (Buchthal and Kahlson, 1944; Saji *et al.*, 1975; Ewald, 1976; Ribeiro, 1977; Akasu *et al.*, 1981; see Stone, 1981). The amplitude of the current induced by ionophoretic application of ACh to the frog skeletal muscle endplate is increased in the presence of ATP, and kinetic analysis has suggested that ATP increases ACh sensitivity by acting on the allosteric site of the receptor-ionic channel complex without changing the affinity of ACh for its recognition site.

## NORADRENALINE AND ATP

It has been known for a number of years that ATP is stored and released together with catecholamines from adrenal chromaffin cells (Douglas and Poisner, 1966; Douglas, 1968; Stevens *et al.*, 1972). It has also been suggested that medullary granule-associated nucleotides may act locally as "co-agonists" with biogenic amines and may additionally provide a circulatory pool of purines for use by heart and lungs (Van Dyke *et al.*, 1977). However, evidence that ATP is released together with NA from adrenergic nerves has not been available until more recently (see Stjärne and Lishajko, 1966; Geffen and Livett, 1971; and below).

### Storage of ATP and its release from adrenergic nerves

#### *Guinea-pig taenia coli*
The first indication that ATP might be released from adrenergic nerves was the demonstration that stimulation of periarterial adrenergic nerves lead to release of tritium from taenia coli preincubated in [$^3$H]-adenosine (which is taken up and converted to [$^3$H]-ATP); both the release of tritium and NA were blocked by guanethidine (Su *et al.*, 1971).

#### *Cat nictitating membrane*
Langer and Pinto (1976) suggested that the substantial residual non-adrenergic, non-cholinergic response of the cat nictitating membrane following depletion of NA by reserpine, may be due to release of the ATP remaining in adrenergic nerves.

#### *Vas deferens*
Westfall and his colleagues have presented evidence that ATP is stored and released as a co-transmitter together with NA from adrenergic nerves supplying the guinea-pig vas deferens (Westfall *et al.*, 1978; Fedan *et al.*, 1981). The initial phasic component of the excitatory response to sympathetic nerve stimulation is preferentially antagonised by arylazido aminopropionyl ATP, which is claimed to be a specific ATP antagonist, while the secondary more tonic component of the response is antagonised by prazosin and reserpine (Fedan *et al.*, 1981).

#### *Some blood vessels*
Su (1975; 1978*a*) used tritium-labelled adenosine and NA to show that ATP is released together with NA from sympathetic nerves supplying the rabbit aorta and portal vein. Coexistence of NA and ATP has also been demonstrated in rabbit ear artery (Head *et al.*, 1977) and in dog basilar artery (Muramatsu *et al.*, 1981).

ATP as well as NA release from guinea-pig portal vein has been shown to be abolished following sympathectomy (Burnstock *et al.*, 1979). Fluorescence in nerves of the rat portal vein following incubation in quinacrine, which binds to ATP (Irvin and Irvin, 1954; Olson *et al.*, 1976), is also abolished by sympathectomy (Crowe, personal communication).

### Adipose tissue and heart

Evidence has been presented that in adipose tissue and heart, stimulation of sympathetic nerves leads to some postjunctional release of adenosine (Fredholm *et al.*, 1979; Hedqvist and Fredholm, 1979).

## Actions of purine nucleotides and nucleosides on adrenergic transmission

### Prejunctional actions

Adenine nucleosides and nucleotides have been shown to inhibit NA release from adrenergic nerves supplying a variety of visceral and vascular tissues including vas deferens, spleen, kidney, heart, subcutaneous adipose tissue and saphenous, tibial, portal, pulmonary and mesenteric vessels (Fredholm, 1974; Kazic and Milosavjevic, 1976; Clanachan *et al.*, 1977; Enero and Saidman, 1977; Verhaeghe *et al.*, 1977; Paton *et al.*, 1978; Ribeiro, 1978; Su, 1978*b*; Hedqvist and Fredholm, 1979; Lokhandwala, 1979; Moylan and Westfall, 1979; Mueller *et al.*, 1979; Vizi, 1979; Nedergaard *et al.*, 1980; Hom and Lokhandwala, 1981; Paton, 1981). Adenosine has also been shown to modulate depolarisation-induced release of NA from slices of rat brain neocortex (Harms *et al.*, 1978). As for cholinergic terminals, the presynaptic receptor that mediates these actions is the $P_1$-purinoceptor, since the inhibitory actions of both ATP and adenosine are blocked by methylxanthines and because slowly degradable analogues of ATP are ineffective (De Mey *et al.*, 1979). It has been suggested that occupation of $P_1$-purinoceptors leads to decrease in $Ca^{2+}$ influx and subsequent reduction in NA release (Wakade and Wakade, 1978). Diminished purinergic modulation of vascular adrenergic neurotransmission has been claimed in spontaneously hypertensive rats (Kamikawa *et al.*, 1980).

### Postjunctional actions

ATP can act directly on $P_2$-purinoceptors in the membranes of smooth muscles supplied by sympathetic nerves (see Burnstock, 1981*b*). It may also have modulatory actions on the postjunctional actions of NA. AMP and adenosine were shown to enhance contractile responses to NA in the guinea-pig vas deferens (Hedqvist and Fredholm, 1976), and it has been suggested that there is a mutual interaction between purinergic and alpha-adrenoreceptor mechanisms (Holck and Marks, 1978). Guanine nucleotides are known to enhance beta-adrenoceptor activation (Mukherjee and Lefkowitz, 1976). Conversely, NA potentiates the responses to ATP in the vas deferens and seminal vesicle (Nakanishi and Takeda, 1973; Holck and Marks, 1978).

## SUMMARY

There is growing evidence that ATP is stored and released from autonomic nerves together with ACh or NA, although there seems to be considerable variation in the proportions of the released ATP and classical transmitters, perhaps as a consequence of variations in physiological needs during evolution. After its release, ATP may act on postjunctional effector cells as a cotransmitter (for example, together with NA in the vas deferens or together with ACh in the urinary bladder), or it is rapidly broken down to AMP and adenosine where it has potent actions on $P_1$-purinoceptors on nerve terminals leading to inhibition of release of the principal transmitter (figure 6.1). There is also evidence that it has

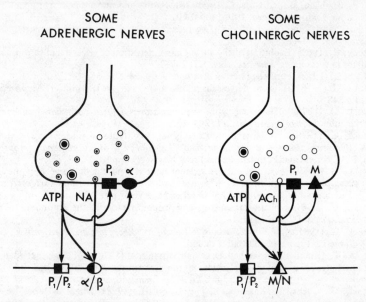

Figure 6.1 Schematic representation of coexistence of ATP and classical transmitters in some adrenergic and cholinergic nerves and their various actions after release, including roles: (1) as transmitters on postjunctional receptors ($P_1$-/$P_2$-purinoceptors, $\alpha$/$\beta$-adrenoceptors and muscarinic (M) and nicotinic (N) cholinergic receptors; (2) as modulators of transmission by both prejunctional inhibition of transmitter release and postjunctional modulation of transmitter action.

modulatory actions on the postjunctional effects of ACh and NA. In view of the evidence that peptides are stored together with ATP in endocrine cells (Fujita and Kobayashi, 1977), the possibility that ATP may also be a cotransmitter in peptidergic nerves should also be explored.

## REFERENCES

Akasu, T., Hirai, K. and Koketsu, K. (1981). Increase of acetylcholine-receptor sensitivity by adenosine triphosphate: a novel action of ATP on ACh-sensitivity. *Br. J. Pharmac.*, **74**, 505–507

Black, I. B., Bohn, M. C., Jonakait, G. M. and Kessler, J. A. (1981). Transmitter phenotypic expression in the embryo. In *Development of the Autonomic Nervous System*, Ciba Foundation Symposium 83, (ed. K. Elliot and G. Lawrenson), Pitman Medical, London, pp. 177–186

Boyne, A. F. (1976). Isolation of synaptic vesicles from *Narcine brasiliensis* electric organ – some influences on release of vesicular acetylcholine and ATP. *Brain Res.*, 114, 481–491

Brănisteanu, D. D., Hăulica, I. D., Proca, B. and Nhue, B. G. (1979). Adenosine effects upon transmitter release parameters in the $Mg^{2+}$-paralyzed neuromuscular junctions of frog. *Naunyn Schmeid. Arch. Pharmac.*, 308, 273–279

Brownstein, M. J., Saavedra, J. M., Axelrod, J., Zeman, G. H. and Carpenter, D. O. (1974). Coexistence of several putative neurotransmitters in single identified neurones of *Aplysia. Proc. natn. Acad. Sci. U.S.A.*, 71, 4662–4665

Buchthal, F. and Kahlson, G. (1944). The motor effect of adenosine triphosphate and allied phosphorus compounds on smooth mammalian muscle. *Acta Physiol. Scand.*, 8, 325–334

Bunge, R., Johnson, M. and Ross, C. D. (1978). Nature and nurture in development of the autonomic neurone. *Science*, 199, 1409–1416

Burn, J. H. and Rand, M. J. (1965). Acetylcholine in adrenergic transmission. *A. Rev. Pharmac.*, 5, 163–182

Burnstock, G. (1969). Evolution of the autonomic innervation of visceral and cardiovascular systems in vertebrates. *Pharmac. Rev.*, 21, 247–324

Burnstock, G. (1972). Purinergic nerves. *Pharmac. Rev.*, 24, 509–581

Burnstock, G. (1976). Do some nerve cells release more than one transmitter? *Neuroscience*, 1, 239–248

Burnstock, G. (1978a). Do some sympathetic neurones release both noradrenaline and acetylcholine? *Progr. Neurobiol.*, 11, 205–222

Burnstock, G. (1978b). A basis for distinguishing two types of purinergic receptor. In *Cell Membrane Receptors for Drugs and Hormones: A Multidisciplinary Approach*, (ed. R. W. Straub and L. Bolis), Raven Press, New York, pp. 107–118

Burnstock, G. (1979). Past and current evidence for the purinergic nerve hypothesis. In *Physiological and Regulatory Functions of Adenosine and Adenine Nucleotides*, (ed. H. P. Baer and G. I. Drummond), Raven Press, New York, pp. 3–32

Burnstock, G. (1981a). Neurotransmitters and trophic factors in the autonomic nervous system. *J. Physiol. Lond.*, 313, 1–35

Burnstock, G. (1981b). (Editor). *Purinergic Receptors: Receptors and Recognition*, Series B, Volume 12, Chapman and Hall, London

Burnstock, G., Campbell, G., Satchell, D. G. and Smythe, A. (1970). Evidence that adenosine triphosphate or a related nucleotide is the transmitter substance released by non-adrenergic inhibitory nerves in the gut. *Br. J. Pharmac.*, 40, 668–688

Burnstock, G., Cocks, T., Kasakov, L. and Wong, H. (1978). Direct evidence for ATP release from non-adrenergic, non-cholinergic ("purinergic") nerves in the guinea-pig taenia coli and bladder. *Eur. J. Pharmac.*, 49, 145–149

Burnstock, G., Crowe, R. and Wong, H. K. (1979). Comparative pharmacological and histochemical evidence for purinergic inhibitory innervation of the portal vein of the rabbit, but not guinea-pig. *Br. J. Pharmac.*, 65, 377–388

Chan-Palay, V., Jonsson, G. and Palay, S. L. (1978). Serotonin and Substance P co-exist in neurones of the rat's central nervous system. *Proc. natn. Acad. Sci. U.S.A.*, 75, 1582–1586

Clanachan, A. S., Johns, A. and Paton, D. M. (1977). Presynaptic inhibitory actions of adenine nucleotides and adenosine on neurotransmission in rat vas deferens. *Neuroscience*, 2, 597–602

Cottrell, G. A. (1976). Does the giant cerebral neurone of *Helix* release two transmitters: ACh and serotonin? *J. Physiol. Lond.*, 259, 44P–45P

Davies, L. P. (1978). ATP in cholinergic nerves – evidence for axonal-transport of a stable pool. *Expl. Brain Res.*, 33, 149–157

De Mey, J., Burnstock, G. and Vanhoutte, P. M. (1979). Modulation of the evoked release of noradrenaline in canine saphenous vein *via* presynaptic receptors for adenosine but not ATP. *Eur. J. Pharmac.*, 55, 401–405

Douglas, W. W. (1968). Stimulus-secretion coupling: the concept and clues from chromaffin and other cells. *Br. J. Pharmac.*, **34**, 451–474

Douglas, W. W. and Poisner, A. M. (1966). On the relation between ATP splitting and secretion in the adrenal chromaffin cell: extrusion of ATP (unhydrolised) during release of catecholamines. *J. Physiol. Lond.*, **183**, 249–256

Dowdall, M. J. (1978). Adenine nucleotides in cholinergic transmission: presynaptic aspects. *J. Physiol. Paris*, **74**, 497–501

Dowdall, M. J., Boyne, A. F. and Whittaker, V. P. (1974). Adenosine triphosphate: a constituent of cholinergic synaptic vesicles. *Biochem. J.*, **140**, 1–12

Dowdle, E. B. and Maske, R. (1980). The effects of calcium concentration on the inhibition of cholinergic neurotransmission in the myenteric plexus of guinea-pig ileum by adenine nucleotides. *Br. J. Pharmac.*, **71**, 245–252

Eccles, J. (1976). From electrical to chemical transmission in the central nervous system. *Notes and Records R. Soc. Lond.*, **30**, 219–230

Enero, M. A. and Saidman, B. O. (1977). Possible feed-back inhibition of noradrenaline release by purine compounds. *Naunyn Schmiedeberg's Arch. Pharmac.*, **297**, 39–46

Ewald, D. A. (1976). Potentiation of postjunctional cholinergic sensitivity of rat diaphragm muscle by high-energy phosphate adenine nucleotides. *J. Membrane Biol.*, **29**, 47–65

Fedan, J. S., Hogaboom, G. K., O'Donnell, J. P., Colby, J. and Westfall, D. P. (1981). Contribution by purines to the neurogenic response of the vas deferens of the guinea-pig. *Eur. J. Pharmac.*, **69**, 41–53

Fredholm, B. B. (1974). Vascular and metabolic effects of theophylline, dibutyryl cyclic AMP and dibutyryl cyclic GMP in canine subcutaneous adipose tissue *in situ*. *Acta Physiol. Scand.*, **90**, 226–236

Fredholm, B. B., Hedqvist, P. and Vernet, L. (1979). Release of adenosine from the rabbit heart by sympathetic-nerve stimulation. *Acta Physiol. Scand.*, **106**, 381–382

Fujita, T. and Kobayashi, S. (1977). Structure and function of gut endocrine cells. *Int. Rev. Cytol.*, suppl., **6**, 187–233

Geffen, L. B. and Livett, B. G. (1971). Synaptic vesicles in sympathetic neurons. *Physiol. Rev.*, **51**, 98–157

Ginsborg, B. L. and Hirst, G. D. S. (1971). Theophylline and adenosine at the neuromuscular junction. *Br. J. Pharmac.*, **43**, 432–433

Ginsborg, B. L. and Hirst, G. D. S. (1972). The effect of adenosine on the release of the transmitter from the phrenic nerve of the rat. *J. Physiol. Lond.*, **224**, 629–645

Gintzler, A. R. and Musacchio, J. M. (1975). Interactions of morphine, adenosine, adenosine-triphosphate and phosphodiesterase inhibitors on field-stimulated guinea-pig ileum. *J. Pharmac. exp. Ther.*, **194**, 575–582

Gustafsson, L., Hedqvist, P., Fredholm, B. B. and Lundgren, G. (1978). Inhibition of acetylcholine release in guinea pig ileum by adenosine. *Acta Physiol. Scand.*, **104**, 469–478

Harms, H. H., Wardeh, G. and Mulder, A. H. (1978). Adenosine modulates depolarization-induced release of $^3$H-noradrenaline from slices of rat-brain neocortex. *Eur. J. Pharmac.*, **49**, 305–308

Hayashi, E., Mori, M., Yamada, S., Kunitomo, M. (1978). Effects of purine compounds on cholinergic nerves – specificity of adenosine and related compounds on acetylcholine-release in electrically stimulated guinea-pig ileum. *Eur. J. Pharmac.*, **48**, 297–307

Hayashi, E., Yamada, S. and Shinozuka, K. (1981). The influence of extracellular $Ca^{2+}$ concentration on the inhibitory effect of adenosine in guinea-pig ileal longitudinal muscles. *Jap. J. Pharmac.*, **31**, 141–143

Head, R. J., Stitzel, R. E., Delaland, I. S. and Johnson, S. M. (1977). Effect of chronic denervation of activities of monoamine-oxidase and catechol-o-methyl transferase and on contents of noradrenaline and adenosine-triphosphate in rabbit ear artery. *Blood Vessels*, **14**, 229–239

Hedqvist, P. and Fredholm, B. B. (1976). Effects of adenosine on adrenergic neurotransmission; prejunctional inhibition and postjunctional enhancement. *Naunyn-Schmiedeberg's Arch. Pharmac.*, **293**, 217–223

Hedqvist, P. and Fredholm, B. B. (1979). Inhibitory effect of adenosine on adrenergic neuroeffector transmission in the rabbit heart. *Acta Physiol. Scand.*, **105**, 120–122

Heller, I. H. and McIlwain, H. (1973). Release of $^{14}$C-adenine derivatives from isolated subsystems of the guinea-pig brain: actions of electrical stimulation and of papaverine. *Brain Res.*, 53, 105–116

Hendry, I. A., Hill, C. E. and Bonyhady, R. E. (1981). Interactions between developing autonomic neurons and their target tissues. In *Development of the Autonomic Nervous System*, Ciba Foundation Symposium 83, (ed. K. Elliot and G. Lawrenson), Pitman Medical, London, pp. 194–206

Hökfelt, T., Lundberg, J. M., Schultzberg, M., Johansson, O., Skirboll, L., Änggård, A., Fredholm, B., Hamberger, B., Pernow, B., Rehfeld, J. and Goldstein, M. (1980). Cellular localization of peptides in neural structures. *Proc. R. Soc. Lond.*, B210, 63–77

Holck, M. I. and Marks, B. H. (1978). Purine nucleoside and nucleotide interactions on normal subsensitive *alpha* adrenoreceptor responsiveness in guinea-pig vas deferens. *J. Pharmac. exp. Ther.*, 205, 104–117

Hom, G. J. and Lokhandwala, M. F. (1981). Effect of dipyridamole on sympathetic nerve function: role of adenosine and presynaptic purinergic receptors. *J. cardiovasc. Pharmac.*, 3, 391–401

Hoyes, A. D., Barber, P. and Martin, B. G. H. (1975). Comparative ultrastructure of ureteric innervation. *Cell Tissue Res.*, 160, 515–524

Irvin, J. L. and Irvin, E. M. (1954). The interaction of quinacrine with adenine nucleotides. *J. biol. Chem.*, 210, 45–56

Israel, M., Lesbats, B., Meunier, F. M. and Stinnakre, J. (1976). Postsynaptic release of adenosine triphosphate induced by single impulse transmitter action. *Proc. R. Soc. Lond.*, B193, 461–468

Israel, M., Lesbats, R., Manaranche, J., Marsal, P., Mastour-Frachan, P. and Meunier, F. M. (1977). Related changes in amounts of ACh and ATP in resting and active *Torpedo* nerve electroplaque synapses. *J. Neurochem.*, 28, 1259–1267

Israel, M., Dunant, Y., Lesbats, B., Manaranche, R., Marsal, J. and Meunier, F. (1979). Rapid acetylcholine and adenosine triphosphate oscillations triggered by stimulation of the *Torpedo* electric organ. *J. exp. Biol.*, 81, 63–73

Israel, M., Lesbats, B., Manarance, R., Meunier, F. M. and Frachon, P. (1980). Retrograde inhibition of transmitter release by ATP. *J. Neurochem.*, 34, 923–932

Kamikawa, Y., Cline, W. H. and Su, C. (1980). Diminished purinergic modulation of the vascular adrenergic neurotransmission in spontaneously hypertensive rats. *Eur. J. Pharmac.*, 66, 347–354

Kazic, T. and Milosavljevic, D. (1976). Influence of adenosine, cAMP and db-cAMP on responses of the isolated terminal guinea-pig ileum to electrical stimulation. *Arch. int. Pharmacodyn. Ther.*, 223, 187–195

Kluge, H., Fischer, H-D., Zahlten, W., Hartmann, W. and Wieczorek, V. (1977). Brain acetylcholine, adenine nucleotides and their degradation products after intraperitoneal and intracerebral adenosine administration. *Acta biol. Med. Germ.*, 36, 1299–1306

Kosterlitz, H. W. and Lees, G. M. (1972). Interrelationships between adrenergic and cholinergic mechanisms. In *Catecholamines, Handbook of Experimental Pharmacology*, 33, (ed. H. Blaschlco and E. Muscholl), Springer, Berlin, pp. 762–812

Kuroda, Y., Saito, M. and Kobayashi, K. (1976). Concomitant changes in cyclic AMP level and postsynaptic potentials of olfactory cortex slices induced by adenosine derivatives. *Brain Res.*, 109, 196–201

Langer, S. Z. and Pinto, J. E. B. (1976). Possible involvement of a transmitter different from norepinephrine in residual responses to nerve stimulation of cat nictitating membrane after pretreatment with reserpine. *J. Pharmac. exp. Ther.*, 196, 697–713

Le Douarin, N. (1981). Plasticity in the development of the peripheral nervous system. In *Development of the Autonomic Nervous System*, Ciba Foundation Symposium 83, (ed. K. Elliot and G. Lawrenson), Pitman Medical, London, pp. 19–46

Leighton, H. J. and Parmeter, L. L. (1977). Presynaptic inhibition of acetylcholine (ACh) and release by adenosine and adenosine analogs. *Fedn Proc.*, 36, 976

Lokhandwala, M. F. (1979). Inhibition of cardiac sympathetic neurotransmission by adenosine. *Eur. J. Pharmac.*, 60, 353–357

MacKenzie, I., Burnstock, G. and Dolly, J. O. (1981). The effects of purified botulinum neurotoxin type A on cholinergic, adrenergic and non-adrenergic, atropine-resistant autonomic neuromuscular transmission. *Neuroscience*, in press

Meunier, F. M. (1978). Effet de la dépolarisation sur la liberation d'ATP pre- et postsynaptique. Nucleotides and Neurotransmission Conf. Neurobiologie de Gif, p.15

Meunier, F. M., Israel, M. and Lesbats, B. (1975). Release of ATP from stimulated nerve electroplaque junctions. *Nature London*, 257, 407–408

Moody, C. and Burnstock, G. (1982). Evidence for the presence of $P_1$-purinoceptors on cholinergic nerve terminals in the guinea-pig ileum. *Eur. J. Pharmac.*, 77, 1–9

Mori, M. I., Yamada, S., Takamura, S. and Hayashi, E. (1973). Effect of purine nucleotides on acetylcholine output from cholinergic nerves in guinea-pig ileum. *Jap. J. Pharmac.*, 23, suppl., 124, 137

Moritoki, H., Kanbe, T., Maruoka, M., Ohara, M. and Ishida, Y. (1978). Potentiation by dipyridamole of inhibition of guinea-pig ileum twitch response caused by adenine-derivatives. *J. Pharmac. exp. Ther.*, 204, 343–350

Moylan, R. D. and Westfall, T. C. (1979). Effect of adenosine on adrenergic neurotransmission in the super-fused rat portal-vein. *Blood Vessels*, 16, 302–310

Mueller, A. L., Mosimann, W. F. and Weiner, N. (1979). Effects of adenosine on neurally mediated norepinephrine release from the cat spleen. *Eur. J. Pharmac.*, 53, 329–333

Mukherjee, C. and Lefkowitz, R. J. (1976). Desensitization of beta-adrenergic receptors by beta-adrenergic agonists in a cell-free system: resensitization by guanosine 5'-(beta, gamma-imino) triphosphate and other purine nucleotides. *Proc. natn. Acad. Sci. U.S.A.*, 73, 1494–1498

Muramatsu, I., Fujiwara, M., Miura, A. and Sakakibara, Y. (1981). Possible involvement of adenine nucleotides in sympathetic neuroeffector mechanisms of dog basilar artery. *J. Pharmac. exp. Ther.*, 216, 401–408

Nakanishi, H. and Takeda, H. (1973). The possible role of adenosine triphosphate in chemical transmission between the hypogastric nerve terminal and seminal vesicle in the guinea-pig. *Jap. J. Pharmac.*, 23, 479–490

Nedergaard, O. A., Husted, S. and Schrold, J. (1980). Presynaptic regulation of noradrenaline release in blood vessels: effects of cholinergic drugs, adenosine and adenine nucleotides. In *Vascular Neuroeffector Mechanisms*, (ed. J. A. Bevan), Raven Press, New York, pp. 139–146

Okamoto, M., Askari, A. and Kuperman, A. S. (1964). The stabilizing actions of adenosine triphosphate and related nucleotides on calcium-deficient nerve. *J. Pharmac. exp. Ther.*, 144, 229–235

Okwuasaba, F. K. and Cook, M. A. (1980). The effect of theophylline and other methylxanthines on presynaptic inhibition of the longitudinal smooth muscle of the guinea pig ileum induced by purine nucleotides. *J. Pharmac. exp. Ther.*, 215, 704–709

Olson, L., Alund, M. and Norberg, K-A. (1976). Fluorescence microscopical demonstration of a population of gastrointestinal nerve fibres with a selective affinity for quinacrine. *Cell Tissue Res.*, 171, 407–423

Paton, D. M. (1981). Presynaptic neuromodulation mediated by purinergic receptors. In *Purinergic Receptors, Receptors and Recognition*, Series B, volume 12, (ed. G. Burnstock), Chapman and Hall, London, pp. 199–219

Paton, D. M., Bar, H. P., Clanachan, A. S. and Lauzon, P. A. (1978). Structure activity relations for inhibition of neurotransmission in rat vas deferens by adenosine. *Neuroscience*, 3, 65–70

Patterson, P. H. (1978). Environmental determination of autonomic neutrotransmitter functions. *A. Rev. Neurosci.*, 1, 1–17

Potter, D. D., Landis, S. C. and Furshpan, E. J. (1981). Adrenergic-cholinergic dual function in cultured sympathetic neurons of the rat. In *Development of the Autonomic Nervous System*, Ciba Foundation Symposium 83, (ed. K. Elliot and G. Lawrenson), Pitman Medical, London, pp. 123–138

Pull, I. and McIlwain, H. (1972). Adenine derivatives as neurohumoral agents in the brain. The quantities liberated on excitation of superfused cerebral tissues. *Biochem. J.*, 130, 975–981

Ribeiro, J. A. (1977). Potentiation of postjunctional cholinergic sensitivity of rat diaphragm muscle by high-energy-phosphate adenine nucleotides. *J. Membrane Biol.*, **33**, 401–402

Ribeiro, J. A. (1978). ATP-related nucleotides and adenosine on neurotransmission. *Life Sci.*, **22**, 1373–1380

Ribeiro, J. A. (1979). Purinergic modulation of transmitter release. *J. theor. Biol.*, **80**, 259–270

Ribeiro, J. A. and Dominguez, M. L. (1978). Mechanisms of depression of neuromuscular transmission by ATP and adenosine. *J. Physiol. Paris*, **74**, 491–496

Ribeiro, J. A. and Walker, J. (1975). The effects of adenosine triphosphate and adenosine diphosphate on transmission at the rat and frog neuromuscular junctions. *Br. J. Pharmac.*, **54**, 213–218

Rose, G. and Schubert, P. (1977). Release and transfer of $^3$H-adenosine derivatives in cholinergic septal system. *Brain Res.*, **121**, 353–357

Saji, Y., Escalona de Motta, G. and del Castillo, J. (1975). Depolarization and potentiation of responses to acetylcholine elicited by ATP on frog muscle. *Life Sci.*, **16**, 945–954

Sawynok, J. and Jhamandas, K. H. (1976). Inhibition of acetylcholine release from cholinergic nerves by adenosine, adenine-nucleotides and morphine-antagonism by theophylline. *J. Pharmac. exp. Ther.*, **197**, 379–390

Scholfield, C. N. (1978). Depression of evoked-potentials in brain-slices by adenosine compounds. *Br. J. Pharmac.*, **63**, 239–244

Silinsky, E. M. (1975). On the association between transmitter secretion and the release of adenine nucleotides from mammalian motor nerve terminals. *J. Physiol. Lond.*, **247**, 145–162

Silinsky, E. M. (1980). Evidence for specific adenosine receptors at cholinergic nerve endings. *Br. J. Pharmac.*, **71**, 191–194

Silinsky, E. M. and Hubbard, J. I. (1973). Release of ATP from rat motor nerve terminals. *Nature London*, **243**, 404–405

Starke, K. (1977). Regulation of noradrenaline release by presynaptic receptor systems. *Rev. Physiol. Biochem. Pharmac.*, **77**, 1–124

Stevens, P., Robinson, R. L., Van Dyke, K. and Stitzel, R. (1972). Studies of the synthesis and release of adenosine triphosphate-8-$^3$H in the isolated perfused cat adrenal gland. *J. Pharmac. exp. Ther.*, **181**, 463–471

Stjärne, L. and Lishajko, F. (1966). Comparison of spontaneous loss of catecholamines and ATP *in vitro* from isolated bovine adrenomedullary, vesicular gland, vas deferens and splenic nerve granules. *J. Neurochem.*, **13**, 1213–1216

Stone, T. W. (1981). Physiological roles for adenosine and adenosine 5′-triphosphate in the nervous system. *Neuroscience*, **6**, 523–555

Su, C. (1975). Neurogenic release of purine compounds in blood-vessels. *J. Pharmac. exp. Ther.*, **195**, 159–166

Su, C. (1978a). Modes of vasoconstrictor and vasodilator neurotransmission. *Blood Vessels*, **15**, 183–189

Su, C. (1978b). Purinergic inhibition of adrenergic transmission in rabbit blood vessels. *J. Pharmac. exp. Ther.*, **204**, 351–361

Su, C., Bevan, J. A. and Burnstock, G. (1971). $^3$H-Adenosine triphosphate: release during stimulation of enteric nerves. *Science*, **173**, 337–339

Takagi, K. and Takayanagi, I. (1972). Effect of N$^6$, 2′-O-dibutyryl 3′5′-cyclic adenosine monophosphate, 3′,5′-cyclic adenosine monophosphate and adenosine triphosphate on acetylcholine output from cholinergic nerves in guinea pig ileum. *Jap. J. Pharmac.*, **22**, 33–36

Van Dyke, K., Robinson, R., Urquilla, P., Smith, D., Taylor, M., Trush, M. and Wilson, M. (1977). Analysis of nucleotides and catecholamines in bovine medullary granules by anion-exchange high pressure liquid chromatography and fluorescence evidence that most of catecholamines in chromaffin granules are stored without associated ATP. *Pharmacology*, **15**, 377–391

Verhaeghe, R. H., Vanhoutte, P. M. and Shepherd, J. T. (1977). Inhibition of sympathetic neurotransmission in canine blood vessels by adenosine and adenine nucleotides. *Circulat. Res.*, **40**, 208–215

Vizi, E. S. (1979). Presynaptic modulation of neurochemical transmission. *Progr. Neurobiol.*, **12**, 181–290

Vizi, E. S. and Knoll, J. (1976). The inhibitory effect of adenosine and related nucleotides on the release of acetylcholine. *Neuroscience*, 1, 391–398

Wakade, A. R. and Wakade, T. D. (1978). Inhibition of noradrenaline release by adenosine. *J. Physiol. Lond.*, 282, 35–49

Westfall, D. P., Stitzel, R. E. and Rowe, J. N. (1978). The postjunctional effects and neural release of purine compounds in guinea-pig vas deferens. *Eur. J. Pharmac.*, 50, 27–38

Wu, P. H. and Phillis, J. W. (1978). Distribution and release of adenosine-triphosphate in rat-brain. *Neurochem. Res.*, 3, 563–571

Zimmerman, H. (1978). Turnover of adenine nucleotides in cholinergic synaptic vesicles of the *Torpedo* electric organ. *Neuroscience*, 3, 827–836

Zimmerman, H. (1979). Commentary: vesicle recycling and transmitter release. *Neuroscience*, 4, 1773–1803

Zimmerman, H. and Bokor, J. T. (1979). 5′-triphosphate recycles independently of acetylcholine in cholinergic synaptic vesicles. *Neurosci. Lett.*, 13, 319–324

Zimmerman, H. and Denston, C. R. (1976). Adenosine triphosphate in cholinergic vesicles isolated from the electric organ of *Electrophorus electricus*. *Brain Res.*, 111, 365–376

Zimmerman, H. and Denston, C. R. (1977). Separation of synaptic vesicles of different functional states from the cholinergic synapses of the *Torpedo* electric organ. *Neuroscience*, 2, 715–730

Zimmerman, H., Dowdall, M. J. and Lane D. A. (1979). Purine salvage at the cholinergic nerve-endings of the *Torpedo* electric organ-central role of adenosine. *Neuroscience*, 4, 979–993

# 7

# Coexistence of neuroactive substances as revealed by immunohistochemistry with monoclonal antibodies

J. V. Priestley and A. C. Cuello (Neuroanatomy Neuropharmacology Group,
University Departments of Pharmacology and Human Anatomy,
South Parks Road, Oxford, UK)

## INTRODUCTION

The idea that neuroactive substances may coexist in neurones is not new and indeed probably goes back as far as the original hypothesis of Burn and Rand (1959) concerning the presence of acetylcholine (ACh) along with noradrenaline (NA) in certain postganglionic sympathetic nerves. Although this hypothesis as originally proposed has not been confirmed it has been shown that autonomic neurones can produce alternatively acetylcholine or noradrenaline (for review, see Patterson, 1978). These early ideas and their implications for present concepts of coexistence have been reviewed by a number of authors (Burnstock, 1976; see also Burnstock, Jaim Etcheverry and Zieher, and Osborne, chapters 6, 8 and 9). Yet it is only recently that the idea that a neurone may contain more than one neuroactive substance has found general acceptance, and this has been largely due to the discovery of peptides in the nervous system and to the application of immunohistochemical techniques for their localisation (for reviews, see Cuello, 1978; Emson 1979; Hökfelt *et al.*, 1980*a*).

Geffen, Livett and their collaborators were the first to apply immunohistochemistry for the localisation of peptides in neurones with studies on chromogranin A and dopamine-$\beta$-hydroxylase in sympathetic neurones (Geffen *et al.*, 1969) followed by work on the localisation of neurophysin-II in the hypothalamo-hypophysial system (Livett *et al.*, 1971). Substance P was the first peptide to be localised by immunohistochemistry in the brain outside the hypothalamic neuroendocrine system (Nilsson *et al.*, 1974) and soon after the first examples of coexistence appeared with somatostatin-like immunoreactivity in some peripheral sympathetic noradrenergic neurones (Hökfelt *et al.*, 1977*a*). In 1978 two groups demonstrated the coexistence of the peptide substance P and the indoleamine 5-hydroxytryptamine (5-HT) in a population of central nervous system (CNS) raphe neurone cell bodies (Chan-Palay *et al.*, 1978; Hökfelt *et al.*, 1978). This particular observation has been confirmed more recently by workers using different immunohistochemical procedures (Chan-Palay, 1979; Priestley *et al.*, 1980; Cuello *et al.*, 1982).

In the past few years there has been a veritable explosion in the application of immunohistochemical techniques and now a very large number of cases of coexistence between peptides or between peptides and other transmitters have been described (Hökfelt *et al.*, 1980*b*; also Chan-Palay, and Hökfelt *et al.*, chapter 4). It thus seems timely to briefly review some of the immunohistochemical procedures which are available for the examination of coexistence situations, to consider the sort of information which can be derived from their applications, and to describe some of the novel approaches which we are developing using monoclonal antibodies to explore problems in this field. This will be illustrated by consideration of the 5-HT and substance P-containing neurones of the raphe nuclei.

## LOCALISATION OF CELL BODIES

Immunohistochemistry is a very suitable technique for examining the distribution in the brain of transmitters, peptides and transmitter markers (see Cuello, 1978; Hökfelt *et al.*, 1980*a*) and the procedures that are now most widely used are the indirect fluorescence procedure (Coons and Kaplan, 1950) or the unlabelled peroxidase antiperoxidase (PAP) procedure (Sternberger, 1979). For the localisation of transmitter markers in cell bodies it is sometimes necessary to first inhibit axonal transport with a drug such as colchicine (Dahlström, 1968; Barry *et al.*, 1973) and this has allowed several detailed maps of the distribution of various peptides and transmitters in cell bodies to be produced (for example, Sar *et al.*, 1978; Ljungdahl *et al.*, 1978; Uhl *et al.*, 1979; Steinbusch, 1981). Comparison of the results of such maps can provide some indication as to where situations of coexistence may occur, but to demonstrate coexistence more sophisticated staining procedures must be used.

If the antigens of interest survive dehydration and embedding, serial paraffin sections can be stained using different antibodies, as applied by Sofroniew (1979) in studies on the coexistence of adrenocorticotrophic hormone (ACTH) and β-endorphin. However, it is often necessary to carry out staining on unembedded sections in which case it may be possible to cut thin (5 $\mu$m) serial cryostat sections and stain these to reveal different antigens using either immunofluorescence (for example, Hökfelt *et al.*, 1978) or immunoperoxidase procedures. We have applied this latter approach to examine the localisation of 5-HT and substance P in neurones of the raphe nuclei (Priestley *et al.*, 1980) (figure 7.1). Our results

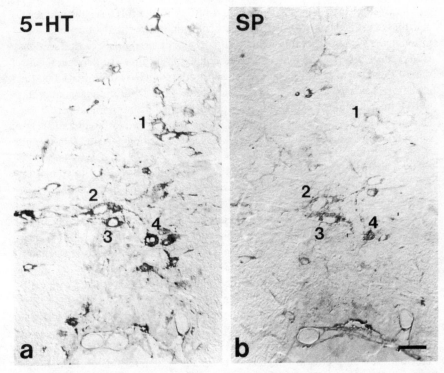

Figure 7.1 Coexistence of 5-HT and substance P (SP) in single neurones of nucleus raphe magnus. *a* and *b* show serial 5 μm cryostat sections stained for either 5-HT (*a*) or substance P (*b*) using the PAP immunocytochemical procedure. Several neurones (1–4) can be identified in both sections and stain for both putative transmitters. Scale bar = 50 μm.

agree very well with those of earlier workers who have used slightly different techniques (Chan-Palay *et al.*, 1978; Hökfelt *et al.*, 1978) and show that the two putative transmitters coexist in many cells of the caudal raphe groups (B1–B3). The cell groups contain neurones which stain only for 5-HT as well as those which stain for both 5-HT and substance P but using series of sections which alternate sections stained for either 5-HT or substance P we have been unable to identify cells which stain only for substance P, although previous workers have reported the existence of such cells (Hökfelt *et al.*, 1978; Chan-Palay, 1979).

Recently Johansson and his colleagues (1981) have combined immunofluorescence staining of serial sections with the antibody elution and restaining procedure of Tramu *et al.* (1978) to show that some 5-HT-containing raphe cells contain thyrotropin releasing hormone (TRH) and that certain cells contain 5-HT, TRH, and substance P. Other putative transmitters found in raphe nuclei include enkephalin (Hökfelt *et al.*, 1977*b*), neurotensin (Snyder, 1980), cholecystokinin (CCK) (Van der Kooy, 1981), γ-aminobutyric acid (GABA) (Belin *et al.*, 1979) and dopamine (Ochi and Shimizu *et al.*, 1978) and of these enkephalin and GABA have been shown to coexist with 5-HT in dorsal raphe nuclei (Basbaum *et al.*, 1980; Belin *et al.*, 1981).

The relationship of most of these transmitters to the 5-HT cells is unknown and there is still much to be discovered concerning coexisting compounds even in the raphe system. The production of thin (5 μm or less) serial cryostat sections is very difficult and the elution and restaining procedures also have problems, one of the main ones being that several transmitter antigens are destroyed by the eluting reagents commonly in use (Vandesande *et al*., 1977; Johansson *et al*., 1981). In an attempt to overcome these problems dual colour immunoperoxidase staining procedures have been developed which permit two different antigens to be stained in a single section without the need for antibody elution (Mason and Sammons, 1978; Joseph and Sternberger, 1979).

However, these methods have not proved generally very useful in studies on the CNS and in particular have not been employed for the examination of coexistence, partly because they produce colour mixing which can be very difficult to interpret. A way round this problem has been explored by Chan-Palay (1979) who has combined autoradiography for 5-HT uptake with substance P immunohistochemistry, thus combining a particulate label (the autoradiogram) with a diffuse stain (immunoperoxidase) (see Chan-Palay, chapter 1). Similarly, Beaudet *et al*. (1980) have described the combination of 5-HT uptake with enkephalin or tyrosine hydroxylase immunohistochemistry. Such procedures also have the advantage over previous methodologies of being potentially applicable at the electron microscopic level (see Priestley and Cuello, 1982). However, the procedures of Chan-Palay (1979) and of Beaudet *et al*. (1980) depend on the fact that neurones possess a high affinity uptake system for one of the transmitters of interest (that is, 5-HT), and therefore are only useful for dual staining studies in which one transmitter can be labelled by uptake autoradiography and in which the radioactive label can be fixed *in situ* under conditions suitable for subsequent immunohistochemistry.

We have therefore explored a more general dual staining procedure involving autoradiography and immunohistochemistry which depends on the combination of two immunohistochemical techniques rather than on immunohistochemistry and transmitter uptake. The hybrid myeloma procedure of Köhler and Milstein (1975) can be used to produce monoclonal antibodies directed against transmitter markers and we have used this technique to produce monoclonal antibodies against substance P (Cuello *et al*., 1979), 5-HT (Consolazione *et al*., 1981) and enkephalin. The antibody-producing clones can be grown in the presence of tritiated amino acids and subsequently produce internally radiolabelled antibodies of high specific activity (Galfre and Milstein, 1981) which can be applied to tissue sections in the same way as in conventional immunohistochemistry and then developed as autoradiograms (Cuello *et al*., 1980). This procedure has been named "radioimmunocytochemistry" and seems to be more sensitive than traditional immunohistochemical techniques (Cuello and Milstein, 1981; Cuello *et al*., 1982). Some results obtained using a [$^3$H]-internally labelled substance P antibody are shown in figure 7.2. Radioimmunocytochemistry can also be combined with other more traditional immunohistochemical approaches such as the

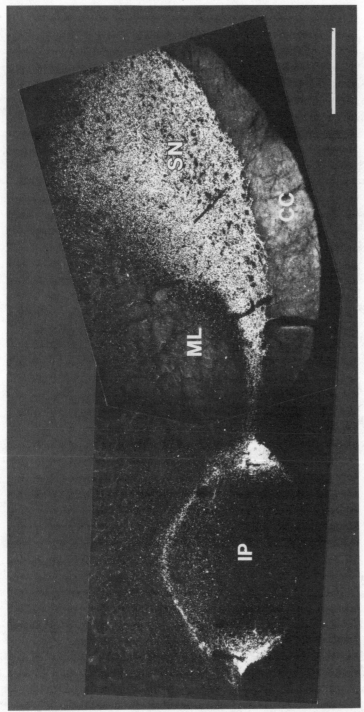

Figure 7.2 Radioimmunocytochemistry using an internally labelled anti substance P antibody ([³H]-NCI/34). Intense staining for immunoreactive substance P is seen in the substantia nigra (SN) and on the borders of the nucleus interpeduncularis (IP). CC, Crus cerebri; ML, medial lemniscus. Scale bar = 100 μm.

PAP procedure allowing the simultaneous localisation in single sections of two different antigens (Cuello *et al.*, 1982). Figure 7.3 shows schematically the general principles involved and figure 7.4 shows applications for the dual localisation of substance P and 5-HT. Recently we have produced a $[^3H]$ - internally labelled 5-HT antibody (Cuello and Milstein, 1981) for the study of raphe neurones (figure 7.5) and this can be applied in combination with PAP for any other transmitter marker to examine a number of possible coexistence situations in the 5-HT system.

The combination of radioimmunocytochemistry and PAP would seem to have great potential, if only because it provides a method of dual localisation at the ultrastructural level of two different transmitter antigens (Cuello *et al.*, 1982; see also discussion below), but it is not without its own particular problems. Light microscopic autoradiograms are generally easy enough to interpret but electron microscopic autoradiograms sometimes may require statistical analysis (Salpeter *et al.*, 1969). In addition, in dual staining studies care has to be taken to prevent any cross reaction of the developing PAP antibodies with the internally labelled primary antibody (Cuello *et al.*, 1982). Becuase of this latter problem we have explored the possibility of using a direct labelled immunoenzyme method in combination with radioimmunocytochemistry, instead of using PAP. The monoclonal antibody technique allows the production of large quantities of a particular antibody which can be easily further purified and concentrated (Galfre and Milstein, 1981). Using such a concentrated pure antibody preparation and using the two-stage glutaraldehyde conjugation procedure (Avrameas and Ternynck, 1971) in collaboration with Drs D. Boorsma and F. Van Leeuwen we have produced peroxidase-labelled monoclonal antibodies of high purity and activity (Boorsma *et al.*, 1982). Such reagents are ideal for immunohistochemistry and figure 7.6 shows the staining obtained using such a directly labelled substance P antibody. We are now applying such reagents in combination with radioimmunocytochemistry and are hopeful that they will prove useful for co-localisation studies.

## LOCALISATION OF FIBRES

The various recent reports on the coexistence of transmitters and peptides almost all refer to co-localisation in neuronal cell bodies and very little about the axonal systems of these neurones has been described. The basis and significance of co-storage in axons and terminals, and the area of innervation of such terminals, is generally unknown. This is because the techniques which have been used for studies on cell bodies, such as serial sectioning and elution with restaining, are inapplicable for studies on axons because of their small size and low antigen content. For example, in the raphe system such techniques can show that substance P and 5-HT are contained in the same fibre bundles (figure 7.7) but cannot show whether the two putative transmitters are contained together in the same axons. Information on coexistence in axons and terminals has had

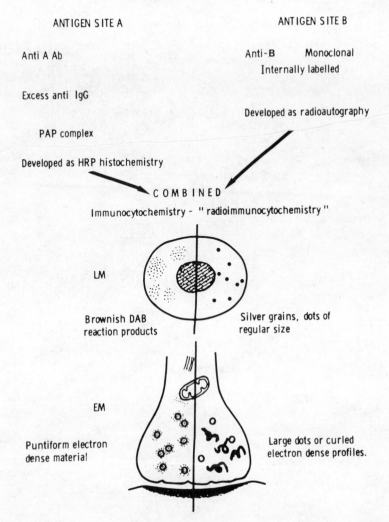

ANTIGEN SITE A

ANTIGEN SITE B

Anti A Ab

Anti-B     Monoclonal
Internally labelled

Excess anti IgG

Developed as radioautography

PAP complex

Developed as HRP histochemistry

COMBINED
Immunocytochemistry - "radioimmunocytochemistry"

LM

Brownish DAB
reaction products

Silver grains, dots of
regular size

EM

Puntiform electron
dense material

Large dots or curled
electron dense profiles.

Figure 7.3 Schematic diagram showing the principles of combined immunocytochemistry and radioimmunocytochemistry allowing the simultaneous localisation of two different antigenic sites. One antigen (site A) is revealed using traditional PAP immunocytochemistry. This uses a peroxidase enzyme (HRP) as marker which will oxidise an electron donor such as diamino benzidine (DAB) to produce an insoluble osmiophilic polymer. DAB can be detected at both light microscopic (LM) and electron microscopic (EM) levels (left hand side of diagram). The second antigen (site B) is revealed with radioimmunocytochemistry using a radioactive internally labelled monoclonal antibody. This is developed as a radioautogram and the clusters of silver grains produced in the photographic emulsion can be visualised at both light and electron microscopic level (right hand side of diagram). Since the two procedures use different and easily distinguishable labels they can be applied together to allow the detection of two different antigens in single profiles at either light or electron microscopic level. Ab, Antibody; IgG, immunoglobulin.

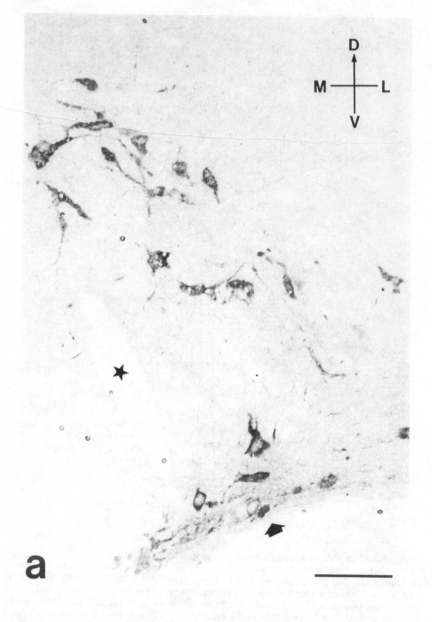

Figure 7.4 Application of combined PAP immunocytochemistry and radioimmunocyto-chemistry for the demonstration of 5-HT and substance P coexistence in single raphe neurones. *a*, 5-HT immunoreactive neurones in one of the lateral wings of nucleus raphe magnus demonstrated using PAP immunocytochemistry. D, L, V, M indicate dorsal, lateral, ventral and medial. Star, blood vessel; arrow, pial surface. Scale bar = 100 μm. *b*, Substance P-immunoreactive neurones in the same area of raphe magnus as shown in *a* and demon-strated using radioimmunocytochemistry. Stained neurones (arrows) are marked by the pre-

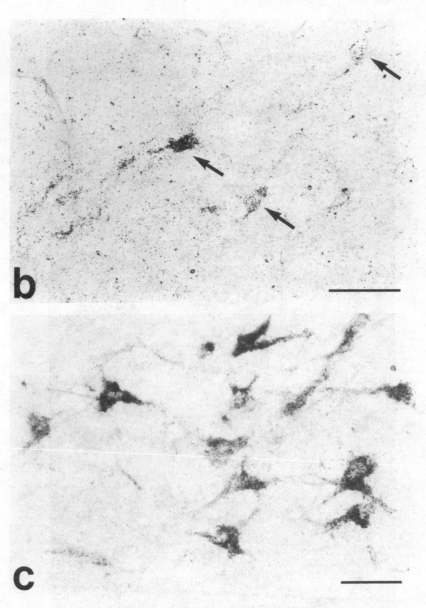

sence of large numbers of small dots and these are formed by silver grains in the developed emulsion of the autoradiogram. Scale bar = 200 μm. *c* Neurones containing both 5-HT and substance P immunoreactivity in the same area of raphe magnus as shown in *a* and *b*. PAP immunocytochemistry for 5-HT in combination with radioimmunocytochemistry for substance P. Neurones show a diffuse PAP immunostaining upon which is superimposed the small dots of the substance P radioimmunocytochemistry. Scale bar = 50 μm.

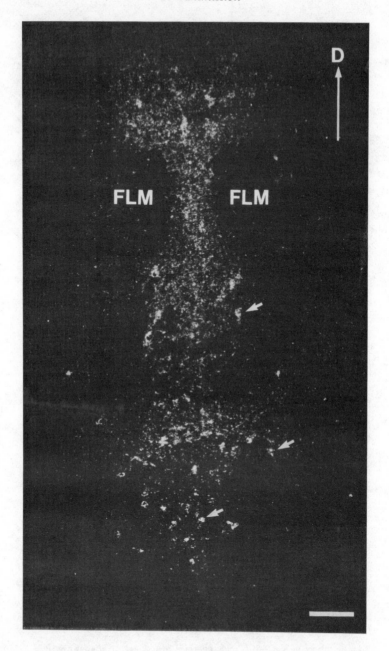

Figure 7.5  Radioimmunocytochemistry using an internally labelled 5-HT antibody ([³H]-
YC5/45). Raphe dorsalis and raphe medialis (groups B7 and B8 of Dahlstrom and Fuxe,
1964). Section shows diffuse staining as well as many labelled cell bodies (arrows). FLM,
Fasiculus longitudinalis medialis; D, dorsal. Dark field illumination. Scale bar = 100 $\mu$m.

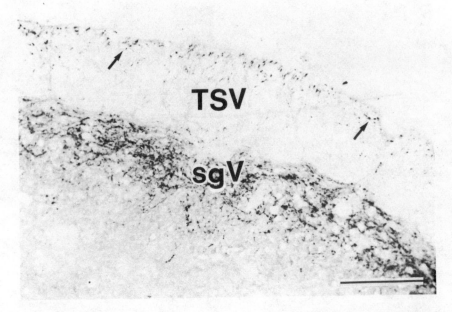

Figure 7.6 Direct labelled peroxidase immunocytochemistry using peroxidase conjugated monoclonal substance P antibody (NCl/34). Substance P immunoreactivity in the substantia gelatinosa (sgV) of the rat spinal trigeminal nucleus. Background staining in the spinal tract (TSV) is minimal and a few transversely cut immunoreactive fibres in the tract are clearly visible (arrows). Scale bar = 100 μm.

to be inferred from comparisons of the distribution of substance P and 5-HT immunostaining in the spinal cord, or from studies on the effect of specific 5-HT neurotoxins on immunostaining (Hökfelt *et al.*, 1978; Johansson *et al.*, 1981; Gilbert *et al.*, 1982; see also Hökfelt *et al.* and Gilbert *et al.* chapter 3).

Recently procedures which enable retrograde tract tracing techniques to be combined with immunohistochemistry have been developed (Ljungdahl *et al.*, 1975; Priestley *et al.*, 1981) and these can provide information on the site of termination of peptidergic raphe cells (Bowker *et al.*, 1981; Van der Kooy *et al.*, 1981). However, with these various procedures it is not possible to look directly at the distribution of coexisting transmitter/peptide terminals, for which it is necessary to be able to stain simultaneously the two compounds in individual fibres. The various dual staining procedures discussed in the previous section have not so far proved very useful for the examination of fibres and so we have explored an alternative approach based on dual colour immunofluorescence staining. The method depends on having two primary antibodies which have been raised in different species and which can be localised using two different secondary antibodies, each of which is labelled with a different fluorochrome. Appropriate combinations of filters allow each fluorochrome to be viewed independantly, and using an epifluorescence illuminator equipped with

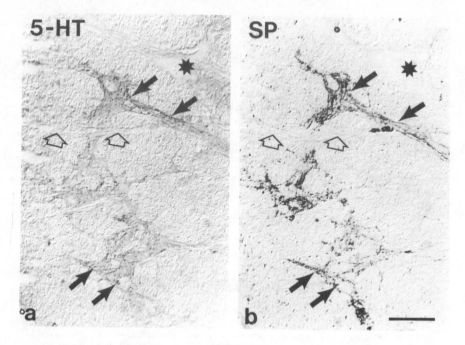

Figure 7.7  Serial cryostat sections PAP immunostained for either 5-HT (*a*) or substance P (SP) (*b*). Certain fibre bundles stain for both compounds (arrows) while other bundles stain for neither (open arrow heads). Star indicates blood vessel. Scale bar = 50 μm.

interchangeable filter block combinations it is possible to view either fluoro-chrome on a labelled section simply by changing the relevant filter block (see Ploem, 1975).

Dual colour immunofluorescence staining has been used quite widely in direct labelled procedures (see Nairn, 1976) but has not been used much for indirect labelled immunohistochemistry because primary antibodies raised in different species are not often available. However, monoclonal techniques produce rat or mouse raised antibodies which can be used in combination with traditional rabbit raised polyclonal antibodes. To examine the distribution of substance P and 5-HT in the spinal cord we have therefore used a monoclonal rat anti-5-HT antibody localised with fluorescein isothiocyanate (FITC) rabbit anti-rat IgG in combination with a rabbit anti-substance P antibody localised with rhodamine-conjugated goat anti-rabbit IgG. Preparations were examined on a Leitz Dialux 20 microscope fitted with Ploemopak vertical illuminator, water immersion objectives, and Leitz filter block N2 for viewing selective rhodamine fluorescence. Various controls were carried out to check for artifactual dual staining and special staining schedules were adopted to prevent the rhodamine anti-rabbit IgG from binding to the FITC rabbit anti-rat IgG.

Figure 7.8*a* and *b* show a dually stained preparation in the region of the central canal of the spinal cord, where there is heavy staining for substance P and 5-HT including a prominant bundle of fibres immediately ventral to the canal which stains only for substance P. In contrast, figure 7.8c and d show an area of the ventral horn in which individual fibres clearly stain for both 5-HT and substance P. Using such preparations areas of coexisting substance P/5-HT fibres can be quickly identified and compared with areas innervated by separate substance P or 5-HT systems. However, although this approach allows two putative transmitters to be localised in single fibres and varicosities it gives no information about the subcellular storage of the two compounds. Such data can only be obtained from electron microscopic immunocytochemical studies.

## ULTRASTRUCTURAL LOCALISATION OF COEXISTING COMPOUNDS

For the localisation of coexisting putative transmitters in single nerve terminals, or for the examination of their subcellular storage sites, immunohistochemical techniques have to be applied at the electron microscopic level. Staining can be carried out either after plastic embedding and thin sectioning (post-embedding staining) or before plastic embedding (pre-embedding staining). The former procedure allows serial sections to be stained for different antigens, in the same manner as described earlier for light microscopy. Recently Pelletier and his collegues (1981) have applied this approach to demonstrate the localisation of 5-HT and substance P in single dense core vesicles of terminals in the spinal cord. However, the post-embedding staining procedure is not widely applicable to studies on the CNS, as most of the relevant antigens do not survive the dehydration and plastic embedding and so pre-embedding staining must be used (Priestley and Cuello, 1982).

Pre-embedding staining allows a single antigen to be localised at the ultrastructural level and can provide some information pertinant to coexistance situations. Such studies on the localisation of substance P in the substantia gelatinosa of the spinal cord and spinal trigeminal have generally shown that the peptide is contained in nerve terminals with a heterogeneous vesicle population consisting of small agranular spherical vesicles and also large dense core vesicles of diameter in the range 60–110 nm (Chan-Palay and Palay, 1977; Pickel *et al.*, 1977; Barber *et al.*, 1979; Priestley, 1981). Immunohistochemical staining is usually most intense on the dense core vesicles and on the membranes of the small granular vesicles. It is known that some substance P terminals in the spinal cord also contain 5-HT but since traditional immunohistochemical pre-embedding techniques do not allow a single terminal to be stained for both a peptide and another transmitter it is not possible to say whether the two types of vesicles reflect storage of two types of transmitter. However, some authors have speculated that while peptides are contained in the large dense core vesicles the small agranular vesicles might contain a coexisting classical transmitter (Pickel *et al.*, 1977; Barber *et al.*, 1979) although it is recognised that a large number of other arrangements are also possible (Chan-Palay, 1979; Hokfelt *et al.*, 1980a;b).

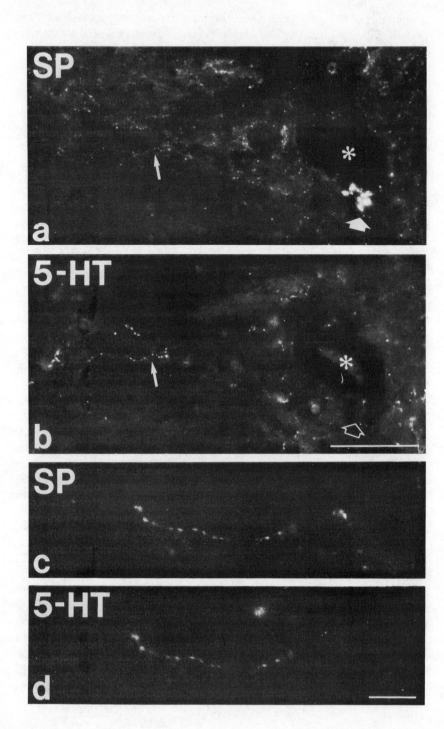

Post-embedding studies on serial section have shown staining for both substance P and 5-HT in large dense core vesicles (Pelletier *et al.*, 1981). If peptides are contained in the dense core vesicles it is possible that they are processed in the same way as are the posterior pituitary hormones oxytocin and vasopressin and their neurophysin carriers which are probably synthesised and packaged into granules in the cell body and then subsequently transported down the axon to the terminals (Gainer *et al.*, 1977; Pickering, 1980). Pre-embedding immunocytochemistry for neurophysin has shown reaction deposit associated mainly with rough endoplasmic reticulum, Golgi saccules, secretory granules and also secondary lysosomes in the supraoptic nucleus cell bodies (Broadwell *et al.*, 1979).

In the CNS vasopressin and oxytocin fibres are thought to be derived from the hypothalamus (Buijs, 1978; Sofroniew and Schrell, 1981) but contain dense core vesicles similar in size to those described for other peptides in the CNS (100 nm) and significantly smaller than those associated with the magnocellular hypothalamo-neurohypophyseal system (Buijs and Swaab, 1979). However, it is possible that the neurohypophyseal projection cells and the extrahypothalamic projection cells of the paraventricular nucleus constitute distinct populations (Hosoya and Matsushita, 1979). It is also possible that some non-granular intra-axonal transport of peptides can take place in the smooth endoplasmic reticulum (Alonso and Assenmacher, 1979), in the same way as may occur for catecholamines (Tranzer, 1972).

Some insight into these various issues as they effect CNS peptides can be obtained from those few ultrastructural immunocytochemical studies which have described the appearance of immunoreactive peptide-containing neuronal cell bodies in the CNS. In the striatum Pickel and her colleagues (1980) have described enkephalin immunoreactivity diffusely throughout nucleus and cytoplasm but with the cells containing many alveolate vesicles, while in sensory ganglia Chan-Palay and Palay (1977) have reported substance P immunoreactivity associated with large (100–300 nm) vesicles contained in so-called "storage vacuoles". Two other reports of interest are those of Johansson and his colleagues showing from light microscopy that somatostatin immunoreactivity in CNS neuronal cell bodies is probably associated with the Golgi apparatus (Johansson,

Figure 7.8 Use of dual colour immunofluorescence staining to demonstrate the coexistence of substance P (SP) and 5-HT in single fibres. *a* and *b*, Area of the rat spinal cord around the aqueduct (asterisk) stained simultaneously for substance P using rhodamine-labelled second antibody and for 5-HT using FITC-labelled second antibody. In *a* a filter combination is used which reveals only the substance P/rhodamine combination, whereas in *b* a filter combination is used which reveals the 5-HT/FITC combination. A prominant bundle of fibres immediately ventral to the aqueduct stains for substance P (arrow head) but not for 5-HT (hollow arrow head). Elsewhere are areas which appear to stain for both substance P and 5-HT (arrow). Scale bar = 100 μm. *c* and *d*, High magnification micrographs of an area of the ventral horn of the spinal cord processed as described for *a* and *b* above. A single fibre with several immunoreactive varicosities is seen stained for both substance P (*c*) and 5-HT (*d*). Scale bar = 20 μm.

1978) and from electron microscopy that TRH immunoreactivity in hypothalamus is found in cytoplasm, various membranes and a few large dense core
(100 nm) vesicles (Johansson *et al.*, 1980). Similarly, Dube and Pelletier (1979)
have shown an increase in numbers of somatostatin-immunoreactive secretory
granules (80-110 nm) in hypothalamic cell bodies following colchicine treatment. These various studies do not include any CNS peptidergic neurones which
also contain a classical transmitter and so we have used pre-embedding ultrastructural immunocytochemistry to examine the localisation of substance P in
raphe neurones. Using this staining methodology it cannot be concluded that the
substance P stained cells necessarily also contain 5-HT but the previous light
microscopic studies indicate that this is highly likely (Hökfelt *et al.*, 1978;
Priestley *et al.*, 1980; Johansson *et al.*, 1981).

To show the peptide in the cell bodies we pretreated rats with 80 $\mu$g colchicine
injected into the IVth ventricle. Figure 7.9 shows the results obtained. At light
microscopic level cells were seen to have strong but rather uneven cytoplasmic
immunostaining. Electron microscopic examination revealed that immunostained
cells contained extensive and slightly fragmented endoplasmic reticulum. Vesicles
were seen accumulated especially at the periphery of the cell body and in axonal
swellings. Similar observations have been described for the effect of colchicine
on hypothalamic neurons (Flament-Durand and Dustin, 1972; Hindelang-Gertner
*et al.*, 1976). Immunoreaction deposit occurred on the membranes of mitochondria and endoplasmic reticulum and also on a few small vesicles but the
most intense staining was on large (80-120 nm) dense core vesicles. Colchicine
causes gross disruption of cellular organisation and in certain circumstances
shows selective neurotoxicity (Goldschmidt and Steward, 1980) and so extra-
polation from these results to obtain an understanding of the normal functioning
of the cell must be carried out with great care. However, it does seem from this
data that in raphe peptidergic neurones substance P is packaged into dense core
vesicles in the cell body and the vesicles are subsequently transported down the
axon to the terminals. However, these studies do not give any information on
the relationship between 5-HT and peptide handling in these cotransmitter cells.

To be able to study the ultrastructural basis of coexistence or to examine the
anatomical basis of interactions between putative transmitter, it is necessary to
be able to stain two different antigens in single electron microscopic sections.
The serial sectioning approach employed by Pelletier and his colleagues (1981)
cannot be widely applied because of the difficulty of using post-embedding procedures in the CNS (Priestley and Cuello, 1982). Elution and restaining protocols
based on two colour immunoenzyme staining (Nakane, 1968; Vandesande *et al.*,
1977; Mason and Sammons, 1978; Joseph and Sternberger, 1979) cannot be
used because of the difficult of distinguishing the two different enzymic reaction
products in the electron microscope (Hanker, 1979). A dual staining procedure is
required which gives two different and easily distinguishable signals for the two
different antigens. Methodologies based on iron-dextran antibody conjugates
(Dutton *et al.*, 1979) or on protein A colloidal gold complexes (Geuze and Slot,

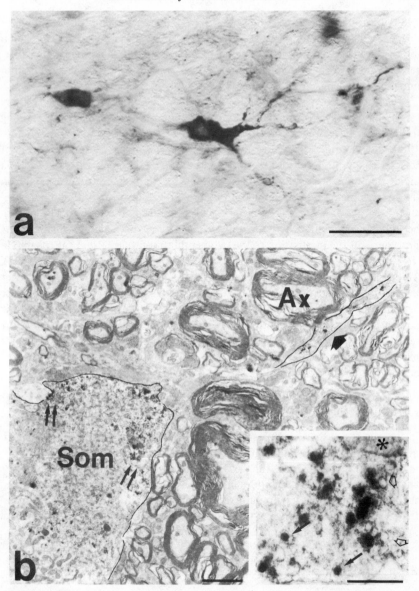

Figure 7.9  Substance P-immunoreactive neurones in the raphe area (nucleus reticularis para-gigantocellularis) of the rat brain stem. Light and electron microscopy. PAP pre-embedding immunocytochemistry. *a*, Light micrograph showing two immunoreactive neurones revealed following colchicine treatment. Scale bar = 50 μm. *b*, Electron micrograph of a neurone similar to those shown in *a*. The cell body (Som) and a single process (black arrow head) are outlined. Accumulations of immunoreactive material can be seen in the neurone (arrows). Ax, Myelinated axon. Scale bar = 2 μm. Inset shows at high magnification the immuno-reactive material in the cell body. Large (100 nm) dense cored vesicles are heavily stained (arrows), whereas other similar sized membrane bound structures are unstained (open arrow heads). Asterisk indicates a mitochondrion. Scale bar = 500 nm.

1980) have been developed but so far have only been applied successfully for post-embedding staining. We have therefore examined the possibility of extending to the ultrastructural level the dual staining procedure described in an earlier section and involving the combination of PAP immunocytochemistry and radio-immunohistochemistry.

The principles involved are outlined in figure 7.3. Radioimmunohistochemistry can be used at the electron microscopic level and involves preembedding staining followed by development of ultrathin sections as autoradiograms (Cuello *et al.*, 1980; Cuello *et al.*, 1982). Figure 7.10a shows an example of the application of this procedure for the localisation of substance P terminals in the substantia nigra. Immunoreactive terminals are marked by the presence of silver grains in the overlying emulsion. Combination of this procedure with PAP immunocyto-chemistry allows a second antigen to be located using the traditional diamino-benzidine osmiophilic reaction deposit. So far we have applied this dual staining procedure for the localisation of the two peptides, substance P and enkephalin, in the substantia gelatinosa of the brain stem (Cuello *et al.*, 1982) (see figure 7.10b). This is a situation in which the two putative transmitters have a very similar localisation but do not coexist and appear rather to be contained in separate neuronal populations (Del Fiacco and Cuello, 1980) which may make synaptic contact with common second order neurones (Priestley, 1981). However, the same methodology can be used for the ultrastructural dual localisation of a number of putative transmitters and we are now applying it in studies on the coexistence of substance P and 5-HT in terminals of the spinal cord.

## CONCLUSIONS

In the past ten years immunohistochemical techniques have made a major contri-bution towards the revolution that has occurred in our understanding of trans-mitter actions in the brain. In particular such techniques have highlighted the widespread occurrence of peptides in neurones of the central nervous system and their coexistence with certain more traditional neurotransmitters. Now, however, the sheer complexity of the system is demanding the development of new and more sophisticated immunohistochemical procedures. Over the coming years it

---

Figure 7.10 Radioimmunocytochemistry using internally labelled substance P antibody ([$^3$H]-NCl/34). Electron microscopy. a, Two large dendrites (d) in the substantia nigra receive synapses (arrow heads) from various terminals. One such terminal (t) is marked by a silver grain cluster (double arrow) indicating the presence of substance P immunoreactivity. Another process is also labelled (arrow). Scale bar = 1 $\mu$m. b, Combination of radioimmuno-cytochemistry for substance P and PAP immunocytochemistry for enkephalin. Substantia gelatinosa of the spinal trigeminal nucleus. A terminal (t$_1$) labelled for substance P by radioimmunocytochemistry and a terminal (t$_2$) labelled for enkephalin by PAP immuno-cytochemistry are in close apposition to a common dendrite (d). Another terminal (t$_3$) and an unidentified process (arrow) are also labelled for substance P. Scale bar = 1 $\mu$m.

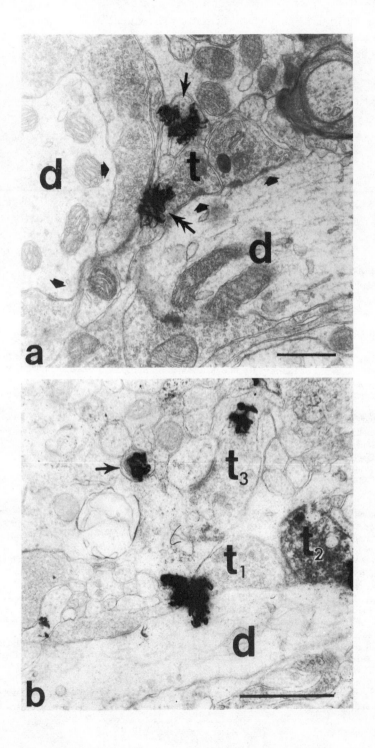

seems likely that immunohistochemistry will continue to play a prominant role in unravelling the transmitter and peptide interactions of the brain and presumably there will be yet more surprises in store for us.

## ACKNOWLEDGEMENTS

J.V.P. is a Beit Memorial Research Fellow and part of this work was done during the tenure of an MRC scholarship. A.C.C. acknowledges grants from the Wellcome Trust, The Medical Research Council (UK) and assistance from the E. P. Abraham Cephalosporin Trust (Oxford). Messers B. Archer and T. Barclay and Miss J. Lloyd are thanked for expert photographic work and the technical assistance of Mr S. Bramwell and secretarial assistance of Mrs E. Iles and Miss J. Ballinger is also gratefully acknowledged. Dr C. Milstein (Cambridge) is thanked for critical discussion and preparation of internally labelled antibodies. Thanks also to Dr P. C. Emson (Cambridge) and Dr R. Miller (Chicago) for generous provision of polyclonal anti-substance P and anti-enkephalin antibodies and to Dr A. Consolazione for contributing figure 7.2.

## REFERENCES

Alonso, G. and Assenmacher, I. (1979). The smooth endoplasmic reticulum in neurohypophysial axons of the rat: possible involvement in transport, storage and release of neurosecretory material. *Cell Tiss. Res.*, 199, 415–429

Avrameas, S. and Ternynck, T. (1971). Peroxidase labelled antibody and Fab conjugates with enhanced intracellular penetration. *Immunochemistry*, 8, 1175–1179

Barber, R. P., Vaughn, J. E., Randall-Slemmon, J., Salvaterra, P. M., Roberts, E. and Leeman, S. E. (1979). The origin, distribution and synaptic relationships of substance P axons in rat spinal cord. *J. comp. Neurol.*, 184, 331–352

Barry, J., Dubois, M. P. and Poulain, P. (1973). LRF-producing cells of the mammalian hypothalamus. *Z. Zellforsch. Mikrosk. Anat.*, 146, 351–366

Basbaum, A. I., Glazer, E. J., Steinbusch, H., and Verhofstad, A. (1980). Serotonin and enkephalin co-exist in neurons involved in opiate and stimulation-produced analgesia in the cat. *Soc. Neurosci. Abstr.*, 6, 540

Beaudet, A., Pickel, V. M., Joh, T. H., Miller, R. J. and Cuenod, M. (1980). Simultaneous detection of serotonin and tyrosine hydroxlase or enkephalin containing neurons by combined radioautorgraphy and immunocytochemistry in the central nervous system of the rat. *Soc. Neurosci. Abstr.*, 6, 353

Belin, M. F., Aguera, M., Tappaz, M., McRae-Degueuroe, A., Bobillier, P. and Pujol, J. F. (1979). GABA-accumulating neurons in the nucleus raphe dorsalis and periaqueductal gray in the rat: a biochemical and radioautographic study. *Brain Res.*, 170, 279–297

Belin, M. F., Nanopoulos, D., Steinbusch, H., Verhofstrad, A., Maitre, M., Jouvet, M. and Pujol, J. F. (1981). Glutamate decarboxylase and serotonin in a single neuron in the nucleus raphe dorsalis of the rat demonstrated by combined immunocytochemical staining method. *C.r. Acad. Sci.*, series D, 293, 337–342

Boorsma, D., Cuello, A. C. and Van Leeuwen, F. (1982). Direct immunocytochemistry with a horseradish peroxidase conjugated monoclonal antibody against substance P. *J. Histochem. Cytochem.*, in press

Bowker, R. M., Steinbusch, H. W. M. and Coulter, J. D. (1981). Serotonergic and peptidergic projections to the spinal cord demonstrated by a combined retrograde HRP histochemical and immunocytochemical staining method. *Brain Res.*, 211, 412–417

Broadwell, R. D., Oliver, C. and Brightman, M. W. (1979). Localization of neurophysin within organelles associated with protein synthesis and packaging in the hypothalamo-neurohypophysial system: an immunocytochemical study. *Proc. natn. Acad. Sci. U.S.A.*, 76, 5999–6003

Buijs, R. M. (1978). Intra- and extrahypothalamic vasopressin and oxytocin pathways in the rat. Pathways to the limbic system, medulla oblongata and spinal cord. *Cell Tiss. Res.*, 192, 423–435

Buijs, R. M. and Swaab, D. F. (1979). Immunoelectronmicroscopical demonstration of vaso-pressin and oxytocin synapses in the limbic system of the rat. *Cell Tiss. Res.*, 204, 355–365

Burn, J. H. and Rand, M. I. (1959). Sympathetic postganglionic mechanism. *Nature London*, 184, 163–165

Burnstock, G. (1976). Do some nerve cells release more than one transmitter? *Neuroscience*, 1, 239–248

Chan-Palay, V. and Palay, S. L. (1977). Ultrastructural identification of substance P and their processes in rat sensory ganglia and their terminals in the spinal cord by immuno-cytochemistry. *Proc. natn. Acad. Sci U.S.A.*,74, 4050–4054

Chan-Palay, V., Jonsson, G. and Palay, S. L. (1978). Serotonin and substance P coexist in neurons of the rat's central nervous system. *Proc. natn. Acad. Sci. U.S.A.*, 75, 1581–1586

Chan-Palay, V. (1979). Combined immunocytochemistry and autoradiography after *in vivo* injections of monoclonal antibody to substance P and $^3$H-serotonin: coexistence of two putative transmitters in single raphe cells and fiber plexuses. *Anat. Embryol. Berlin*, 156, 241–254

Consolazione, A., Milstein, C., Wright, B. and Cuello, A. C. (1981). Immunocytochemical detection of serotonin with monoclonal antibodies. *J. Histochem. Cytochem.*, 29, 1425–1430

Coons, A. H. and Kaplan, M. H. (1950). Localisation of antigens in tissue cells: II Improve-ments in a method for the detection of antigen by means of fluorescent antibody. *J. exp. Med.*, 91, 1–9

Cuello, A. C. (1978). Immunocytochemical studies of the distribution of neurotransmitters and related substance in CNS. In *Handbook of Psychopharmacology*, 9 (ed. L. L. Iversen, S. D. Iversen and S. H. Snyder), Plenum Press, New York, pp. 69–137

Cuello, A. C., Galfre, G. and Milstein, C. (1979). Detection of substance P in the central nervous system by a monoclonal antibody. *Proc. natn. Acad. Sci. U.S.A.*, 76, 3532–3536

Cuello, A. C., Milstein, C. and Priestley, J. V. (1980). Use of monoclonal antibodies in immunocytochemistry with special reference to the central nervous system. *Brain Res. Bull.*, 5, 575–587

Cuello, A. C. and Milstein, C. (1981). Use of internally labelled monoclonal antibodies. In *Physiological Peptides and New Trends in Radioimmunology* (ed. Ch. A. Bizollon) Elsevier, Amsterdam, pp. 293–305

Cuello, A. C., Priestley, J. V. and Milstein, C. (1982). Immunocytochemistry with internally labelled monoclonal antibodies. *Proc. natn. Acad. Sci. U.S.A.*, 79, 665–669

Dahlström, A. (1968). Effect of colchicine on transport of amine storage granules in sympa-thetic nerves of rat. *Eur. J. Pharmac.*, 5, 111–113

Dahlström, A. and Fuxe, K. (1964). Evidence for the existence of monoamine-containing neurons in the central nervous system. I. Demonstration of monoamines in the cell bodies of brainstem neurons. *Acta Physiol. Scand.*, 62, suppl. 232, 1–55

Del Fiacco, M. and Cuello, A. C. (1980). Substance P and enkephalin-containing neurones in the rat trigeminal system. *Neuroscience*, 5, 803–815

Dube, D. and Pelletier, G. (1979). Effect of colchicine on the immunohistochemical localiz-ation of somatostatin in the rat brain: light and electron microscopic studies. *J. Histo-chem. Cytochem.*, 27, 1577–1581

Dutton, A. H., Tokuyasu, K. T. and Singer, S. J. (1979). Iron-dextran antibody conjugates: general method for simultaneous staining of two components in high resolution immuno-electron microscopy. *Proc. natn. Acad. Sci. U.S.A.*, 76, 3392–3396

Emson, P. C. (1979). Peptides as neurotransmitter candidates in the mammalian CNS. *Progress in Neurobiology*, 13, 61–116

Flament-Durand, J. and Dustin, P. (1972). Studies on the transport of secretory granules in the magnocellular hypothalamic neurons. I. Action of colchicine on axonal flow and neurotubules in the paraventricular nuclei. *Z. Zellforsch.*, 130, 440–454

Gainer, H., Sarne, Y. and Brownstein, M. J. (1977). Biosynthesis and axonal transport of rat neurohypophyseal proteins and peptides. *J. Cell Biol.*, 73, 366–381

Galfre, G. and Milstein, C. (1981). Preparation of monoclonal antibodies, strategies and procedures. *Methods in Enzymology*, 73, 3–46

Gaffen, L. B., Livett, B. G. and Rush, R. A. (1969). Immunohistochemical localization of protein components of catecholamine storage vesicles. *J. Physiol. Lond.*, 204, 593–605

Geuze, J. J. and Slot, J. W. (1980). Double-labelling and quantitative immunoelectron microscopy on utrathin frozen sections. In *EMBO Practical Course Immunocytochemistry* (abstract).

Gilbert, R. F. T., Emson, P. C., Hunt, S. P., Bennett, G. W., Marsden, C. A., Sandberg, B.E.B., Steinbusch, H. W. M. and Verhofstad, A. A. J. (1982). The effects of monoamine neurotoxins on peptides in the rat spinal cord. *Neuroscience*, 7, 69–87

Goldschmidt, R. B. and Steward, O. (1980). Preferential neurotoxicity of colchicine for granule cells of the dentate gyrus of the adult rat. *Proc. natn. Acad. Sci. U.S.A.*, 77, 3047–3051

Hanker, J. S. (1979). Osmiophilic reagents in electronmicroscopic histocytochemistry. *Prog. Histochem. Cytochem.*, 12, (1), 1–85

Hindelang-Gertner, C., Stoeckel, M. E. and Stutinsky, F. (1976). Colchicine effects on neurosecretory neurons and other hypothalamic and hypophysial cells, with special reference to changes in the cytoplasmic membranes. *Cell Tiss. Res.*, 170, 17–41

Hökfelt, T., Elfvin, L., Elde, R., Schultzberg, M., Goldstein, M. and Luft, R. (1977a). Occurrence of somatostatin-like immunoreactivity is some peripheral sympathetic noradrenergic neurons. *Proc. natn. Acad. Sci. U.S.A.*, 74, 3587–3591

Hökfelt, T., Ljungdahl, A., Terenius, L., Elde, R. and Nilsson, G. (1977b). Immunohistochemical analysis of peptide pathways possibly related to pain and analgesia: enkepahlin and substance P. *Proc. natn. Acad. Sci. U.S.A.*, 74, 3081–3085

Hökfelt, T., Ljungdahl, A., Steinbusch, H., Verhofstad, A., Nilsson, G., Brodin, E., Pernow, B. and Goldstein, M. (1978). Immunohistochemical evidence of substance P-like immunoreactivity in some 5-hydroxytryptamine-containing neurons in the rat central nervous system. *Neuroscience*, 3, 517–538

Hökfelt, T., Johansson, O., Ljungdahl, A., Lundberg, J. M. and Schultzberg, M. (1980a). Peptidergic neurones. *Nature London*, 284, 515–521

Hökfelt, T., Lundberg, J. M., Schultzberg, M., Johansson, O., Ljungdahl, A. and Rehfeld, J. (1980b). Coexistence of peptides and putative transmitters in neurons. In *Neural Peptides and Neuronal Communication* (ed. E. Costa and M. Trabucchi), Raven Press, New York, pp. 1–23

Hosoya, Y. and Matsushita, M. (1979). Identification and distribution of the spinal and hypophyseal projection neurons in the paraventricular nucleus of the rat. A light and electron microscopic study with the horseradish peroxidase method. *Expl Brain Res.*, 35, 315–331

Johansson, O. (1978). Localization of somatostatin-like immunoreactivity in the golgi apparatus of central and peripheral neurons. *Histochemistry*, 58, 167–176

Johansson, O., Hökfelt, T., Jeffcoate, N. White, N. and Sternberger, L. A. (1980). Ultrastructural localisation of TRH-like immunoreactivity. *Expl Brain Res.*, 38, 1–10

Johansson, O., Hökfelt, T., Pernow, B., Jeffcoate, S. L., White, N., Steinbusch, H. W. M., Verhofstad, A. A. J., Emson, P. C. and Spindel, E. (1981). Immunohistochemical support for three putative transmitters in one neuron: coexistence of 5-hydroxytryptamine, substance P- and thyrotropin releasing hormone-like immunoreactivity in medullary neurons projecting to the spinal cord. *Neuroscience*, 6, 1857–1881

Joseph, S. A. and Sternberger, L. A. (1979). The unlabelled antibody method. Contrasting colour staining of β-lipotropin and ACTH-associated hypothalamic peptides without antibody removal. *J. Histochem. Cytochem.*, 27, 1430–1437

Köhler, G. and Milstein, C. (1975). Continuous cultures of fused cells secreting antibody of predefined specificity. *Nature London*, 256, 495–497

Livett, B. G., Uttenthal, L. O. and Hope, D. B. (1971). Localization of neurophysin-II in the hypothalamo-neurohypophysial system of the pig by immunofluorescence histochemistry. *Phil. Trans. R. Soc. Lond.*, B261, 371–378

Ljungdahl, A., Hökfelt, T., Goldstein, M. and Park, D. (1975). Retrograde peroxidase transport tracing of neurons combined with transmitter histochemistry. *Brain Res.*, 84, 313–319

Ljungdahl, A., Hökfelt, T. and Nilsson, G. (1978). Distribution of substance P-like immunoreactivity in the central nervous system of the rat. I. Cell bodies and nerve terminals. *Neuroscience*, 3, 861–943

Mason, D. Y. and Sammons, R. (1978). Alkaline phosphatase and peroxidase for double immunoenzymatic labelling of cellular constituents. *J. clin. Path.*, 31, 454–460

Nairn, R. C. (1976). *Fluorescent Protein Tracing*. Fourth edition, Churchill Livingstone, Edinburgh.

Nakane, P. K. (1968). Simultaneous localisation of multiple tissue antigens using the peroxidase-labelled antibody method: a study on pituitary glands of the rat. *J. Histochem. Cytochem.*, 16, 557–560

Nilsson, G., Hökfelt, T. and Pernow, B. (1974). Distribution of substance P-like immunoreactivity in the rat central nervous system as revealed by immunohistochemistry. *Med. Biol.*, 52, 424–427

Ochi, J. and Shimizu, K. (1978). Occurrence of dopamine-containing neurons in the midbrain raphe nuclei of the rat. *Neurosci. Lett.*, 8, 317–320

Patterson, P. H. (1978). Environmental determination of autonomic neurotransmitter function. *A. Rev. Neurosci.*, 1, 1–17

Pelletier, G., Steinbusch, H. W. M. and Verhofstad, A. A. J. (1981). Immunoreactive substance P and serotonin present in the same dense-core vesicles. *Nature London*, 293, 71–72

Pickel, V. M., Reis, D. J. and Leeman, S. E. (1977). Ultrastructural localisation of substance P in neurons of rat spinal cord. *Brain Res.*, 122, 534–540

Pickel, V. M., Sumal, K. K., Beckley, S. C., Miller, R. J. and Reis, D. J. (1980). Immunocytochemical localization of enkephalin in the neostriatum of rat brain: a light and electron microscopic study. *J. comp. Neurol.*, 189, 721–740

Pickering, B. T. (1980). Lessons from a peptidergic neurone. *Nature London*, 288, 117

Ploem, J. S. (1975). General introduction to Fifth International Conference on Immunofluorescence and Related Staining Techniques. *Ann. N. Y. Acad. Sci.*, 254., 4–20

Priestley, J. V., Consolazione, A. and Cuello, A. C. (1980). Identification of substance P and serotonin containing neurones in the CNS with monoclonal antibodies. In *Abstracts VIth International Histochemistry and Cytochemistry Congress*. Royal Microscopical Society, Oxford, p. 310

Priestley, J. V. (1981). Ultrastructural localisation of substance P and enkephalin in the substantia gelatinosa of the spinal trigeminal nucleus. *Br. J. Pharmac.*, 74, 893P

Priestley, J. V., Somogyi, P. and Cuello, A. C. (1981). Neurotransmitter specific projection neurons revealed by combining PAP immunohistochemistry with retrograde transport of HRP. *Brain Res.*, 220, 231–240

Priestley, J. V. and Cuello, A. C. (1982). Electron microscopic immunocytochemistry: CNS transmitters and transmitter markers. In *IBRO Handbook Methods in the Neurosciences: Immunohistochemistry* (ed. A. C. Cuello), Wiley, Chichester, UK, in press

Salpeter, M. M., Bachmann, L. and Salpeter, E. E. (1969). Resolution in electron-microscopic radioautography. *J. Cell Biol.*, 41, 1–20

Sar, M., Stumpf, W. C., Miller, R. J., Chang, K.-J. and Cuatrecasas, P. (1978). Immunohistochemical localisation of enkephalin in rat brain and spinal cord. *J. comp. Neurol.*, 182, 17–38

Sofroniew, M. V. (1979). Immunoreactive β-endorphin and ACTH in the same neuron of the hypothalamic arcuate nucleus in the rat. *Am. J. Anat.*, 154, 283–288

Sofroniew, M. V., and Schrell, U. (1981). Evidence for a direct projection from vasopressin neurons in the hypothalamic paraventricular nucleus to the medulla oblongata: immunohistochemical visualization of both the horseradish peroxidase transported and the peptide produced by the same neurons. *Neurosci. Lett.*, 22, 211–217

Snyder, S. H. (1980). Peptide neurotransmitters with possible involvements in pain perception. In *Pain: Association for Research in Nervous and Mental Disease* 58, (ed. J. J. Bonica), Raven Press, New York, pp. 233–243

Steinbush, J. W. M. (1981). Distribution of serotonin-immunoreactivity in the central nervous system of the rat-cell bodies and terminals. *Neuroscience*, 6, 557–618

Sterngerger, L. A. (1979). *Immunocytochemistry*. Second edition, Wiley, Chichester, UK.

Tramu, G., Pillez, A. and Leonardelli, J. (1978). An efficient method of antibody elution for the successive or simultaneous localization of two antigens by immunocytochemistry. *J. Histochem. Cytochem.*, **26**, 322–324

Tranzer, J. P. (1972). A new amine storing compartment in adrenergic axons. *Nature New Biol.*, **237**, 57–58

Uhl, G. R., Goodman, R. R. and Snyder, S. H. (1979). Neurotensin-containing cell bodies, fibres and nerve terminals in the brain stem of the rat: immunohistochemical mapping. *Brain Res.*, **167**, 77–91

Van der Kooy, D., Hunt, S. P., Steinbusch, H. W. M. and Verhofstad, A. J. (1981). Separate populations of cholecystokinin and 5-hydroxytryptamine-containing neuronal cells in the dorsal raphe, and their contribution to the ascending raphe projections. *Neurosci. Lett.*, **26**, 25–30

Vandesande, F., Dierickx, K. and DeMey, J. (1977). The origin of the vasopressinergic and oxytocinergic fibres of the external regions of the median eminence of the rat hypothalamus. *Cell Tiss. Res.*, **180**, 443–452

# 8

# Coexistence of monoamines in peripheral adrenergic neurones

Guillermo Jaim-Etcheverry and Luis Maria Zieher (Instituto de Biologia
Celular, Facultad de Medicina, Paraguay 2155, 1121 Buenos
Aires, Argentina)

## INTRODUCTION

The suggestion that we made in 1968 that noradrenaline and serotonin (5-hydroxy-tryptamine) were not only present in the same sympathetic fibres innervating the pineal gland of the rat but might also coexist in their storage vesicles (Jaim-Etcheverry and Zieher, 1968b), was received with skepticism and regarded as a curiosity of nature. However, since then the possibility of the coexistence of putative transmitters in neurones has been more seriously considered and experimental evidence supporting that mechanism accumulated over the years. Such data, in addition to its theoretical implications, have been the subject of several review articles and commentaries (Burnstock, 1976, 1978; Osborne, 1979, 1981; Dismukes, 1979). Nowadays, mainly due to the explosive growth of our knowledge about the localisation of various peptides both in the CNS and in the periphery, the coexistence in neurones of several molecules active in cellular communication, is considered to represent an important mechanism in the regulation of that process (Hökfelt et al., 1980a and b). The articles gathered in this volume bear witness to the profound changes that took place in the ideas that prevailed not long ago.

The evidence obtained from the study of several experimental systems favouring the coexistence hypothesis, is thoroughly analysed in the various chapters of this book. Therefore, it is our purpose to briefly describe the evolution of the investigations carried out in our laboratory on the coexistence of monoamines in peripheral sympathetic neurones since this exemplifies a

189

mechanism somewhat different to that resulting in the coexistence described in other systems. As will be seen, although much indirect evidence has been obtained during the past decade in favour of the proposed mechanism of amine coexistence, our ultimate goal, to demonstrate that a single nerve vesicle contains more than one active substance, remains as feasible as it looked at the onset of these investigations.

## ULTRASTRUCTURAL LOCALISATION OF MONOAMINES IN PINEAL SYMPATHETIC NERVES

The pineal gland of the rat is richly innervated by sympathetic fibres, terminal arborisations of noradrenergic neurones which have their cell bodies in the superior cervical ganglia (Ariëns Kappers, 1960). These sympathetic nerves contain noradrenaline (NA), and several histochemical, pharmacological and biochemical studies have shown that they also store serotonin. Although the adrenergic nerves have the enzymatic machinery responsible for NA synthesis, they take up serotonin from the surrounding medium. As shown in figure 8.1, serotonin is present in the parenchymal cells of the gland where it serves as the precursor for melatonin synthesis or is deaminated by monoamine oxidase. Part of the serotonin, however, leaves the pinealocyte and is taken up by sympathetic nerves. This is due to the relative unspecificity of the process of NA re-uptake that takes place physiologically all along the membrane of these endings, thus making them unique in that they store NA and serotonin (Pellegrino de Iraldi *et al.*, 1963, 1965; Bertler *et al.*, 1964; Owman, 1964; Neff *et al.*, 1969).

The presence of two monoamines within a single type of nerve terminal provided a good experimental system to analyse the nature of the mechanisms responsible for their storage. Ultrastructural studies had shown that the osmiophilic cores present in the synaptic vesicles, characteristic of sympathetic nerve endings were the morphological correlates of the presence of NA in these vesicles (Pellegrino de Iraldi and De Robertis, 1961; Grillo, 1966; Hökfelt, 1968). However, little was known about the storage sites of serotonin in pineal nerves.

In 1967, Wood described a cytochemical procedure that differentiated catecholamines from serotonin under the light microscope. Since this method could help to elucidate the nature of the serotonin storage sites in pineal nerves, we undertook a study of its specificity at the ultrastructural level using isolated rabbit blood platelets as a test system. In these experiments, monoamine stores in the platelets were pharmacologically manipulated and the changes in the levels of these compounds as well as in the ultrastructure of the platelets, were analysed. Whereas fixation with glutaraldehyde before treatment with potassium dichromate (GD reaction) demonstrated cellular sites containing both catecholamines and serotonin, the fixation of the tissues with formaldehyde before treatment with glutaraldehyde and dichromate (FGD reaction), selectively revealed serotonin-containing sites (Jaim-Etcheverry and Zieher, 1968*a*).

Having characterised the specificities of the cytochemical procedures at the

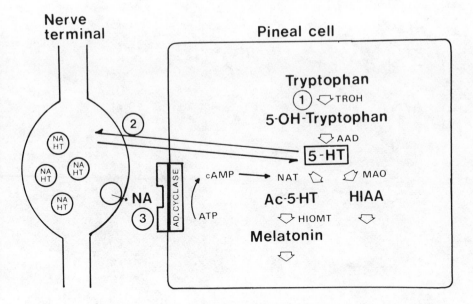

Figure 8.1 Diagram showing the metabolic relationship between parenchymal cells and adrenergic nerve terminals in the pineal gland of the rat. In the pinealocytes, the pathway of indole metabolism is described. Tryptophan, incorporated from the circulation, is converted by tryptophan-hydroxylase (TROH) into 5-OH-tryptophan which is decarboxylated to serotonin (5-HT) by aromatic-L-amino acid decarboxylase (AAD). Serotonin can be N-acetylated by N-acetyltransferase (NAT) to N-acetyl-serotonin which is converted by hydroxyindole-O-methyl transferase (HIOMT) to melatonin which then leaves pineal cells. Serotonin can also be metabolised to 5-hydroxyl-indoleacetic acid (HIAA) by monoamine oxidase (MAO) or, alternatively, leave the pineal cell and be taken up by the adrenergic nerve terminals where it is stored in vesicles apparently with noradrenaline (NA). When NA is released it acts on a $\beta$-adrenergic receptor in the membrane of the pinealocyte which activates adenylate cyclase that converts adenosine triphosphate to cyclic AMP; this activates NAT. The numbers in circles show the site of action of compounds used in the experiments described in the text which act on the synthesis of serotonin (1), its uptake by nerve terminals (2) and the $\beta$-adrenergic receptor (3).

ultrastructural level, these methods were applied to the pineal gland and other structures in an attempt to localise the amines stored in the sympathetic fibres innervating these organs. Conventional procedures had shown that sympathetic nerves have a mixed population of vesicles characterised by an osmiophilic content: small (400–600 Å in diameter) and large (800–1000 Å in diameter) granular vesicles (figure 8.2*a*) (see Jaim-Etcheverry and Zieher, 1971*a*). In pineal nerves, reactive sites corresponding to the dense cores of both small and large vesicles were observed after processing the tissue with the GD as well as with the FGD methods (figure 8.2*b*). This confirmed that serotonin in pineal sympathetic fibres was localised in the cores of both types of vesicles. On the contrary, in the fibres innervating the vas deferens, a positive reaction

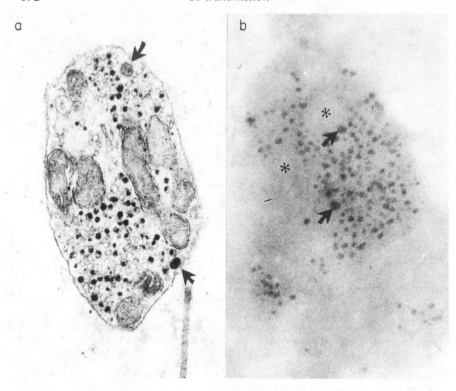

Figure 8.2 Electron micrographs of adrenergic nerve terminals in the perivascular space of the pineal gland of normal rats. In a, the tissue has been conventionally processed with aldehyde fixation, followed by osmium tetroxide and lead staining of the thin section. Apart from mitochondria, small dense-cored vesicles are observed as well as some larger vesicles (arrows) also containing a dense core. (× 50,000). In b, the tissue was processed with the formaldehyde-glutaraldehyde-dichromate sequence for the demonstration of serotonin storage sites. Small and large deposits corresponding to the cores observed in small and large (arrows) granular vesicles as well as the negative image of mitochondria (asterisk) are observed. (× 60,000.)

was only observed when the tissue was processed according to the GD sequence and not after prefixation with formaldehyde, confirming the presence of catecholamines but not of serotonin in the vesicles of these nerves (Jaim-Etcheverry and Zieher, 1968b, 1974; Pellegrino de Iraldi *et al.*, 1971).

At that time, we were also investigating the ultrastructural localisation of serotonin in some endocrine cells belonging to the APUD system described by Pearse (1969). The beta cells of the endocrine pancreas of the guinea-pig and the C cells of the thyroid gland of the sheep, normally contain serotonin in addition to the peptide hormone that they synthesize, insulin and thyrocalcitonin respectively. By combining pharmacological treatments with ultrastructural cytochemistry and biochemical determinations of the concentration of monoamines, it was shown that in these cells serotonin is stored in the same granules which contain the hormone that they produce, results that were later confirmed by using other experimental approaches (Jaim-Etcheverry and Zieher, 1968*c, d*).

Apart from its significance for the interpretation of the process of peptide hormone storage in endocrine cells, the observation of the coexistence of two active molecules, a polypeptide and a monoamine, in the same storage structure, strengthened the possibility that NA and serotonin found in pineal nerves were in fact present in the same storage vesicle. Such a mechanism of amine storage had been previously suggested on the basis of the distribution of reactive sites in the endings since all electron micrographs consistently showed that almost all the surface of pineal nerve terminals was occupied by cores reacting with the procedure revealing serotonin storage sites (Jaim-Etcheverry and Zieher, 1968*b*). These leads prompted the initiation in 1968 of a series of studies aimed at the experimental analysis of the coexistence hypothesis.

## SEROTONIN UPTAKE AS A GENERAL PROPERTY OF PERIPHERAL SYMPATHETIC FIBRES

Are pineal sympathetic nerves unique in their ability to store serotonin? Can other adrenergic terminals, when exposed to concentrations of serotonin similar to those found in the pineal, incorporate the amine into their vesicles? These were the questions that we attempted to answer in a series of studies that we have performed using the rat vas deferens as an experimental model. At that time it was known that the adrenergic nerves of the rat vas deferens could take up exogenous serotonin given in tracer doses (Taxi and Droz, 1966; Eccleston *et al.*, 1968; Taxi, 1969; Thoa *et al.*, 1969). We were, however, interested in establishing if the presence of serotonin around these adrenergic terminals could convert them into fibres "cytochemically" identical to those of the pineal, that is, containing cytochemically demonstrable serotonin in their vesicles.

The initial attempts to show the presence of serotonin in the nerves of the vas deferens by cytochemistry after injecting serotonin into the rats, failed even after using high doses of the exogenous amine. However, if the nerves were depleted of their NA, the same dose of serotonin that did not produce serotonin-positive cores in intact endings, could replenish the empty vesicles (Jaim-Etcheverry and Zieher, 1969*a*). Thus, we assumed that both the nerve terminal and its vesicles, were able to incorporate serotonin but that the concentration of the amine around the terminals achieved after its injection was insufficient to displace the endogenous transmitter from the vesicles in such a way as to make the content cytochemically positive for serotonin. To further explore this possibility, slices of vas deferens were incubated "*in vitro*" with increasing concentrations of serotonin. In these conditions, there was a concentration-dependent depletion of endogenous NA and, once a certain concentration of serotonin has been reached in the medium a positive cytochemical reaction was observed in the nerves (Zieher and Jaim-Etcheverry, 1971). Subcellular fractionation studies showed that in the microsomal fraction derived from vas deferens slices, the content of serotonin was increased whereas that of NA diminished after incubation in the presence of exogenous serotonin, changes that were directly related to the concentration of the amine in the medium (Zieher and Jaim-Etcheverry, 1971).

From these studies, it was concluded that not only pineal fibres but also other sympathetic nerves, when studied in conditions that mimic those found around the fibres innervating the pineal gland, have the ability to incorporate exogenous serotonin. The amine can gradually displace endogenous NA from the vesicles in a concentration-dependent manner and thus give a positive cytochemical reaction once it reaches a high intravesicular concentration.

## DEPLETION OF NEURONAL SEROTONIN FOR PROBING MONOAMINE COEXISTENCE IN PINEAL NERVES

In 1969 octopamine was identified as a naturally occurring amine in mammalian adrenergic nerves and the nature of the mechanisms responsible for its synthesis, storage and release, lead to the suggestion that it may serve as a "cotransmitter", a similar role to that proposed for serotonin in the pineal (Molinoff and Axelrod, 1969, 1972; Molinoff *et al.*, 1969). Since octopamine is present at a relatively high concentration in the pineal gland of the rat (Molinoff and Axelrod, 1972), its coexistence with the other amines in the vesicles was considered feasible. Pineal nerves would thus contain the neurotransmitter NA synthesised in them; octopamine also formed there due to the relative lack of specificity of the enzymes responsible for NA synthesis and serotonin, incorporated as a result of the lack of specificity of the NA uptake mechanism. The "co-transmitters", once in the axoplasm, can be incorporated by the vesicles and stored in them.

The experiments that we carried out during that period of our research, were based on the assumption that the depletion of serotonin from pineal nerves, would leave available storage space in the vesicles and that this could result in increased levels of pineal NA and octopamine. The concentration of serotonin in the gland was already known to change as a consequence of NA depletion (Zweig and Axelrod, 1969).

In an attempt to minimise the influence of other potential actions of the compounds used for lowering neuronal serotonin in the interpretation of the results, two entirely different methods were used to deplete serotonin from pineal nerves (Neff *et al.*, 1969). One was the administration of *p*-chlorophenyla-lanine (PCPA) that interferes with the synthesis of serotonin (Deguchi and Barchas, 1972). Since both the parenchymal and the neuronal compartments are in equilibrium, this procedure should result in the depletion of serotonin from the nerves (site 1 in figure 8.1). The other approach consisted of the injection of desmethylimipramine (DMI), a blocker of the NA re-uptake mechanism, at the level of the nerve terminal membrane. In this case, serotonin disappears from the nerves due to the blockade of its entry but is not depleted from the gland because its synthesis is not affected (site 2 in figure 8.1).

When pineal nerves of rats were examined cytochemically 24 h after the injection of either PCPA or DMI, it was found that the cores that normally react with the procedure revealing the presence of serotonin had disappeared. If the glands were processed with the method demonstrating catecholamines, the usual positive reaction was observed, confirming the effectiveness of both treatments to deplete neuronal serotonin (figure 8.3).

The content of NA and of octopamine markedly increased in the pineals of rats treated with PCPA or DMI (figure 8.4). This elevation was exclusively found in the pineal gland since none of the compounds modified the levels of NA and octopamine in the salivary glands which, like the pineal, receive their sympathetic innervation from the superior cervical ganglia (Jaim-Etcheverry and Zieher, 1971*b*, 1975*a*).

The fact that serotonin is transported into pineal adrenergic nerves by the same carrier responsible for NA re-uptake, has been recently confirmed. Whereas DMI blocks the NA transport system and increases NA levels in the pineal gland, fluoxetine, a specific inhibitor of the system responsible for serotonin uptake, does not affect pineal NA concentration (Fuller and Perry, 1977).

Thus, by using compounds depleting neuronal serotonin through two entirely different mechanisms, the concentration of NA and octopamine was markedly and selectively increased in the pineal gland. Apparently, then, as is schematically summarised in figure 8.5, due to the relative lack of specificity of the processes of NA synthesis and re-uptake, other molecules may be stored together with the neurotransmitter in the vesicles of adrenergic fibres.

But other substances apart from monoamines might be present in pineal nerves. Recent studies have identified several peptides coexisting with NA in the cell bodies of some sympathetic neurones in peripheral ganglia. Thus, somatostatin-like and enkephalin-like peptides have been demonstrated in neurones of the superior cervical ganglia (Hökfelt *et al.*, 1977, 1980*a, b*; Schultzberg *et al.*, 1979). It is not yet known if the terminal portions of these neurones also contain the peptides present in the cell bodies. If this turns out to be the case, pineal nerves could thus contain these or other peptides in addition to the monoamines. A recent study has identified the presence of the vasoactive intestinal peptide (VIP) in pineal nerves of various species but not in those of the rat (Uddman *et al.*, 1980). Although little is yet known about the presence of peptides in peripheral nerves classically regarded as noradrenergic, it is possible that examples of this type of coexistence will be described in the future. The subcellular localisation of these peptides is unknown but since large dense-cored vesicles apparently contain a protein apart from the amine (Jaim-Etcheverry and Zieher, 1969*b*), they could be the site of peptide storage. Moreover, such a possibility is supported by the finding of peptides

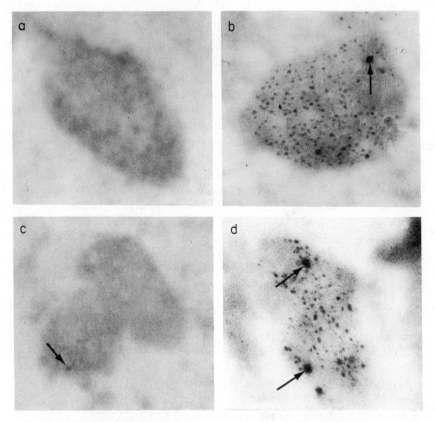

Figure 8.3 Sympathetic fibres in the perivascular space of the pineal gland from rats treated with PCPA (3 × 350 mg/kg intraperitoneally, 72 h) in *a* and *b* and with desmethyl-imipramine (20 mg/kg intraperitoneally 72 h) in *c* and *d*. Nerves in *a* and *c* correspond to pineals processed with the technique for the demonstration of serotonin reactive sites which in normal pineal shows precipitates of different sizes (see figure 8.2*b*). After both treatments, the reaction is negative, showing that they are effective in depleting serotonin. NA shown by the glutaraldehyde-dichromate reaction performed on the other half of the same glands (*b* and *d*), remains after both treatments. *a* and *b*, × 48,000; *c* and *d*, × 52,000. (From Jaim-Etcheverry and Zieher, 1971*b*, with permission.)

in large dense-cored vesicles in the central nervous system by immunocyto-chemistry (see Goldsmith, 1977; Hökfelt *et al.*, 1980*a, b*) as well as by the co-existence of polypeptides and monoamines in endocrine cells (Jaim-Etcheverry and Zieher, 1968*c, d*) where they are present in the same granule.

## MECHANISMS RESPONSIBLE FOR NA ELEVATION IN PINEAL NERVES AFTER DEPLETION OF NEURONAL SEROTONIN

Another aspect of the proposed mechanism of coexistence that we explored was the nature of the processes responsible for the increase of pineal NA follow-

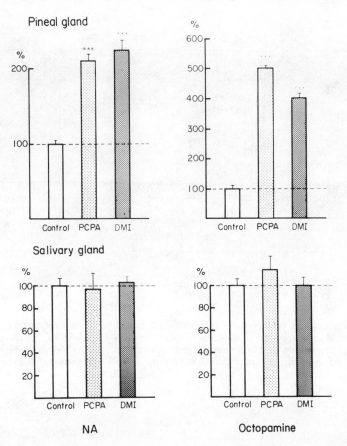

Figure 8.4 Changes in the content of NA and octopamine in the pineal and salivary glands of rats treated with PCPA and DMI as described in the legend to figure 8.3. Absolute control values (mean ± s.e.m.): pineal NA 4.34 ± 0.16 ng/pineal; octopamine 0.31 ± 0.03 ng/pineal. Salivary glands NA 1.60 ± 0.09 µg/g and octopamine 0.20 ± 0.01 µg/g. $P < 0.001$. (Data from Jaim-Etcheverry and Zieher, 1971*b*, 1975*a*.)

ing depletion of neuronal serotonin. The working hypothesis on which these studies were based is diagrammatically shown in figure 8.6. It was assumed that when serotonin disappears from the vesicles, extravesicular NA enters in the partially depleted vesicles. This would free tyrosine hydroxylase (TH) from the negative influence exerted by extravesicular NA on its activity (see Weiner, 1970; Weiner *et al.*, 1972). This would then increase until a new equilibrium is reached when the vesicles are filled with NA, resulting in the higher levels of NA found in the gland. The extravesicular accumulation of NA once the vesicles are filled, would turn the activity of TH off again.

As shown in figure 8.7, the experiments performed to analyse this possibility

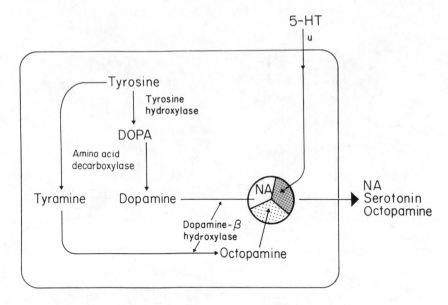

Figure 8.5  Diagram showing the processes that can lead to the storage of several mono-amines in the same vesicle in pineal adrenergic nerves. Whereas the lack of specificity of the re-uptake process (u) is responsible for the accumulation of serotonin in the terminal, the lack of specificity of the enzymes responsible for NA synthesis results in the formation of octopamine.

demonstrated that, after the injection of PCPA, the content of pineal serotonin decreased very rapidly while NA was gradually elevated. Concomitantly with this elevation, tyrosine hydroxylase activity determined in the intact gland, was maximally elevated 4 h after PCPA injection and returned to pretreatment levels at 6 h, a time at which NA was markedly elevated. Supporting the hypothesis on which these experiments were based, the results showed that the increased TH activity was not due to an increase in enzyme protein and it was unrelated to the depletion of pineal serotonin produced by PCPA. This elevation of tyrosine hydroxylase activity after PCPA was observed only in the pineal because, if anything, enzyme activity decreased in other sympathetically innervated organs such as the atria (Rubio *et al.*, 1977).

Thus, when serotonin concentration decreases in pineal nerves, tyrosine hydroxylase activity is enhanced until a new equilibrium is reached, a mechanism that most probably explains the selective increase observed in pineal NA in that situation.

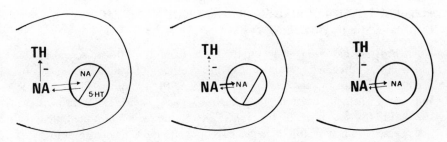

Figure 8.6 Diagram showing the possible changes that take place in a pineal terminal following depletion of neuronal serotonin. Whereas in normal conditions the activity of TH is negatively controlled by the concentration of extravesicular NA as in *a*, the loss of serotonin leaves storage space in the vesicles and results in the incorporation of NA into them, thus releasing TH from the negative control as in *b*. The new equilibrium is shown in *c*, where the vesicle is filled with NA and the extravesicular amine again controls TH activity.

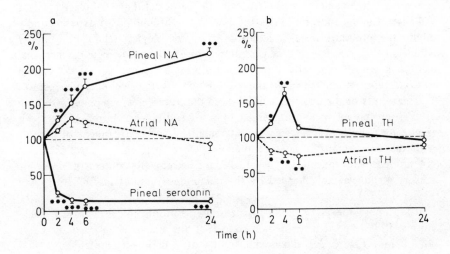

Time (h)

Figure 8.7 In *a*, changes in the content of NA in the pineal gland and in the atria and of serotonin in the pineal of rats injected with *p*-chlorophenylalanine 300 mg/kg intraperitonally at different times before killing. Absolute control values were (mean ± s.e.m.): pineal NA 14.47 ± 0.91 pmol/pineal; pineal serotonin 318.9 ± 11.91 pmol/pineal; atrial NA 7.41 ± 0.78 nmol/g. In *b*, changes in the activity of TH in the presence of 0.1 mM DMPH$_4$ in intact pineals of rats injected at different time intervals with PCPA as described in *a*. Absolute control values (mean ± s.e.m.) for TH activity: pineal 309 ± 20 d.p.m. DOPA formed/pineal/20 min; atria 8.76 ± 2.12 × 10$^3$ d.p.m. DOPA formed/g/20 min. *$P < 0.05$; **$P < 0.001$; ***$P < 0.001$ when compared with control values. (From Rubio *et al.*, 1977, with permission.)

## POSSIBLE PHYSIOLOGICAL SIGNIFICANCE OF MONOAMINE COEXISTENCE IN PINEAL NERVES

Much progress has been made on the understanding of the mechanisms by which pineal adrenergic nerves control the synthesis of indole compounds by parenchymal cells, mainly due to the efforts of the groups of Julius Axelrod and David Klein in Bethesda (see Axelrod, 1974; Klein, 1974; Brownstein, 1975). Briefly, as shown in figure 8.1, these studies demonstrated that the NA released from sympathetic nerves acts upon a $\beta$-adrenergic receptor localised in the membrane of the pinealocytes that in turn stimulates adenylate cyclase. The cyclic adenosine monophosphate formed, activates the enzyme $N$-acetyl-transferase that converts serotonin into $N$-acetyl-serotonin which serves as the substrate of hydroxyindole-$O$-methyl-transferase to form melatonin. Through this mechanism, adrenergic stimulation causes an important reduction in the content of serotonin in the gland.

Up to this point, we had studied the changes in pineal NA in situations in which serotonin was depleted by non-physiological procedures such as the interference with its synthesis or with its incorporation by the adrenergic nerves. Although we could assume that the changes observed had their physiological counterpart in the elevation of NA levels in the pineal that take place at night when serotonin concentration is the lowest, we attempted to experimentally mimic the processes brought about by the physiological stimulation of the adrenergic receptor. By injecting isoproterenol we sought to deplete parenchymal serotonin and subsequently its neuronal stores, by enhancing its conversion to $N$-acetyl-serotonin through the stimulation of the $\beta$-adrenergic receptor.

The results of these experiments showed that the decrease in pineal serotonin after isoproterenol was accompanied by a marked increase in pineal NA levels (figure 8.8). Both changes were counteracted by the pretreatment of the rats with the adrenergic $\beta$-blocker propranolol. Once again, the changes in pineal NA produced by isoproterenol were selective because the content of NA in the salivary gland was not changed by the compounds used (Jaim-Etcheverry and Zieher, 1975$b$).

To propose the participation of neuronal serotonin in phsyiological mechanisms, it is important to demonstrate that the amine is released by nerve stimulation. Figure 3.9 shows the results of experiments initiated in 1969 that we have recently concluded, indicating that when the preganglionic nerves to both superior cervical ganglia were electrically stimulated, the reactive cores characteristic of pineal nerve vesicles almost totally disappear from the small vesicles but remain in the larger ones. Cores reacting cytochemically for serotonin as well as those giving a positive reaction for NA were depleted by stimulation (Jaim-Etcheverry and Zieher, 1980$a$).

Thus, both the transmitter and the "co-transmitter", seem to be released by nerve impulses, a finding consistent with the hypothesis that they are stored together within nerve vesicles. The analysis of this experimental situation, which

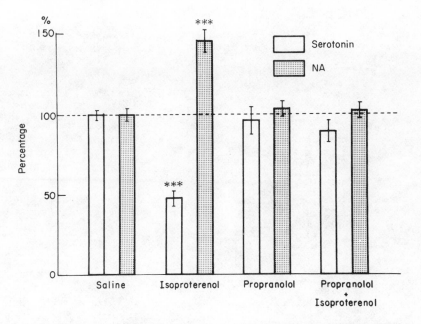

Figure 8.8 Changes in the content of serotonin and NA in the pineal gland of rats injected with isoproterenol (15 mg/kg intraperitoneally, 8 h; 10 mg/kg, 4.5 h and 2 h before killing), propranolol (3 × 30 mg/kg intraperitoneally either alone or 30 min before isoproterenol). Absolute control values were (mean ± s.e.m.): serotonin 329 ± 9.62 pmol/pineal; NA 26.07 ± 1.10 pmol/pineal. ***$P < 0.001$ when compared with control values. (From Jaim-Etcheverry and Zieher, 1975*b*, with permission.)

is being currently pursued in our laboratory, is providing interesting clues with respect to the process of recovery of synaptic vesicles after nerve stimulation (Jaim-Etcheverry and Zieher, 1980*b*).

On the basis of the evidence so far accumulated, we have suggested that the presence of serotonin in pineal nerves could provide an efficient mechanism for the regulation of the control exerted by pineal adrenergic nerves on indole metabolism in the parenchyma (Jaim-Etcheverry and Zieher, 1974, 1975*b*; Rubio *et al.*, 1977). During the day, when levels of serotonin are higher and those of NA lower than at night, the release of the content of the nerve vesicles, could result in a reduced stimulation of the adrenergic receptor. At night, due to the increased firing of noradrenergic neurones and to the supersensitivity developed in the β-adrenergic receptors, the conversion of serotonin to melatonin is enhanced. This decreases serotonin in the pinealocytes as well as in the nerves and, as a consequence, tyrosine hydroxylase activity is enhanced and pineal NA increased. All these changes have been reported to occur in physiological conditions. In this manner, amine coexistence could provide a mechanism for dampening the effects of nerve activity during the day through

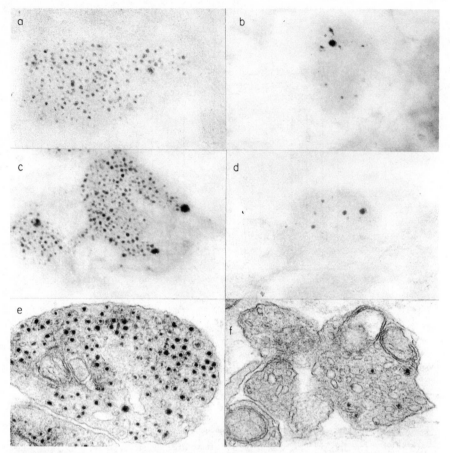

Figure 8.9 Sympathetic nerve endings in the pineal gland of the rat. The nerves in *a, c* and *e*, correspond to sham-stimulated animals, whereas those in *b, d* and *f* corresponds to rats in which both preganglionic trunks to the superior cervical ganglia were electrically stimulated with square pulses (25 Hz, 1 ms duration, 20 min, supramaximal voltage). Tissue in *a* and *b* (× 50.000) was processed with the cytochemical procedure for the demonstration of serotonin; pineals in *c* (× 52,000) and *d* (× 60,000), were processed with glutaraldehyde-dichromate for the demonstration of catecholamines and indoleamines while glands in *e* (× 52,000) and *f* (× 60,000) were fixed with aldehyde before dichromate treatment, osmium tetroxide fixation and lead staining of the thin sections. Note that nerve stimulation almost completely depletes small serotonin reacting cores as well as similar catecholamine reactive sites, leaving unaffected the sites corresponding to the cores of large vesicles. In conventionally processed tissue, the cores have also disappeared from small vesicles but remain in the larger ones. Note the change in size and shape of stimulated vesicles in *f*. (From Jaim-Etcheverry and Zieher, 1980*a*, with permission.)

a local feedback loop. In this scheme, it is not necessary to postulate direct or indirect effects of the "co-transmitter' or modulator serotonin on post-synaptic receptors because it could act by simply modifying the amount of NA released by the nerve impulse.

## EXCHANGE OF SIGNALING MOLECULES BETWEEN NEURONES AS A POSSIBLE MODULATORY MECHANISM OF SYNAPTIC TRANSMISSION

Some years ago we suggested that the described mechanism of coexistence might also modulate synaptic communication in the CNS (Jaim-Etcheverry and Zieher, 1974; Bloom, 1974). Central catecholamine containing neurones have the capacity to take up exogenous serotonin (Lichtensteiger *et al.*, 1967) whereas serotonergic neurones can incorporate catecholamines (Barrett and Balch, 1971). The phenomena results from the relative lack of specificity of monoamine re-uptake processes in central monoaminergic neurones, similar to that described in the periphery (Shaskan and Snyder, 1970). This situation might also take place in physiological conditions and, for example, noradrenergic terminals impinging upon serotonergic cell bodies or dendrites, could take up serotonin if the amine released from these sites (figure 8.10*a*). Alternatively, serotonin could diffuse from its sites or release and be taken up by noradrenergic endings present in their vicinity (figure 8.10*b*). In both cases,

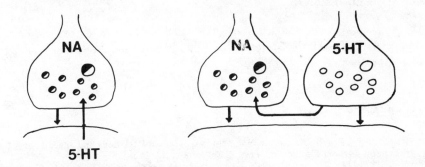

Figure 8.10 Diagrammatic representation of the suggested interactions between a serotonin (5-HT) containing cell body or dendrite and a noradrenergic ending impinging upon them (*a*) or between two neighbouring terminals containing NA and 5-HT respectively (*b*).

the net effect of noradrenergic nerve activity could be markedly modified through this mechanism. Since active molecules achieve very high concentrations at their sites of release, their "non-specific" uptake by other endings in the vicinity of these sites is not so improbable and the exchange of these molecules between neighbouring terminals could be a much more common phenomenon than is generally assumed. The dendritic release of active molecules as well as the non-synaptic liberation of monoamines, possibilities that are being increasingly considered (see Cuello and Iversen, 1978; Dismukes, 1979; Osborne, 1981), could provide the missing links in the chain of events participating in this form of modulation of synaptic communication.

The one described would constitute a special case for co-transmission that does not require the presence of the enzymatic machinery necessary for the synthesis of all the active molecules found in a given ending. This type of coexistence results from the peculiar anatomical and biochemical milieu surrounding a given terminal. Therefore, different endings of the same neurone would not necessarily contain similar active molecules. Moreover, even the molecular signaling system of a given ending, may change with time, depending on the activities of the surrounding neuronal elements.

This brief overview of more than a decade of research into the problem of amine coexistence in peripheral adrenergic neurones as well as the contemporary developments in the field, support the statement made by Geoffrey Burnstock (1978) in a recent review: ". . . there must be many different ways to solve the problems of nervous communication in the body at pre- as well as post-junctional levels and we would be in error to close our minds to these possibilities, even if it means challenging the earlier hypotheses that provide such valuable leads in the study of the nervous system".

## ACKNOWLEDGEMENTS

The original work on which this article is based has been supported by grants from CONICET, SECYT, Secretaria de Salud Pública, and the Cargill Foundation, Argentina.

## REFERENCES

Ariëns Kappers, J. (1960). The development, topographical relations and innervation of the epiphysis cerebri in the albino rat. *Z. Zellforsch.*, **52**, 163-215

Axelrod, J. (1974). The pineal gland: a neurochemical transducer. *Science*, **184**, 699-714

Barrett, R. E. and Balch, T. St. (1971). Uptake of catecholamines into serotonergic nerve cells as demonstrated by fluorescence histochemistry. *Experientia*, **27**, 633-4

Bertler, A. B., Falck, B. and Owman, C. (1964). Studies on 5-hydroxytryptamine stores in pineal gland of the rat. *Acta physiol. Scand.*, **63**, Suppl., 239

Bloom, F. E. (1974). Dynamics of synaptic modulation: perspectives for the future. In *The Neurosciences: Third Study Program*, (ed. F. O. Schmitt and F. G. Worden), MIT Press, Cambridge, Mass achusetts, p. 989

Brownstein, M. (1975). The pineal gland. *Life Sci.*, **16**, 1363-74

Burnstock, G. (1976). Do some nerve cells release more than one transmitter? *Neuroscience*, **1**, 239-48

Burnstock, G. (1978). Do some sympathetic neurones synthesize and release both noradrenaline and acetylcholine? *Progr. Neurobiol.*, **11**, 205-22

Cuello, A. C. and Iversen, L. L. (1978). Interactions of dopamine with other neurotransmitters in the rat substantiz nigra. A possible functional role for dendritic dopamine. In *Interactions between Putative Transmitters in the Brain*, (ed. S. Garattini, J. F. Pujol and R. Samamin), Raven Press, New York, pp. 127-49

Deguchi, T. and Barchas, J. (1972). Effect of p-chlorophenylalanine on hydroxylation of tryptohpan in pineal and brain of rats. *Molec. Pharmac.*, **8**, 770-9

Dismukes, R. K. (1979). New concepts of molecular communication among neurons. *Behav. Brain Sci.*, **2**, 409-48

Eccleston, D., Thoa, N. B. and Axelrod, J. (1968). Inhibition by drugs of the accumulation in vitro of 5-hydroxytryptamine in guinea pig vas deferens. *Nature Lond.*, **217**, 846-7

Fuller, R. W. and Perry, K. W. (1977). Increase of pineal noradrenaline concentration in rats by desipramine but not fluoxetine: implications concerning the specificity of these uptake inhibitors. *J. Pharm. Pharmac.*, 29, 710–11

Goldsmith, P. C. (1977). Ultrastructural localization of some hypothalamic hormones. *Fedn. Proc.*, 36, 1968–72

Grillo, M. A. (1966). Electron microscopy of sympathetic tissues. *Pharmac. Rev.*, 19, 387–99

Hökfelt, T. (1968). In vitro studies on central and peripheral monamine neurons at the ultrastructural level. *Z. Zellforsch.*, 91, 1–74

Hökfelt, T., Elfvin, L. G., Elde, R., Schiltzberg, M., Goldstein, M. and Luft, R. (1977). Occurrence of somatostatin-like immunoreactivity in some peripheral sympathetic noradrenergic neurons. *Proc. natn. Acad. Sci. U.S.A.*, 74, 3597–91

Hökfelt, T., Johansson, O., Ljungdahl, A., Lundberg, J. M. and Schultzberg, M. (1980a). Peptidergic neurones. *Nature Lond.*, 284, 515–21

Hökfelt, T., Lundberg, J. M., Schultzberg, M., Johansson, O., Ljungdahl, A. and Rehfeld, J. (1980b). Coexistence of peptides and putative transmitters in neurons. In *Neural Peptides and Neuronal Communication* (ed. E. Costa and M. Trabucchi), Raven Press, New York, p. 1

Jaim-Etcheverry, G. and Zieher, L. M. (1968a). Cytochemistry of 5-hydroxytryptamine at the electron microscope level. Study of the specificity of the reaction in isolated blood platelets. *J. Histochem. Cytochem.*, 16, 162–71

Jaim-Etcheverry, G. and Zieher, L. M. (1968b). Cytochemistry of 5-hydroxytryptamine at the electron microscope level. II. Localization in the autonomic nerves of rat pineal gland. *Z. Zellforsch.*, 86, 393–400

Jaim-Etcheverry, G. and Zieher, L. M. (1968c). Electron microscopic cytochemistry of 5-hydroxytryptamine (5-HT) in the beta cells of guinea pig endocrine pancreas. *Endocrinol*, 83, 917–23

Jaim-Etcheverry, G. and Zieher, L. M. (1968d). Cytochemical localization of monoamine stores in sheep thyroid gland at the electron microscope level. *Experientia*, 24, 593–5

Jaim-Etcheverry, G. and Zieher, L. M. (1969a). Ultrastructural cytochemistry and pharmacology of 5-hydroxytryptamine in adrenergic nerve endings. II. Localization of exogenous 5-hydroxytryptamine in the autonomic nerves of the rat vas deferens. *J. Pharmac. exp. Ther.*, 166, 264–71

Jaim-Etcheverry, G. and Zieher, L. M. (1969b). Selective demonstration of a type of synaptic vesicle by phosphotungstic acid staining. *J. cell Biol.* 42, 855–60

Jaim-Etcheverry, G. and Zieher, L. M. (1971a). Ultrastructural aspects of neurotransmitter storage in adrenergic nerves. *Adv. Cytopharmac.*, 1, 343–61

Jaim-Etcheverry, G. and Zieher, L. M. (1971b). Ultrastructural cytochemistry and pharmacology of 5-hydroxytryptamine in adrenergic nerve endings. III. Selective increase of norepinephrine in the rat pineal gland consecutive to depletion of neuronal 5-hydroxytryptamine. *J. Pharmac. exp. Ther.*, 178, 42–8

Jaim-Etcheverry, G. and Zieher, L. M. (1974). Localizing serotonin in central and peripheral nerves. In *The Neurosciences: Third Study Program* (ed. F. O. Schmitt and F. G. Worden), MIT Press, Cambridge, Massachusetts, p. 917

Jaim-Etcheverry, G. and Zieher, L. M. (1975a). Octopamine probably coexists with noradrenaline and serotonin in vesicles of pineal adrenergic nerves. *J. Neurochem.*, 25, 915–17

Jaim-Etcheverry, G. and Zieher, L. M. (1975b). Stimulation of beta-adrenergic receptors in the pineal gland increases the noradrenaline stores of its sympathetic nerves. *Naunyn Schmied. Arch. Pharmac.*, 290, 425–31

Jaim-Etcheverry, G. and Zieher, L. M. (1980a). Stimulation-depletion of serotonin and noradrenaline from vesicles of sympathetic nerves in the pineal gland of the rat. *Cell Tissue Res.*, 207, 13–20

Jaim-Etcheverry, G. and Zieher, L. M. (1980b). Stimulation depletes serotonin and noradrenaline from vesicles of pineal sympathetic nerves. *Soc. Neurosci. Abstr.*, 6, 445

Klein, D. J. (1974). Circadian rhythms in indole metabolism in the rat pineal gland. In *The Neurosciences: Third Study Program* (ed. F. O. Schmitt and F. G. Worden), MIT Press, Cambridge, Massachusetts, p. 509

Lichtensteiger, W., Mutzner, U. and Langemann, H. (1967). Uptake of 5-hydroxytryptamine and 5-hydroxytryptophan by neurons of the central nervous system normally containing catecholamines. *J. Neurochem.*, 14, 489–97

Molinoff, P. B. and Axelrod, J. (1969). Octopamine: normal occurrence in sympathetic nerves of rats. *Science*, **164**, 428–9

Molinoff, P. B. and Axelrod, J. (1972). Distribution and turnover of octopamine in tissues. *J. Neurochem.*, **19**, 157–63

Molinoff, P. B., Landsberg, L. and Axelrod, J. (1969). An enzymatic assay for octopamine and other beta-hydroxylated phenylethylamines. *J. Pharmac. exp. Ther.*, **170**, 253–61

Neff, N. H., Barrett, R. E. and Costa, E. (1969). Kinetic and fluorescent histochemical analysis of the serotonin compartments in rat pineal gland. *Eur. J. Pharmac.* **5**, 348–56

Osborne, N. N. (1979). Is Dale's principle valid? *Trends Neurosci.*, **2**, 73–5

Osborne, N. N. (1981). Communication between neurones: current concepts. *Neurochem. Internat.*, **3**, 3–16

Owman, C. (1964). Sympathetic nerves probably storing two types of monoamines in the rat pineal gland. *Int. J. Neuropharmac.*, **2**, 105–12

Pearse, A. G. E. (1969). The cytochemistry and ultrastructure of polypeptide hormone producing cells of the APUD series and the embryologic, physiologic and pathologic implications of the concept. *J. Histochem. Cytochem.*, **17**, 303–13

Pellegrino de Iraldi, A. and De Robertis, E. (1961). Action of reserpine on the submicroscopic morphology of the pineal gland. *Experientia*, **17**, 122–3

Pellegrino de Iraldi, A., Gueudet, R. and Suburo, A. M. (1971). Differentiation between 5-hydroxytryptamine and catecholamines in synaptic vesicles. *Progr. Brain. Res.*, **34**, 161–70

Pellergrino de Iraldi, A., Zieher, L. M. and De Robertis, E. (1963). 5-hydroxytryptamine content and synthesis of normal and denervated pineal gland. *Life Sci.*, **1**, 691–6

Pellegrino de Iraldi, A., Zieher, L. M. and De Robertis, E. (1965). Ultrastructural and pharmacological studies of nerve endings of the pineal gland. *Progr. Brain Res.*, **10**, 389–421

Rubio, M. C., Jaim-Etcheverry, G. and Zieher, L. M. (1977). Tyrosine hydroxylase activity increases in adrenal sympathetic nerves after depletion of neuronal serotonin. *Naunyn Schmied. Arch. Pharmac.*, **301**, 75–8

Schultzberg, M., Hökfelt, T., Terenius, L., Elfvin, L. G., Lundberg, J. M., Brandt, J., Elde, R. P. and Goldstein, M. (1979). Enkephalin immunoreactive nerve fibres and cell bodies in sympathetic ganglia of the guinea-pig and rat. *Neuroscience*, **4**, 249–70

Shaskan, E. G. and Snyder, S. H. (1970). Kinetics of serotonin accumulation into slices from rat brain: relationship to catecholamine uptake. *J. Pharmac. exp. Ther.*, **175**, 404–18

Taxi, J. (1969). Morphological and cytochemical studies on the synapses in the autonomic nervous system. *Progr. Brain Res.*, **31**, 5–20

Taxi, J. and Droz, B. (1966). Etude de l'incorporation de noradrenaline-[3]H (NA-[3]H) et de 5-hydroxytryptophane-[3]H (5-HTP-[3]H) dans les fibres nerveuses du canal deferent et de l'intestin. *C. r. Hebd. Seances Acad. Sci. Paris*, **263**, 1237–40

Thoa, N. B., Eccleston, D. and Axelrod, J. (1969). The accumulation of C[14]-serotonin in the guinea-pig vas deferens. *J. Pharmac. exp. Ther.*, **169**, 68–73

Uddman, R., Alumets, J., Håkanson, R., Lorén, I. and Sundler, F. (1980). Vasoactive intestinal peptide (VIP) occurs in the nerves of the pineal gland. *Experientia*, **36**, 1119–20

Weiner, N. (1970). Regulation of norepineprine biosynthesis. *A. Rev. Pharmac.*, **10**, 273–90

Weiner, N., Cloutier, G., Bjur, R. and Pfeffer, R. I. (1972). Modification of norepinephrine synthesis in intact tissue by drugs and during short term adrenergic nerve stimulation. *Pharmac. Rev.*, **24**, 203–21

Wood, J. G. (1967). Cytochemical localization of 5-hydroxytryptamine (5-HT) in the central nervous system (CNS). *Anat. Rec.*, **157**, 343

Zieher, L. M. and Jaim-Etcheverry, G. (1971). Ultrastructural cytochemistry and pharmacology of 5-hydroxytryptamine in adrenergic nerve endings. II. Accumulation of 5-hydroxytryptamine in nerve vesicles containing norepinephrine in rat vas deferens. *J. Pharmac. exp. Ther.*, **178**, 30–41

Zweig, M. and Axelrod, J. (1969). Relationship between catecholamines and serotonin in sympathetic nerves of the rat pineal gland. *J. Neurobiol.* **1**, 87–97

# 9

# Coexistence of neurotransmitter substances in a specifically defined invertebrate neurone

Neville N. Osborne, (Nuffield Laboratory of Ophthalmology, University of Oxford, Oxford OX2 6AW, UK)

## INTRODUCTION

Whether some neurones utilise more than one neurotransmitter is a question which has attracted considerable attention in the past ten years (see Burnstock, 1976, 1978; Osborne, 1979, 1981). This interest was sparked off by biochemical studies on isolated invertebrate neurones (Brownstein *et al.*, 1974; Hanley *et al.*, 1974; Osborne, 1977), and also through the development of specific immuno-histochemical procedures to visualise transmitter-specific neurones (Chan-Palay *et al.*, 1978; Hökfelt *et al.*, 1977a,b, 1980 see also, chapters 1 and 4). Before this era it was generally accepted that each neurone had the ability to synthesise, store and release only one transmitter substance. This belief, widely known as Dale's principle, was based on a vast quantity of experimental data but was consistently questioned due to the lack of conclusive proof, for example, the cholingergic link in adrenergic transmission (Burn and Rand, 1965; Koelle, 1962).

One of the major reasons for the inability to test Dale's principle is the limited amount of suitable, practically amenable nervous systems where it is possible for the neurobiologist to discover the exact function(s) of substances specific to the neurone-type. In this respect certain invertebrate nervous systems (for example, gastropod molluscs) offer many advantages over the vertebrates (Osborne, 1974, 1980). Not only are the perikarya of gastropod nervous systems fewer and much larger than in a mammal, but the neurones can also overcome slight environmental changes which could prove disastrous to vertebrate cells. The neurones also retain their functional activity for several hours or even days.

In practice, the technical advantages of gastropod nervous systems enable workers to record from single identified neurones and their follower neurones and to test the effects of different substances on identified follower neurones and the synaptic connections. This makes it possible to detect transmitter release from single neurones. The large size of the neurones also allows the dissection and biochemical analysis of the cell. It is therefore possible to correlate bio-chemical, morphological and electrophysiological data on individually defined neurones, thus increasing the potential for discovering the transmitter(s) used by a neurone.

The purpose of this article is to gather and analyse the data which have been compiled about one particular giant neurone situated in each metacerebral ganglion of the gastropod CNS. This neurone, known as the giant serotonin cell (GSC), because it contains serotonin (5-hydroxytryptamine) (see Cottrell, 1977; Osborne and Neuhoff, 1980) was originally discovered by Kunze (1921) and noted for its large size and accessibility for electrophysiological studies by Kandel and Tauc (1966). The results would seem to suggest that the GSCs may indeed utilise more than one substance as a chemical messenger.

## MORPHOLOGY AND HISTOLOGY OF GSCs

The morphology and histology of the GSCs in pulmonate (for example, *Helix*, the garden snail) and opisthobranch (for example, *Aplysia*, Tritonia) molluscs have been subjected to intensive analysis (Cottrell, 1977; Osborne 1978; Weinreich *et al.*, 1973) and shown to be, in general, the same. The amine-fluorescence histochemical procedure (Falck and Owman 1965), revealed that each meta-cerebral ganglion of the snail (*Helix*) brain contained a large yellow fluorescing neurone (Osborne and Cottrell 1971a; Cottrell and Osborne, 1970), measuring about 120 μm across its major axis (figure 9.1). Subsequent electromicroscopical studies showed that the neurone's cytoplasm contains many dense-core vesicles together with large lysosome-like bodies (Cottrell and Osborne 1970; Osborne 1973a), as in figure 9.2. The vesicles have a mean diameter of about 100 nm, are present throughout the cell and have electron-dense cores in osmium-fixed tissue. These electron-dense deposits stained positively when tissues were pro-cessed by the method of Wood (1965, 1966) (figure 9.2) and prior injection of reserpine into animals greatly reduced the number of reactive granules in the GSCs. It was therefore concluded that serotonin is sequestered in the small granular vesicles.

The pathway taken by the axons of the GSC has been studied in depth by Pentreath *et al.* (1973). Injection of either procion yellow (Cottrell, 1971; Cottrell and Macon, 1974) or radiolabelled serotonin (Pentreath *et al.*, 1973) directly into the GSC somata of *Helix* followed by electrophysiology and/or autoradiography were the main procedures used to study the geometry and axonal branching of the neurone. It was found that the GSC had three main branches (see figure 9.3), with two of the branches apparently making contact

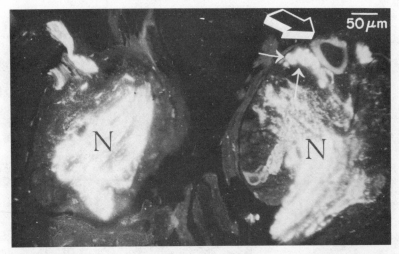

Figure 9.1 Section through the cerebral ganglia of *Helix* processed by formaldehyde histochemical method for localising monoamines. The GSC fluoresces yellow and can be seen clearly in one ganglion (arrow). Near the large neurone are a number of green-fluorescing dopamine cells (small arrows). A number of fluorescing terminals in the neuropile (N) is seen throughout both ganglia.

with three neurones situated in either buccal ganglion. Moreover, the autoradiographical data of Pentreath (1976) showed clearly that the radiolabelled serotonin was transported down the axons of the GSCs.

## EVIDENCE THAT THE GSC CONTAINS SEROTONIN

Although serotonin was identified in animal tissues in 1949 (Rapport) it was not until 1957 that Brodie and Shore (1957) suggested it could be a neurotransmitter substance. The evidence for serotonin being a neurotransmitter in various nervous systems is now accepted (see Osborne, 1982). The initial indication that the GSCs contained serotonin came from fluorescence-histochemical studies, as already mentioned, although confirmation of this had to await chromatographic analysis of isolated GSCs. Isolated GSCs were first homogenised, their extracts dansylated and the dansylated products fractionated by microchromatography (Osborne and Cottrell, 1971*b*; Osborne 1972). Serotonin was identified in the GSCs but was found to be absent from control cells which did not exhibit any amine-specific fluorescence (see figure 9.4).

It has been demonstrated that *Helix* GSCs also take up radiolabelled 5-hydroxytryptophan (5-HTP) (Pentreath and Cottrell, 1973) and convert it to serotonin, both *in vivo* (Osborne, 1972) and *in vitro* (Cottrell and Powell, 1971). In contrast, tryptophan is accumulated by nervous tissues of the snail in a nonselective manner (Osborne, 1973*b*; Pentreath and Cottrell, 1973); the GSCs, however, seem to have the specific capacity for metabolising it to form serotonin and 5-HTP (Osborne, 1973*b*). Pretreatment of snails with *p*-chlorophenylalanine,

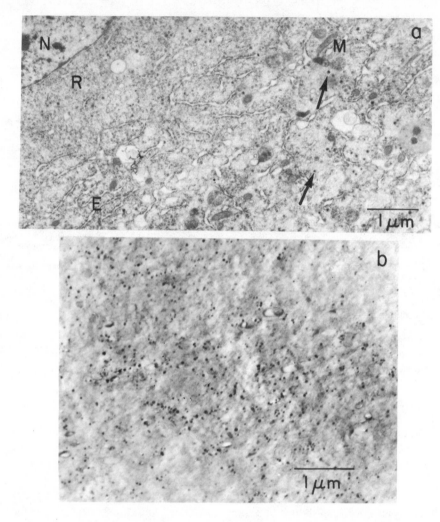

Figure 9.2 Electron micrograph showing the inclusion of the GSC cytoplasm *a*. N, nucleus; M, mitochondrion; E, endoplasmic reticulum; R, ribosomes. Arrows point to some dense-cored vesicles. A portion of the GSC cytoplasm processed by the method of Wood for the demonstration of amines is shown in *b*. There is a close agreement between the distribution and size of the reacting sites, which are the only electron-dense structures visible, and the distribution of vesicle cores shown in *a*.

which inhibits tryptophan hydroxylase (Koe and Weissmann, 1966), did not interfere with the uptake of tryptophan into the GSCs but prevented the formation of 5-HTP or serotonin (Osborne, 1973*b*). The enzyme tryptophan-hydroxylase (that is, the enzyme converting tryptophan to 5-HTP) is present in the GSCs and is the enzyme responsible for determining the rate of formation of serotonin.

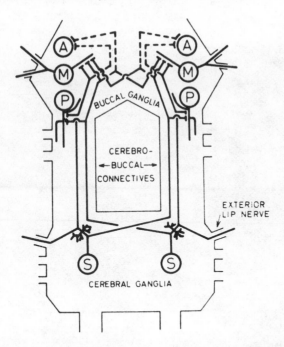

Figure 9.3 Diagrammatic representation of the cerebral and buccal ganglia of *Helix pomatia* showing the position of the GSCs and the neurones with which they make contact. The neurones in the buccal ganglia that receive synaptic input from the GSCs are called anterior (A), medial (M), and posterior (P) cells. None of the three giant buccal cells contains mono-amines as determined by fluorescence microscopy. The processes from the different cells were traced either by dye injection or by electrophysiological methods. GSCs are marked S. (After Cottrell, 1971.)

## EVIDENCE THAT SEROTONIN IS UTILISED AS A TRANSMITTER BY THE GSCs

There is impressive evidence supporting the opinion that the serotonin within the GSCs is used as a transmitter substance (see Cottrell, 1977; Osborne, 1978; Osborne and Neuhoff, 1980; Pentreath *et al.*, 1982). The cytochemical studies which implied that serotonin in the GSCs is situated in synaptic-type vesicles have already been discussed (see figure 9.3). These are corroborated by other studies which showed that when radioactive serotonin is injected directly into the GSCs it is rapidly taken up in the particulate form (vesicles?) and is thus transported from the cell body to the terminals (Schwartz, 1979; Goldman and Schwartz, 1974). Neurones that do not contain amine lack this capacity. The transport of radioactive serotonin along the axons of the GSCs is in the form of discrete peak followed by a relatively low smooth trail. Goldberg *et al.* (1976) concluded from their studies that the velocity of the serotonergic vesicles is positively dependent on the local concentration of vesicles.

**a**

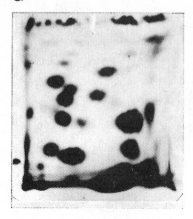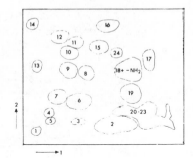

**b**

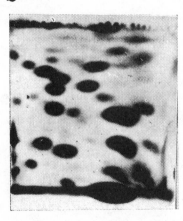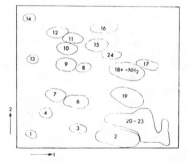

Figure 9.4 *a*, Autoradiograms of microchromatograms of extracts of GSCs from *Helix pomatia* which had been reacted with [$^{14}$C]-dansyl-chloride, developed in two solvent systems in order to separate most dansyl derivatives. The direction of chromatography is indicated by the arrows: first direction, water/formic acid (100:3); second direction, benzene/ acetic acid (9:1). Identification keys are presented to assist in the interpretation of dansyl derivatives on the microchromatograms: 1, starting point; 2, dansyl-OH; 3, N-tyrosine; 4, tryptophan; 5, unknown; 6, *bis*-ornithine; 7, *bis*-lysine; 8, methionine; 9, phenylalanine; 10, leucine; 11, isoleucine; 12, unknown; 13, *bis*-tyrosine; 14, 5-hydroxyindole; 15, valine; 16, proline; 17, ethanolamine; 18, alanine; 19, glycine; 20, glutamic acid; 21, aspartic acid; 22, glutamine, serine and threonine; 23, arginine, ε-lysine, cystine and α-amino-histidine; 24, γ-aminobutyric acid; 25, N-serotonin; 26, *bis*-serotonin; ?, 5-hydroxytryptophan.

*b*, Autoradiograms of microchromatograms from extracts of buccal neurones (posterior giant buccal cells) from *Helix pomatia* after having been reacted with [$^{14}$C]-dansyl-chloride and separated in two solvent systems. The spot numbers on the identification keys and the conditions of chromatography are as explained in *a*.

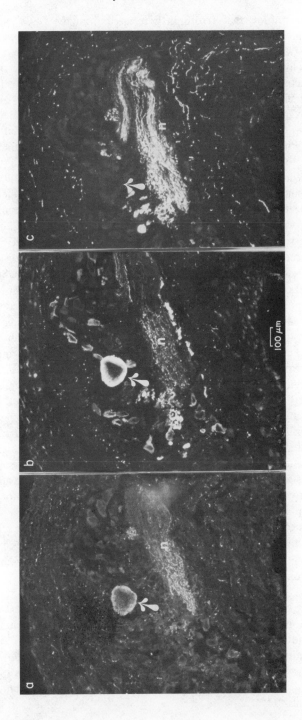

Figure 9.5 Series of consecutive sections taken through a single GSC (arrows): *a* processed for visualising serotonin; *b* for CCK; *c* for substance P. It can be seen that the cytoplasm of the GSC reacts positively for serotonin and CCK but not for substance P. Note that fibres in the neuropile (N) and other somata react positively for each of the substances. (For details see Osborne *et al.*, 1981.)

The demonstration that serotonin is released from the GSCs' endings and exerts an influence on the postsynaptic cell so that single impulses can continue between the two cells would be unambiguous proof that serotonin has a transmitter role. This has been achieved. Cottrell and collaborators have shown that the GSCs make monosynaptic contact with the middle buccal cells (see figure 2.3) in the snail CNS (Cottrell and Macon, 1974; Cottrell *et al.*, 1974; Cottrell, 1970). For example, when the GSC is made to evoke an action potential, individual e.p.s.p.s of 500–600 ms duration could be observed in both left and right buccal cells. With repetitive stimulation of the GSC, the e.p.s.p.s were facilitated to give rise to an action potential. Injection of the GSC with tetraethylammonium, which prolongs the action potential, increased the amplitude of the e.p.s.p.s (presumably by increasing transmitter release: Katz and Miledi, 1967), and high concentrations of calcium, which blocks polysynaptic transmission, did not interfere with transmission between the GSCs and the middle buccal cells. The hypothesis that the GSCs make monosynaptic contact with the middle buccal cells seems therefore highly probable. The next step is to show that serotonin is released at the synapse or the contacts between the GSC and the middle buccal cells. It was shown by iontophoretic experiments that the middle buccal cells possess serotonin receptors, that the serotonin-induced potentials can be blocked by drugs (for example, morphine), and that the receptors are rapidly desensitized by serotonin. The substance that reversibly abolished the middle buccal cell potential (that is, morphine) was also effective in antagonising transmission from the GSCs to the middle buccal cell. Moreover, decreasing the sodium concentration of the medium diminished the size of the serotonin-induced potential and the GSCs' elicited e.p.s.p.s. in the middle buccal cells.

The work by Cottrell and collaborators summarised above and reviewed by Cottrell himself (1977) has, in general, been confirmed for *Aplysia* as well (Gerschenfeld and Paupardin-Tritsch, 1974). The latter have also supplied proof of the endogenous release of serotonin from the endings of the GSCs in *Aplysia*. These authors stimulated single GSCs and were able to measure the endogenous release of serotonin from the endings, provided the uptake inhibitor chlorimipramine was present (Gerschenfeld *et al.*, 1978).

The evidence for the GSCs utilising serotonin as a transmitter substance is most convincing and may be summarised as follows:

(a)  The neurone can form serotonin from tryptophan.
(b)  Serotonin in the neurone is situated in synaptic-type vesicles.
(c)  Serotonin is transported from perikarya to endings.
(d)  Stimulation of the GSCs specifically shows endogenous serotonin is released by the endings of the cells.
(e)  Stimulation of the GSCs specifically elicits a response on follower buccal cells. This response remains unaltered by high concentrations of calcium, suggesting there are monosynaptic contacts between GSCs and follower buccal cells.

(f) Response elicited on follower buccal cells after stimulation of the GSCs can be mimicked by iontophoretic application of serotonin to the buccal cells. All responses could be antagonised by classical serotoninergic blockers.

(g) Evidence exists that exogenous serotonin is specifically taken up by GSCs' endings, suggesting that serotonin is inactivated by a re-uptake mechanism.

## EVIDENCE THAT THE GSCs ALSO UTILISE ACETYLCHOLINE AS A TRANSMITTER

The first suggestion that the GSC may be a cholinergic neurone came from studies by Emson and Fonnum (1972). These authors biochemically analysed isolated *Helix* GSCs and concluded that some choline acetyltransferase (ChAT), an enzyme involved in acetylcholine synthesis, activity was present. In a follow-up study, the same group showed that the ChAT activity was much greater than previously indicated and that 21 pmol authentic acetylcholine is synthesised per cell per hour (Hanley *et al.*, 1974). These results lead the authors to speculate that the GSCs utilise acetylcholine as a second transmitter.

Osborne (1974) had consistently pointed out, however, that care has to be taken in the interpretation of biochemical data from hand-dissected isolated neurones, especially in the case of invertebrates, whose neurones have many glial investments which penetrate deep into the cell body, and also many adhering satellite cells. A biochemical analysis of hand-dissected neurones should immediately prompt the question: How "clean" were the neurones? Is it possible, moreover, to dissect a "clean" neurone without damaging its surface? These problems have all been discussed elsewhere (Osborne, 1974, 1979). The data published by Hanley *et al.* (1974), that *Helix* GSCs contain large quantities of ChAT, must be questioned, especially since an analysis of *Aplysia* GSCs yielded negative results (Weinreich *et al.*, 1973; Brownstein *et al.*, 1974).

In a re-analysis of the GSCs from *Helix*, Osborne (1977) showed that trace amounts of a number of substances (histamine, dopamine, choline acetyltransferase) seem to be present in the cells (table 9.1). In this study, great care was taken with the dissection and yet Osborne (1977) considered that the trace quantities of substance were exogenous. This conclusion was based on results showing that other neurones also contained trace amounts of these substances (the GSC contained, additionally, a huge amount of serotonin), whereas a "cholinergic" neurone had enormous quantities of ChAT instead. Moreover, it was shown that the GSCs could only produce serotonin from [$^{14}$C]-tryptophan (table 9.2).

The observation that not all the vesicles in the neurone have electron-dense deposits and that some are clear (see figure 9.2), argues in favour of the GSCs possibly utilising acetylcholine as a transmitter. It is known that cholinergic neurones are clear, when viewed at electron level, even when tissues have been fixed with osmium tetroxide. It could be maintained equally well that the clear vesicles are merely "empty" serotonergic vesicles.

Table 9.1  Transmitter candidates in GSCs and cell 21 of *Helix pomatia*

| Substance | Concentration (M) | |
|---|---|---|
| | In GSCs | In cell 21 |
| Serotonin | $3.8 \times 10^{-4}$ | $2 \times 10^{-8}$ |
| Histamine | $2 \times 10^{-8}$ | $10^{-8}$ |
| Octopamine | ND | ND |
| Dopamine | $8\text{-}10^{-9}$ | $3 \times 10^{-8}$ |
| Noradrenaline | ND | ND |
| ChAT | $0.2$ pmol cell$^{-1}$ h$^{-1}$ | $61$ pmol cell$^{-1}$ h$^{-1}$ |
| Glutamate | $6 \times 10^{-4}$ | $3 \times 10^{-4}$ |
| Aspartate | $7 \times 10^{-5}$ | $9 \times 10^{-5}$ |
| Glycine | $5 \times 10^{-4}$ | $5.9 \times 10^{-4}$ |
| Taurine | $6 \times 10^{-6}$ | $6 \times 10^{-6}$ |

The total volume of each cell type was estimated by measuring the diameters of a number of cells (mean diameter of both cell types, 120–140 $\mu$m) under light microscopy. It was found that the GSCs and cell 21 had volumes of 1.2 nl. The molarity (results reported for five to seven determinations; in each experiment four neurones were pooled) of each substance in the two neurone types could then be calculated.
ND, not detected.
Note that cell 21 is situated in the suboesophageal ganglion.
(From Osborne, 1977.)

Much more convincing evidence for the GSCs being cholinergic neurones comes from electrophysiological studies. It was shown (Cottrell, 1976, 1977) that hexamethonium, the acetylcholine antagonist, was effective in changing the nature of the GSCs' elicited response to follower cells in the buccal ganglia. Stimulation of the GSCs to high frequencies of activity (up to 12 Hz) resulted in the appearance of biphasic depolarising potentials in the follower buccal cells. These were not blocked by high calcium, indicating that they were mediated by a monosynaptic pathway. Hexamethonium selectively antagonised the first phase of the response, whereas the second was less affected. Furthermore, when serotonin was iontophoretically applied to the follower cells which were exposed to hexamethonium, the response was unaltered, whereas in the case of acetylcholine, its normal depolarising effect was completely blocked. These results, together with the demonstration with bioassay procedures that acetylcholine is actually present in the GSCs (Hanley and Cottrell, 1974), provided Cottrell with evidence that the GSCs are cholinergic (Cottrell, 1977).

Are the serotonergic neurones, especially in the case of the GSC, "cholinergic"?. The biochemical evidence leaves much to be desired (Osborne, 1979, 1981); even the demonstration of acetylcholine in the GSCs is questionable, since bioassay procedures are often unreliable. Moreover, the electrophysiological

Table 9.2  [$^3$H]-acetylcholine and [$^3$H]-serotonin formed from 30 μm [$^3$H]-choline or [$^3$H]-tryptophan

| | [$^3$H]-acetylcholine (fmol) | | 5-[$^3$H]-serotonin (fmol) | |
|---|---|---|---|---|
| | Without eserine | With eserine | Without pargyline | With pargyline |
| Per GSC | 0.2 ± 0.2$^‡$ | 0.5 ± 0.2$^‡$ | 9 ± 0.9 | 9 ± 1 |
| | (12) | (12) | (5) | (5) |
| Per cell 21 | 18 ± 3$^‡$ | 56 ± 6$^‡$ | 0.2 ± 0.2$^†$ | 0.2 ± 0.2$^†$ |
| | (12) | (12) | (5) | (5) |
| Per cerebral ganglion | 3000 ± 105 | 4900 ± 195 | 71 ± 4 | 69 ± 5 |
| | (3) | (3) | (3) | (3) |

All values are ± s.e.m. with the number of determinations (in each determination, four neurones were pooled) in parentheses. Values were calculated by taking into consideration the specific activity of the [$^3$H]-choline and [$^3$H]-tryptophan. [$^3$H]-amine neurotransmitters were fractionated from other substances by two-dimensional chromatography on 5 × 5 cm precoated silica gel plates (Osborne, 1977), whereas [$^3$H]-acetylcholine was separated from [$^3$H]-choline by one-dimensional chromatography on 5 × 5 cm precoated cellulose plates using the solvent system butanol-ethanol-acetic acid-water (8:2:1:3 v/v). [$^3$H]-acetylcholine was visualised by iodine vapour and eluted from the chromatogram with methanol; the absolute amount of [$^3$H]-acetylcholine was calculated by assuming the specific activity to be equal to [$^3$H]-choline added to the ganglia at the start of the incubation. Recovery of [$^3$H]-choline and [$^3$H]-acetylcholine was 85 per cent.
(From Osborne, 1977.)
†Not significantly different from blank values (Student's $t$ test; $P < 0.05$).
‡Significantly different from experiments without eserine and with blank values (Student's $t$ test; $P < 0.05$).

evidence would be more convincing if other anticholinergic drugs could be used to support the data on hexamethonium. It is known, for example, that tubocurarine affects serotonin and acetylcholine receptors (Gerschenfeld, 1973). The data reported by Cottrell (1976, 1977) rely heavily on the fact that hexamethonium has no effect on serotonin receptors and that the GSC makes monosynaptic contact with certain buccal cells (M neurones).

The data would be more persuasive if it were possible to influence the serotonin or apparent acetylcholine levels drastically in the giant serotoninergic neurones and then analyse the "release" of these substances from the monosynaptic follower cells in the buccal ganglia. For example, Tauc *et al.* (1974) showed that cholinergic transmission in the snail can be abolished by injection of acetylcholinesterase into the presynaptic neurones; this should not influence the serotonin levels.

## EVIDENCE THAT THE GSCs CONTAIN A CHOLECYSTOKININ-LIKE PEPTIDE WHICH COULD BE A TRANSMITTER SUBSTANCE

A number of neuroactive peptides have been identified in central neurones of a variety of animals and they are thought to be neurotransmitters or neuromodulators. One of these groups of peptides is the cholecystokinin (CCK) which is widely distributed in the vertebrate brain and gut tissues (Pearse, 1976; Dockray, 1979; Larsson and Rehfeld, 1979). CCK has been characterised in the intestine as peptides of 33 to 39 residues. The biologically active C-terminal octapeptide (CCK-8) has also been isolated from brain tissue (Dockray *et al.*, 1978). There is growing evidence that CCK-8 has a transmitter role in the vertebrate CNS. Immunohistochemical studies have shown that it is localised in nerve fibres and nerve endings (Vanderhaeghen *et al.*, 1980; Larsson and Rehfeld, 1979). There is also evidence for its release by a calcium-dependent mechanism (Dodd *et al.*, 1980) and for the presence of specific receptors (Innis and Snyder, 1980). There is clearly substantial evidence that CCK is a likely transmitter in the vertebrate CNS and it was therefore of great interest to show that the GSCs contain a CCK-like peptide (Osborne *et al.*, 1981).

An antiserum raised against synthetic C-terminal tetrapeptide of CCK (Dockray *et al.*, 1981) was used. Alternate sections taken through the GSC were processed to localise CCK-like immunoreactivity, substance P-like immuno-reactivity or serotonin-like immunoreactivity. Monoclonal antibodies were used to establish the presence of substance P and serotonin immunoreactivity (Cuello *et al.*, 1979; Consolazione *et al.*, 1981). As shown in figure 9.5, the GSC stained positively for serotonin and CCK but not substance P. Other neurones in the ganglia also stain for serotonin but none of these was shown to contain CCK-like immunoreactivity. None of the perikarya containing substance P immuno-reactivity in the cerebral ganglia gave positive indication of serotonin or CCK-like immunoreactivity.

It would seem that the GSC which utilises serotonin also contains a CCK-like peptide. It does not contain substance P-immunoreactive material as illustrated in figure 9.5. Unpublished data have also confirmed that the GSC does not contain bombesin, vasoactive intestinal peptide or enkephalin immunoreactivity, yet immunoreactive material towards all three substances exists in other neurones within the snail's ganglionic mass.

Since the antiserum used for localising CCK immunoreactivity reacts similarly with human heptadecapeptide gastrin (G17), CCK-8 and with their common C-terminal tetrapeptide (G4) (Dockray *et al.*, 1981), it was important to establish immunochemically whether a CCK-like peptide in the snail CNS is similar to its mammalian counterpart. Separation of ganglia extracts by gel filtration on Sephadex G50 revealed a major peak of activity eluting between G17 and CCK-8 (figure 9.6), and so probably of a size intermediate between these peptides. In addition, minor peaks of activity earlier and later than the main one may be bio-synthetic precursors or side-products of the main peak.

The specific peptide demonstrated in the GSC is therefore distinguishable from the main forms of mammalian gastrin and CCK. The material is also dif-ferent from molluscan peptide (FMRF amid) isolated from *Macrocallistra* ganglia (Price and Greenberg, 1977), and bearing a slight resemblance to the C-terminal tetrapeptide of CCK. Thus, although the GSC's peptide structure needs to be established, it does show some similarity to the mammalian CCK counterpart, especially in the C-terminal regions.

The fact that the GSC contains a specific peptide is of great interest, but it must first be isolated before physiological studies can determine whether the substance has a transmitter role in the GSC.

## CONCLUSIONS

The evidence in favour of the opinion that the GSC utilises serotonin as a neurotransmitter is excellent. The essential features of a neurotransmitter are that it (a) is located in the neurone, (b) is released from the neurone under physiological levels of stimulation, and (c) induces an effect on the membrane potential of the postsynaptic cells. As discussed above, the large size and position of the GSC and its known synaptic connections with follower buccal cells have enabled us to demonstrate that the GSC's serotonin carries all the features of a neurotransmitter. The evidence that the GSC also uses another transmitter, that is, acetylcholine, is not as persuasive, although it does provide the best example in neurobiology of the possibility of a neurone utilising more than one transmitter. The major arguments against accepting acetylcholine as a transmitter in the GSC are: (a) it has not been unequivocally established that the cell contains acetylcholine or its major synthesising enzyme, ChAT; (b) the release data for acetycholine from the GSC accumulated by Cottrell and collaborators (see Cottrell, 1977) rely exclusively on hexamethonium having no effect on serotonin receptors.

The findings that the GSC contains a specific peptide may prove of immense importance. Literature now quotes quite a few cases of the coexistence of a classical neurotransmitter and a peptide (see Osborne 1981 and other chapters in this book) molecule in specific neurone types. Whether these peptides also function as neurotransmitters or whether they are neuromodulators is a moot point. The distinction between neuromodulator and neurotransmitter is not clear, overlapping in many areas, and this has caused some authors to coin the term "neuroregulator" to cover both. What is understood as a "neuromodulator" and "neurotransmitter" at either extreme is reasonably unambiguous and perhaps these two terms should be maintained. It is now theoretically possible for the first time to find out the function of a specific peptide in a neurone, for example, if the CCK-like peptide acts as a neuromodulator or neurotransmitter in the GSC. The GSC, with its known synaptic connections, makes it physiologically possible to undertake the required experiments. However, before this can be achieved, it is necessary to identify and purify sufficient quantities of the CCK-like peptide. There is now an exciting opportunity ahead to test effectively the validity of Dale's principle.

## ACKNOWLEDGEMENTS

I thank the Stiftung Volkswagenwerk for financing part of this research; and Mrs Joy Shirley for technical assistance.

# REFERENCES

Brodie, B. B. and Shore, P. A. (1957). A concept for a role of Serotonin and norepinephrine as chemical mediators in the brain. *Ann. N.Y. Acad. Sci.*, 66, 631–42

Brownstein, M. J., Saavedra, J. M., Axelrod, J., Zeman, G. H. and Carpenter, D. O. (1974). Coexistence of several putative neurotransmitters in single identified neurons of *Aplysia*. *Proc. natn. Acad. Sci. U.S.A.*, 7, 4662–5

Burn, J. H. and Rand, M. J. (1965). Acetylcholine in adrenergic transmission. *A. Rev. Pharmac.*, 5, 163–82

Burnstock, G. (1976). Do some nerve cells release more than one transmitter? *Neuroscience*, 1, 239–48

Burnstock, G. (1970). Do some sympathetic neurones synthesise and release both noradrenaline and acetylcholine? *Progr. Neurobiol.*, 11, 205–22

Chan-Palay, V., Jonsson, G. and Palay, S. L. (1978). Serotonin and substance-P coexist in neurons of the rat's central nervous system. *Proc. natn. Acad. Sci. U.S.A.*, 75, 1582–6

Consolazione, A., Milstein, C., Wright, B. and Cuello, A. C. (1981). The immunohistochemical detection of serotonin with monoclonal antibodies. *J. Histochem. Cytochem.*, in the press

Cottrell, G. A. (1970). Direct postsynaptic responses to stimulation of serotonin-containing neurons. *Nature*, 225, 1060–2

Cottrell, G. A. (1971). Synaptic connections made by two serotonin-containing neurons in the snail (*Helix pomatia*) brain. *Experientia*, 27, 813–5

Cottrell, G. A. (1976). Does the giant cerebral neurone of *Helix* release two transmitters, acetylcholine and serotonin. *J. Physiol. Lond.*, 259, 44–5P

Cottrell, G. A. (1977). Identified amine-containing neurones and their synaptic connexions. *Neuroscience*, 2, 1–18

Cottrell, G. A. and Macon, J. B. (1974). Synaptic connections of two symmetrically placed giant serotonin-containing neurones. *J. Physiol. Lond.*, 236, 434–64

Cottrell, G. A. and Osborne, N. N. (1970). Subcellular localisation of serotonin in an identified serotonin-containing neuron. *Nature*, 225, 470–2

Cottrell, G. A. and Powell, B. (1971). Formation of serotonin by isolated serotonin-containing neurons and by isolated monoamine-containing neurons. *J. Neurochem.*, 18, 1695–997

Cottrell, G. A., Berry, M. S. and Macon, J. B. (1974). Synapses of a giant serotonin neuron and a giant dopamine neuron: Studies using antagonists *Neuropharmacology*, 13, 431–39

Cuello, A. C., Galfre, G. and Milstein, C. (1979). Detection of substance P in the central nervous system by a monoclonal antibody *Proc. natn. Acad. Sci. U.S.A.*, 76, 3532–6

Dockray, G. J. (1979). Evolutionary relationships of the gut hormones. *Fedn. Proc.*, 38, 2295–301

Dockray, G. J., Gregory, R. A., Hutchinson, J. B., Harris, J. I. and Runswick, M. J. (1978). Isolation, structure and biological activity of two cholecystokinin octopeptides from sheep brain. *Nature*, 274, 711–3

Dockray, G. J., Vaillant, C., and Hutchison, J. B. (1981). Immunochemical characterisation of peptides in endocrine cells and nerves with particular reference to gastrin and cholecystokinin. In *The Cellular Basis of Chemical Messengers in the Digestive System*, (ed. M. I. Grossman, M. A. B. Brazier and J. Lechago), Academic Press, New York, in the press

Dodd, P. R., Edwardson, J. A. and Dockray, G. J. (1980). The depolarization induced release of cholecystokinin C-terminal octapeptide (CCK-8) from rat synaptosomes and brain slices. *Regulatory Peptides*, 1, 17–29

Emson, P. C. and Fonnum, F. (1972). Choline acetyltransferase, acetylcholinesterase and aromatic-L-amino acid decarboxylase in single identified nerve cell bodies from snail *Helix aspersa*. *J. Neurochem.*, 22, 1079, 1088

Falck, B. and Owman, Ch. (1965). A detailed methodological description of the fluoresence method for the cellular demonstration of biogenic monoamines. *Acta Univ. Lund.*, 11 (7), 1, 23

Gerschenfeld, H. M. (1973). Chemical transmission in invertebrate central nervous systems and neuromuscular junctions. *Physiol. Rev.*, 53, 1–119

Gerschenfeld, H. M. and Paupardin-Tritsch, D. (1974). On the transmitter functions of 5-hydroxyhyptamine at excitatory and inhibitory monosynaptic junctions. *J. Physiol. Lond.*, **243**, 457–81

Gershenfeld, H. M., Hamon, M. and Paupardin-Tritisch, D. (1978). Release of endogenous serotonin from two identified serotonin-containing neurones and the physiological role of serotonin uptake. *J. Physiol. Lond.*, **274**, 265–78

Goldberg, D. J., Goldman, J. E. and Schwartz, J. H. (1976). Alterations in amounts and rates of serotonin transported in an axon of the giant cerebral neurone of *Aplysia californica. J Physiol. Lond.*, **259**, 473–90

Goldman, J. E. and Schwartz, J. H. (1974). Cellular specificity of serotonin storage and axonal transport in identified neurons of *Aplysia californica. J. Physiol. Lond.*, **242**, 61–76

Hanley, M. R. and Cottrell, G. A. (1974). Acetylcholine activity in an identified 5-hydroxy-tryptamine-containing neurone. *J. Pharm. Pharmac.*, **26**, 980

Hanley, M. R., Cottrell, G. A., Emson, P. C. and Fonnum, F. (1974). Enzymatic synthesis of acetylcholine by a serotonin-containing neurone from *Helix. Nature New Biol.*, **251**, 631–3

Hökfelt, T., Elfvin, L-C., Schultzberg, M., Goldstein, M. and Nilsson, G. (1977*a*). On the occurrence of substance P-containing fibres in sympathetic ganglia: immunohistochemical evidence. *Brain Res.*, **132**, 29–41

Hökfelt, T., Elfvin, L-G., Elde, R., Schultzberg, M., Goldstein, M. and Lufe, R. (1977*b*). Occurrence of somatostatin-like immunoreactivity in some peripheral sympathetic noradrenergic neurons. *Proc. natn. Acad. Sci. U.S.A.*, **74**, 3587–91

Hökfelt, T., Lundberg, J. M., Schultzberg, M., Johansson, O., Ljumdahl, A. and Rehfeld, J. (1980). Coexistence of peptides and putative transmitters in neurons. In *Neural Peptide and Neuronal Communication* (ed. E. Costa and M. Trabuchi), Raven Press, New York, pp. 1–23

Innis, R. B. and Snyder, S. H. (1980). Cholecystokinin receptor binding in brain and pancreas regulation of pancreatic binding by cyclic and acyclic quanine nucleopeptides. *Eur. J. Pharmac.*, **65**, 123–4

Kandel, E. R. and Tauc, L. (1966). Input organization of two symmetrical giant cells in the snail brain. *J. Physiol. Lond.*, **183**, 269–86

Katz, B. and Miledi, R. (1967). A study of synaptic transmission in the absence of impulses. *J. Physiol. Lond.*, **192**, 407–36

Koelle, G. B. (1962). A new general concept of the neurohumoral functions of acetylcholine and acetylcholinesterase. *J. Pharm. Pharmac.*, **14**, 65–90

Koe, B. K. and Weissman, A. (1966). p-Chlorophenylalanine, a specific depletor of brain serotonin. *J. Pharm. exp. Therap.*, **154**, 499–516

Kunze, H. (1921). Zur Topographie und Histologie des Zentral-nerven-systems von *Helix pomatia. Z. Wiss. Zool.*, **118**, 25–203

Larsson, L.-L. and Rehfeld, J. F. (1979). Localization and molecular heterogeneity of cholecystokinin in central and peripheral nervous systems. *Brain Res.*, **165**, 201–18

Osborne, N. N. (1972). The *in vivo* synthesis of serotonin in an identified serotonin-containing neuron of *Helix pomatia. Int. J. Neurosci.*, **3**, 215–19

Osborne, N. N. (1973*a*). Micro-biochemical and physiological studies on an identified serotonergic neuron in the snail *Helix pomatia. Malacologia*, **14**, 97–106

Osborne, N. N. (1973*b*). Tryptophan metabolism in characterised neurons of *Helix. Br. J. Pharmac.*, **48**, 546–9

Osborne, N. N. (1974). *Microchemical Analysis of Nervous Tissues*, Pergamon Press, Oxford and New York

Osborne, N. N. (1977). Do snail neurones contain more than one transmitter? *Nature*, **270**, 622–3

Osborne, N. N. (1978). The neurobiology of a serotonergic neuron. In *Biochemistry of Characterised Neurones* (ed. N. N. Osborne), pp. 47–80

Osborne, N. N. (1979). Is Dale's principle valid? *Trends Neurosci.*, **2**, 73–5

Osborne, N. N. (1980). Reasons for using the snail brain in pharmacological research. *Trends Pharmac.*, **1**, 290–2

Osborne, N. N. (1981). Communication between neurones: current concepts. *Neurochem. Int.*, **3**, 3–16

Osborne, N. N. (1982). *Biology of Serotonergic Transmission*, Wiley, Chichester, in the press

Osborne, N. N. and Cottrell, G. A. (1971*a*). Distribution of biogenic amines in the slug *Limax maximum. Z. Zellforsch.*, 112, 15–30

Osborne, N. N. and Cottrell, G. A. (1971*b*). Amine and amino acid microanalysis of two identified snail neurones with known characteristics. *Experientia*, 27, 656–8

Osborne, N. N. and Neuhoff, V. (1980). Identified serotonergic neurones. In *International Review of Cytology*, 67 (ed. G. H. Bourne and J. F. Danielli), Academic Press, New York, pp. 259–290

Osborne, N. N., Cuello, A. C. and Dockray, G. J. (1981). The localization of substance P and cholecystokinin-like peptides in specific neurones of the snail *Helix* and the coexistence of cholecystokinin and substance P in a defined giant neurone (GSC). *Science*, in the press

Pentreath, V. W. (1976). Ultrastructure of the terminals of an identified 5-hydroxytryptamine-containing neurone marked by intracellular injection of radioactive 5-hydroxytryptamine. *J. Neurocytol.*, 5, 43–61

Pentreath, V. W. and Cottrell, G. A. (1973). Uptake of serotonin, 5-hydroxytryptophan and tryptophan by giant serotonin-containing neurones and other neurones in the central nervous system of the snail (*Helix pomatia*). *Z. Zellforsch.*, 143, 21–35

Pentreath, V. W., Osborne, N. N. and Cottrell, G. A. (1973). Anatomy of giant serotonin-containing neurones in the cerebral ganglia of *Helix pomatia*, and *Limax maximus Z. Zellforsch.*, 143, 1–20

Pentreath, V. W., Berry, M. S. and Osborne, N. N. (1982). The serotonergic cerebral cells in gastropods. In *Biology of Serotonergic Transmission* (ed. N. N. Osborne), Wiley, Chichester, in the press

Pearse, A. G. E. (1976). Peptides in brain and intestine. *Nature*, 262, 92–3

Price, D. A. and Greenberg, M. J. (1977). Structure of a molluscan cardioexcitatory neuropeptide. *Science*, 197, 670–1

Rapport, M. M. (1949). Serum vasoconstrictor (serotonin) V. presence of creatinine in the complex. A proposed structure of the vasoconstrictor principle. *J. biol. Chem.*, 180, 961–69

Schwartz, J. H. (1979). Axonal transport: components, mechanism and specificity. *A. Rev. Neurosci.*, 2, 467–504

Tauc, L., Hoffman, A., Tsuji, S., Hinzen, D. H. and Faille, L. (1974). Transmission abolished at a cholinergic synapse after injection of cholinesterase into the presynaptic neurone. *Nature*, 250, 496–98

Vanderhaeghen, J. J., Lotsfra, F., de Mey, J. & Giles, C. (1980). Immunohistochemical localization of cholecystokinin and gastrin-like peptides in brain and hypophysis of the rat. *Proc. natn. Acad. Sci. U.S.A.*, 77, 1190–4

Weinreich, D., McCaman, W., McCaman, R. E. & Vaughn, J. E. (1973). Chemical enzymatic and ultra-structural characterisation of 5-hydroxytryptamine-containing neurons from the ganglion of *Aplysia californica* and *Tritonia diomedia. J. Neurochem.*, 20, 969–76

Wood, J. G. (1965). Electron microscopic localisation of 5-hydroxytryptamine (5-HT). *Tex. Rep. biol. Med.*, 23, 828–37

Wood, J. G. (1966). Electron microscopic localisation of amines in central nervous tissue. *Nature*, 209, 1131–3

# 10

# The diffuse neuroendocrine system: an extension of the APUD concept

A. G. E. Pearse (Royal Postgraduate Medical School, Hammersmith Hospital, Du Cane Road, London W12 OHS, UK)

## INTRODUCTION

The diffuse neuroendocrine system (DNES) is constituted by the 40+ peptide and amine-secreting cells of the so-called APUD series. APUD is an acronym for "amine precursor uptake and decarboxylation", signifying not only the amine-handling characteristics which the APUD cells share with neurones, but a number of other cytochemical and ultrastructural characteristics common to all members of the series. For many of the cells there is a clear association with elements of the autonomic nervous system but direct innervation is nevertheless not usual.

The DNES has two divisions: central and peripheral. The first of these comprises the neuroendocrine cells of the hypothalamo-pituitary-pineal complex, whereas the second division contains all those neuroendocrine cells located outside these regions, whether they occur together in organised glands or are diffusely distributed in different organs and tissues.

The majority of cells in the second division of the DNES are found in the gastrointestinal tract and pancreas but a minority are much more widely distributed, particularly in the embryo and foetus, being present in the respiratory and urogenital tracts, in the thyroid, parathyroid and thymus glands, in the adrenal medulla and accessory chromaffin tissue, and in the sympathetic nervous system itself.

## THE APUD CONCEPT

In a long series of papers, with widely differing titles, the Austrian pathologist Friedrich Feyrter (1895-1973) described a system of clear cells (*Helle Zellen*) which constituted in his view a "diffuse endokrine epitheliale Organe" (1946, 1953). The natural, but not direct successors of the *Helle Zellen* are the cells of the APUD series (Pearse, 1968, 1969). These are indeed clear cells, by both light and electron microscopy, since unless specifically stimulated they lack the basophilic and osmiophilic granular endoplasmic reticulum which characterises typical protein-exporting cells (Caro and Palade, 1964).

The earliest reports on the subject (Pearse, 1966a and b) had indicated that a small series of endocrine and presumptively endocrine cells, whose primary function seemed to be the production of a polypeptide hormone, possessed a number of cytochemical and ultrastructural characteristics in common. It was postulated that these characteristics, particularly those connected with the synthesis and secretion of amines, might indicate a common origin of the cells from neuroectoderm. Alternatively, it was suggested that they were derived "from a cell of neural origin, perhaps coming from the neural crest". For the next few years an essentially similar view was maintained but later the concept was restored, more or less to its original form and the "common" derivation of the APUD cells was expressed as being "from neuroendocrine-programmed ectoblast" (Pearse, 1975, 1977). There is, of course, no a priori reason why neuroendocrine characteristics and products should not be acquired, through retrograde differentiation, by cells derived from the two other principal germ layers, that is to say from stem cells normally determined for non-neuronal differentiation. Nevertheless, if only for academic reasons, experiments designed to test the validity of the APUD concept have been carried out in a number of laboratories.

By 1969 the list of APUD cells had grown to 14, five of which, including the newly named C (for calcitonin) cell of the thyroid and ultimobranchial glands (Bussolati and Pearse, 1967), had been shown to be responsible for the synthesis and secretion of known peptide hormones. Within the next few years it became evident, however, from the "biological marker" studies of Le Douarin and Le Lièvre (1970) and Le Douarin and Teillet (1973), supported by studies made by Pearse and Polak (1971), Andrew (1974) and Pictet *et al.* (1976), that only six or seven of the APUD cells, by that time numbering at least 40, could be regarded as direct derivatives of the definitive neural crest. Indeed it became virtually certain that that ephemeral structure could not and did not give rise to the APUD cells of the avian gastrointestinal tract or of the pancreas (Fontaine and Le Douarin, 1977). Since this was considered probably true for all vertebrate species, the remaining 33 cells of the series were further divided, into a group for which derivation from neural or potentially neural ectoderm was considered acceptable and a second group for which no such origin could be sustained by the available experimental evidence.

Notwithstanding these contradictions, it was and is still postulated that the cells of the APUD series constitute a diffuse endocrine or neuroendocrine system which is to be regarded as a third division of the nervous system (Pearse, 1975a). By this token its individual cells can be expected to subserve a number of different functions, including the modulation of the activities of the autonomic division, the initiation of afferent impulses to the somatic division, and the control of the secretory functions of individual members of the series.

## PRESENT STATUS OF THE DNES

The present status of the diffuse neuroendocrine system is expressed in tables 10.1 and 10.2, in which are listed all the cells belonging to the APUD series. Omitted are the many groups of cortical and subcortical neurones whose cytochemical characteristics and peptide products would allow them to be regarded as APUD cells. As recorded by Louis (1970) for rat brain, some 60 per cent of cortical neurones and virtually all the subcortical ones are able to take up and decarboxylate 5-hydroxytryptophan.

The cells of the central division of the DNES are listed in table 10.1; and for each subgroup, in the central and right hand columns, appear their peptide and amine products. The largest single group of products is represented by the pituitary peptides among which, in brackets, appear three for which pituitary status has been claimed but not fully substantiated.

Table 10.1  The central division of the DNES

| Cell type | Peptide products | Amine products |
|---|---|---|
| Pineal | AVT, LRH, TRH, α-MSH | MT, 5-HT |
| Hypothalamic m.c. | AVT, AVP, SST | DA, NA, 5-HT |
| Hypothalamic p.c. | RHs, RIFs, β-LPH, ACTH, NT, α-MSH, Ins, AVP, PP, Subs P | DA, NA, 5-HT |
| Pituitary pars distalis | FSH, LH, TSH, STH, PRL, ACTH, α-MSH, β-LPH, β-endorphin (gastrin, NT, calcitonin) | DA, NA, 5-HT N-term. Trp |
| Pituitary pars intermedia | β-LPH, ACTH, α-MSH, β-endorphin, met/leu-enkephalin (calcitonin) | (T) H, N-term. Trp |

AVT, arginine vasotocin; AVP, arginine vasopressin;
SST, somatostatin; LRH, lutropin releasing hormone;
TRH, thyrotropin releasing hormone; RHs, releasing hormones;
RIFs, release inhibiting factors; NT, neurotensin;
PP, pancreatic polypeptide; MT, melatonin;
NA, noradrenalin; DA, dopamine; T, tyramine;
H, histamine; N-term Trp, N-terminal tryptophyl peptides;
m.c., magnocellular; p.c., parvocellular.

The anterior hypophysis (pars distalis and pars intermedia), regarded by some embryologists as being of placodal rather than stomodeal ectodermal origin, was considered by Takor-Takor and Pearse (1975) to be derived from the neuroectoderm of the ventral neural ridges. Recent studies (Cocchia and Miani, 1980; Nakajima *et al.*, 1980) have shown that the brain-specific S-100 protein is localised in the stellate (non-endocrine) cells of the adeno-hypophysis, indicating that these are certainly of neuroectodermal origin and glial nature, as are the pituicytes of the pars nervosa. Although these observations do not prove that the adenohypophysis is derived from neuroectoderm, they give strong support to such a contention. The remaining components of the central division are indisputably neuroectodermal.

The cells of the peripheral division of the DNES are listed in table 10.2. First come the seven members of the division which are proven derivatives of the neural crest, together with a further four cells (lung, K; urogenital tract, U and EC; skin, Merkel) whose provenance remains uncertain, though all are commonly recorded as having this origin. Against the melanocyte, in the amine column, appears its non-amine, non-peptide but nevertheless fluoro-genic product cysteinyl-DOPA. Normal melanocytes are not recorded as having any identifiable biologically active peptide.

The remaining cells of the peripheral division are then listed in the second part of table 10.2. All are localised either in the gastrointestinal tract or in the pancreas, for these an origin from neural crest has been shown to be impossible.

## PRESENT STATUS OF THE APUD CONCEPT

For the origin of the APUD cells there are essentially only two possibilities. Either they are all neuroendocrine-programmed derivatives of the early embryonic ecto(epi) blast, and hence all are neuroectodermal, or else one half of the series originates in this manner and the other half from a multipotential endodermal stem cell.

If the APUD concept is correct then the precursor cells of the series are committed to neuroendocrine status at very early stages in the embryo, even if for half the series the initial event (neuroendocrine determination) is considered as occurring in a cell in the definitive endoderm. After the onset of determination the cells would supposedly vary their function and products in response to microenvironmental factors, only with respect to the nature and balance of these peptide and amine products.

The alternative explanation of the facts for the APUD cells of the gastro-intestinal tract, is known as the "unitarian" concept (Cheng and Leblond, 1974). It postulates their origin from a single endodermal precursor, the crypt base cell of the intestine. For the pancreas, the basal stem cell of the ductular system is the usually accepted equivalent (Pictet and Rutter, 1972). From this all four endocrine cell types, as well as duct cells and acinar cells are considered to arise.

Table 10.2　The peripheral division of the DNES

| Cell type | | Peptide products | Amine products |
|---|---|---|---|
| Adrenomedullary | A, NA | Met-enkephalin, NT | A, NA |
| Sympathetic | Ganglion | VIP, SST | NA, DA |
| | SIF | – | NA |
| Carotid body | Type 1 | Met-enkephalin | DA, NA |
| Thyroid/UB | C | Calcitonin, SST | 5-HT |
| Skin | Melanocyte | – | Cys-DOPA |
| | Merkel | (Met-enkephalin) | – |
| Lung | K | Bombesin | DA, NA |
| UG tract | U | – | – |
| | EC | – | 5-HT |
| Pancreas | B, A | Insulin, Glucagon | 5-HT, DA |
| | D, PP(F) | SST, PP | – |
| | | (β-endorphin, TRH, LRF) | – |
| Stomach | GA | Gastrin 17, met-enkephalin | – |
| | AL | Glucagon | – |
| | EC1 | Substance P | 5-HT |
| | ECL | – | – |
| | D | SST | – |
| Intestine | EC1 | Substance P | 5-HT |
| | M, EC2 | Motilin, promotilin | –, 5-HT |
| | GI | Gastrin 34 | – |
| | L, S | Glicentin, secretin | – |
| | I, BN | CCK, bombesin | – |
| | D, K | SST, GIP | – |
| | NT | Neurotensin | – |

VIP, vasoactive intestinal peptide;
GIP, gastric inhibitory peptide; CCK, cholecystokinin;
Cys-DOPA, cysteinyl-dihydroxyphenylalanine;
LRF, lutropin releasing factor.
For other abbreviations, see footnote to table 10.1.

These considerations are not merely semantic. The real questions concern the potency, or potential, of APUD cell precursors and the timing and manner of their determination as neuroendocrine. It is difficult to obtain convincing experimental evidence which bears on these two points, but evidence for the neuroendocrine status of the APUD cells is confidently derived from the study of markers.

## NEUROENDOCRINE MARKERS AND THE APUD CELLS

During the past two decades the search for specific markers for neural and neuroendocrine function, and for neural and neuroendocrine determination, has been carried out in a number of biochemical and histochemical laboratories. Only relatively recently has there been other than limited success in this important field. Table 10.3 provides a list of some of the markers whose identification has been made in both neurones and neuroendocrine (APUD) cells.

Table 10.3   Molecular markers for neurons and APUD cells

|  | Non-specific | |
| --- | --- | --- |
| Restricted | | General |
| Carcinoembryonic antigen | | Acetylcholinesterase |
| Estrogen receptor protein | | Non-specific esterases |
| Chromomembrin B (cytochrome b-561) | | L-Amino acid decarboxylase |
| Histaminase | | Amine precursor uptake |
| | | Chloroquin/Quinacrin uptake |

|  | Specific | |
| --- | --- | --- |
| | Restricted | |
| Serotonin-binding protein | | Tryptophan hydroxylase |
| Indolamine 2,3-dioxygenase | | Phenylethanolamine N-methyl transferase |
| Dopamine β-hydroxylase | | Nicotine-atropine uptake |
| Tyrosine hydroxylase | | N-terminal Trp-peptides |

|  | Neuronal | |
| --- | --- | --- |
| | Neuron-specific enolase ($\gamma$-isomer) | |

Restricted: positive in a minority of APUD cells; general: positive in the majority of APUD cells; neuronal: positive in neurons and in all APUD cells.

In the "restricted" section of the upper part of table 10.3, only two markers require additional description. CEA, unexpectedly, has been shown to be present in normal as well as hyperplastic and neoplastic thyroid C cells (Kodama *et al.*, 1980). It has not been demonstrated, however, in any other normal APUD cell, and its status as a marker is doubtful. The chromaffin granule membrane protein chromomembrin B, now shown to be identical with cytochrome b-561 (Winkler and Westhead, 1980), is a potential marker for APUD cell granule membranes since, as shown by Hörtnagl *et al.* (1973), it is present also in the membranes of sympathetic neuronal catecholamine-storing vesicles.

Note in the "general" section of the table, that although the appearance of acetylcholinesterase is established as a sensitive marker for differentiation of neurones in tissue culture it is by no means a specific indicator for this process in other conditions. It cannot be a marker for neuronal determination. Cholinesterases appear in many cell types in the embryo, often as a transient phenomenon (Drews, 1975). Their precise biochemical function is not known and, at best, they can only be ancillary markers for neuroendocrine differentiation. In this section, despite its lack of biochemical specificity, the best APUD marker is the presence of amino acid decarboxylase, usually demonstrated as following the more specific uptake of either of the two amine precursors, L-DOPA and L-5-hydroxytryptophan. It seems that all APUD cells, at some states of their development, possess the acronymous amine-handling capacity even if, in some cases, only for a period of a few days.

The "restricted" list of markers in the lower half of table 10.3 contains several which are certainly specific for neurons and neuroendocrine cells, the majority of these being connected with the synthesis of catecholamines or indolamines. Another marker (nicotine–atropine uptake) is associated with inhibitor functions and yet another (N-tryptophyl peptides) with the pre or pre-pro segments of hormonal peptides.

Within the past two years the concept of a "neural" origin for the APUD cells has received support from their invariable possession of an enolase at one time considered to be restricted to neurones. This enzyme (neurone-specific enolase, NSE), an isomer of the glycolytic enzyme 2-phospho-D-glycerate hydroxylase (EC 4.2.1.11) was characterised by Fletcher *et al.* (1976) and later shown by Marangos *et al.* (1978) to be present in nerve cells as the $\gamma\gamma$ isomer. The other two forms of the enzyme are the $\alpha\alpha$ isomer (liver and most other tissues) and the $\beta\beta$ isomer (skeletal muscle). For APUD cells their possession of the neuronal form of the enzyme was first demonstrated immunocytochemically by Schmechel *et al.* (1978) who reported, for man and monkey, that it was present in some of the cells belonging to both central and peripheral divisions of the DNES. Among the cells demonstrated by this means were those of the adrenal medulla, the endocrine pancreas, the pituitary and pineal glands, and the thyroid C cells. The list has been extended to the endocrine cells of foetal lung (Wharton *et al.*, 1981) and to those of the gastrointestinal tract and pancreas (Pearse *et al.*, 1980; Bishop *et al.*, 1981). As far as has been determined, all the APUD cells listed in tables 10.1 and 10.2 contain NSE, almost certainly in association with the non-neuronal enolase ($\alpha\alpha$ isomer), perhaps as the $\alpha\gamma$ hybrid molecule. This feature they share with many interneurones, but the majority of neurones contain only the $\gamma\gamma$ isomer.

The presence of NSE in a neurone is presently regarded as an expression of its neural differentiation, on the basis of assays indicating that during this process a switch takes place from the $\alpha\alpha$ to the $\gamma\gamma$-isomer (Schmechel *et al.*, 1980) which is consistent with dependence on the making of full synaptic contacts, or perhaps on cessation of mitosis. The presence of NSE in an APUD cell is neither a sign of maturity, nor of the making of synaptic contacts. It may reflect a fall in the rate of mitosis to the low level found in mature APUD cells but this seems unlikely to be the case in embryos as young as those in which NSE is found in APUD cells (8–10 weeks in the human foetus).

In APUD cells of proved neuroectodermal origin the presence of NSE will be taken to indicate neuroendocrine determination if it can be shown to precede specific peptide production. The same connotation necessarily applies to the

APUD cells of gut, and pancreas, irrespective of whether they are finally shown to be neuroectodermal or endodermal in origin. If they are indeed endodermal it becomes necessary to postulate dedifferentiation (retrograde differentiation) of a non-neuronally determined precursor cell, to express the gene coding for the neural isoenzyme. If their precursor has neuroendocrine determination, only modulation (transformation) is required to produce the full range of products.

## FUNCTIONS OF APUD CELLS

"The prime function of the neurally derived, or neurally determined, APUD cell is to apply, to neighbouring or distant cells, chemical activators or inhibitors which are best described as hormones. For the activity of cells acting on neighbouring cells it may be expedient to use the term paracrine (Feyrter, 1938, 1953); in other instances the activity of the cells is truly neuroendocrine (neurosecretory) and in yet others "purely endocrine" (Pearse, 1975*b*). These different routes of secretion by APUD cells were subsequently amplified (Pearse, 1977) to include two more unusual modes of delivery characterising the melanocyte (epicrine) and anuran cutaneous peptide-secreting cells (exocrine). Secretion by one neurone to another without axonal delivery was called neurocrine but that term is perhaps best retained (Leibson, 1979) as a general description for secretory nerve cells (that is, as an abbreviation of neuroendocrine). Secretion between neurone and neurone via soma or dendrites is encompassed by the term paracrine (see also Jaim-Etchverry and Zieher, this volume).

Although the various terms, listed above, describe adequately the modes by which APUD cell products are delivered, they fail completely to elucidate the quality, or nature of the response at the effector site. Can any simple and single term embrace the whole range of activities of such products? Probably the answer must be no, but it may be worthwhile to make the attempt.

The great majority of APUD cells clearly respond to more than one type of input stimulus. This is especially true for the cells in the peripheral division where there is always a close association with the autonomic nervous system, either in its classical adrenergic and cholinergic forms, or in one or other of the newer peptidergic forms, or in one or other of the mixed adrenergic/peptidergic or cholinergic/peptidergic forms.

Perhaps one of the simplest examples is the uncomplicated response of one of the latest members of the APUD series, the Merkel cell, to touch (pressure). These cells have no efferent nerve supply. During development they become associated with the ingrowing sensory nerves to the skin, forming neurite-Merkel cell complexes (Scott *et al.*, 1981), and their nerve supply is thus strictly afferent. Merkel's original notion (Merkel, 1880), transcribed by Munger (1977), was that his cells were acting as transducers of mechanical to neural information, that is to say as mechanosensory effectors. A purely sensory activity can reasonably be attributed to other APUD cells. The type 1 cells of the carotid body are chemosensory effectors, transmitting their information by way of glossopharyngeal afferents to the central nervous system.

In a broad sense, the responses of many other APUD cells can be brought into this group of sensory effectors. The thyroid C cell, though capable of responding to many different stimuli, effectively secretes calcitonin in response to a meal and thus effects a direct diversion of the incoming flow of calcium ions into bone fluid (Talmage *et al.*, 1980). Such an activity is clearly sensory but not neurosensory since in this case no information is transferred to the nervous system.

## CONCLUSIONS

Full elucidation of the activities of each individual APUD cell will require much time and effort. Already a great mass of data is available and attempts to simplify the matter by imposing a stamp of functional uniformity on the whole series are probably without profit. Yet it is still possible to sustain the proposition that the APUD cells constitute a third, endocrine or neuroendocrine division of the nervous system, and also the corresponding proposition that they are all possessors of an inbuilt neuroendocrine program, originating from the embryonic ectoblast. As such, they are to be considered as independent self-reproducing entities, possessing a large measure of functional independence even from their close associates, the neurites of the second, autonomic division of the nervous system.

The DNES has been established as a system of paramount importance for the maintenance of an extensive range of bodily functions. Its status in this respect is not dependent on proofs of any particular origins for its independent but closely interrelated components. Realisation of this fact may save a great deal of wasted time and effort.

## REFERENCES

Andrew, A. (1974). Further evidence that enterochromaffin cells are not derived from the neural crest. *J. Embryol. exp. Morph.*, 31, 589–98

Bishop, A. E., Polak, J. M., Facer, P., Ferri, G-L., Marangos, P. J. and Pearse, A. G. E. (1981). Neuron-specific enolase: general marker for the diffuse neuroendocrine system in the gut and pancreas. *Gastroenterology*, in the press

Bussolati, G. and Pearse, A. G. E. (1967). Immunofluorescent localization of calcitonin in the 'C' cells of pig and dog thyroid. *J. Endocrinol.*, 37, 205–9

Caro, L. G. and Palade, G. E. (1964). Protein synthesis, storage and discharge in the pancreatic exocrine cell. *J. cell. Biol.*, 20, 473–95

Cheng, H. and Leblond, C. P. (1974). Origin, differentiation and renewal of the four main epithelial cell types in the mouse small intestine: V Unitarian theory of the origin of the four epithelial cell types. *Am. J. Anat.* 141, 537–62

Cocchia, D. and Miani, N. (1980). Immunocytochemical localization of the brain-specific S-100 protein in the pituitary gland of adult rat. *J. Neurocytol.*, 9, 771–82

Drews, U. (1975). Cholinesterase in embryonic development. *Progr. Histochem. Cytochem.*, 7, No. 3, 1–52

Feyrter, F. (1938). *Über Diffuse Endokrine Epitheliale Organe*, J. A. Barth, Leipzig
Feyrter, F. (1946). Über die These von peripheren endokrinen Drüsen. *Wiener Zeit. Innere Med.*, 27, 9–38
Feyrter, F. (1953). *Über die Peripheren Endokrinen (Parakrinen) Drüsen des Menschen*, W. Maudrich, Wien
Fletcher, L., Rider, C. C. and Taylor, C. B. (1976). Chromatographic and immunological characteristics of rat brain enolase. *Biochem. Biophys. Acta*, 452, 245–52
Fontaine, J. and Le Douarin, N. M. (1977). Analysis of endoderm formation in the avian blastoderm by the use of quail-chick chimaeras: the problem of the neuroectodermal origin of the cells of the APUD series. *J. Embryol. exp. Morph.*, 41, 209–22
Hörtnagl, H., Winkler, H. and Lochs, H. (1973). Immunological studies on a membrane protein (chromomembrin B) of catecholamine-storing vesicles. *J. Neurochem.*, 20, 977–85
Kodama, T., Fujino, M., Endo, Y., Obara, T., Fujimoto, Y., Oda, T. and Wada, T. (1980). Identification of carcinoembryonic antigen in the C-cell of the normal thyroid. *Cancer*, 45, 98
Le Douarin, N. and Le Lièvre, C. (1970). Démonstration de l'origine neurale des cellules à calcitonine du corps ultimobranchial chez l'embryon de Poulet. *C. r. Acad. Sci., Paris*, série D, 270, 3095–98
Le Douarin, N. M. and Teillet, M.-A. (1973). The migration of neural crest cells to the wall of the digestive tract in avian embryo. *J. Embryol. exp. Morph.*, 30, 31–48
Leibson, L. (1979). Endocrinology, evolution and evolutionary endocrinology. *Perspect. biol. Med.*, 23, 25–43
Louis, C. J. (1970). Autoradiographic localization of [$^3$H]5-hydroxytryptophan uptake by rat neurons in vivo and in tissue culture. *Histochem. J.*, 2, 29–32
Marangos, P. J., Athanasios, P., Zis, A. P., Clark, R. L. and Goodwin, F. K. (1978). Neuronal, non-neuronal and hybrid forms of enolase in brain: structural, immunological and functional comparisons. *Brain Res.*, 150, 117–33
Merkel, F. (1880). *Uber die Endigungen der Sensiblen Nerven in der Haut der Wirbeltiere*, Schmidt, Rostock
Munger, B. L. (1977). Neural-epithelial interactions in sensory receptors. *J. invest. Dermatol.*, 69, 27–40
Nakajima, T., Yamaguchi, H. and Takahashi, K. (1980). S-100 protein in folliculostellate cells of the rat pituitary anterior lobe. *Brain Res.*, 191, 523–31
Pearse, A. G. E. (1966a). 5-Hydroxytryptophan uptake by dog thyroid C cells and its possible significance in polypeptide hormone production. *Nature Lond.*, 211, 598–600
Pearse, A. G. E. (1966b). Common cytochemical properties of cells producing polypeptide hormones, with particular reference to calcitonin and the thyroid C cells. *Vet. Rec.*, 79, 587–90
Pearse, A. G. E. (1968). Common cytochemical and ultrastructural characteristics of cells producing polypeptide hormones (the APUD series) and their relevance to thyroid and ultimobranchial C cells and calcitonin. *Proc. R. Soc. Lond.*, B170, 71–80
Pearse, A. G. E. (1969). The cytochemistry and ultrastructure of polypeptide hormone producing cells of the APUD series, and the embryologic, physiologic and pathologic implications of the concept. *J. Histochem. Cytochem.*, 17, 303–13
Pearse, A. G. E. (1975a). The endocrine division of the nervous system: a logical extension of the APUD concept. *Folia Anat. Iugoslav.*, 4, 5–20
Pearse, A. G. E. (1975b). Neurocristopathy, neuroendocrine pathology and the APUD concept. *Z. Krebsforsch.*, 84, 1–18
Pearse, A. G. E. (1977). The diffuse endocrine (paracrine) system: Feyrter's concept and its modern history. *Verh. Dtsch. Ges., Path.*, 61, 2–6
Pearse, A. G. E. and Polak, J. M. (1971). Cytochemical evidence for the neural crest origin of mammalian ultimobranchial C cells. *Histochemie*, 27, 96–102
Pearse, A. G. E., Polak, J. M., Facer, P. and Marangos, P. J. (1980). Neuron specific enolase in gastric and related endocrine cells. *Hepatogastroenterologia*, 27, 78
Pictet, R. and Rutter, W. J. (1972). Development of the embryonic endocrine pancreas. In *The Endocrine Pancreas*, Handbook of Physiology, 1 (ed. D. F. Steiner and N. Freinkel), Williams Wilkins, Baltimore, pp. 25–66

Pictet, R. L., Rall, L. B., Phelps, P. and Rutter, W. J. (1976). The neural crest and the origin of the insulin-producing and other gastrointestinal hormone-producing cells. *Science*, 191, 191–2

Schmechel, D., Marangos, P. J. and Brightman, M. (1978). Neurone-specific enolase is a molecular marker for peripheral and central neuroendocrine cells. *Nature Lond.*, 276, 834

Schmechel, D. E., Brightman, M. W. and Marangos, P. J. (1980). Neurons switch from non-neuronal enolase to neuron-specific enolase during differentiation. *Brain Res.*, 190, 195–214

Scott, S. A., Cooper, E. and Diamond, J. (1981). Merkel cells as targets of the mechano-sensory nerves in salamander skin. *Proc. R. Soc. Lond.*, B211, 455–70

Takor-Takor, T. and Pearse, A. G. E. (1975). Neuroectodermal origin of avian hypothalamo-hypophyseal complex: the role of the ventral neural ridge. *J. Embryol. exp. Morph.*, 34, 311–25

Talmage, R. V., Grubb, S. A., Norimatsu, H. and Van der Wiel, C. J. (1980). Evidence for an important physiological role for calcitonin *Proc. natn. Acad. Sci. U.S.A.*, 77, 609–13

Wharton, J., Polak, J. M., Cole, G. A., Marangos, P. and Pearse, A. G. E. (1981). Neuron-specific enolase as an immunocytochemical marker for the diffuse neuroendocrine system in human foetal lung. *J. Histochem. Cytochem.*, in press

Winkler, H. and Westhead, E. (1980). The molecular organization of adrenal chromaffin granules. *Neuroscience*, 5, 1803–23

# 11

# Neuropharmacological and neurophysiological consequences of the co-release of neurotransmitters

R. W. Ryall (Department of Pharmacology, University of Cambridge, Cambridge, UK)

## INTRODUCTION

When two or more transmitters are liberated at different synapses on the same neurone and the sites of action are restricted to the immediately adjacent sub-synaptic membrane, they may mutually interact as a consequence of their postsynaptic effects. Depolarisations arising from selective conductance increases at different parts of the neurone may be synergistic at the sites of impulse generation, although the summation may be less than additive if the sites of origin of the depolarising effects are so close together that an increase conductance, at one synapse, short-circuits the depolarising currents produced at other synapses. Similarly, the conductance shunts and hyperpolarisations produced by inhibitory neurotransmitters may reduce excitatory potentials to levels at which the threshold for impulse initiation is not reached. Excitatory and, presumably, inhibitory transmission may also be attenuated by presynaptic inhibition in which axo-axonic synapses liberate transmitters which reduce the output of transmitter from the primary afferent and possibly higher order fibres. Such may be considered to be the classical mechanisms of synaptic transmission in which the effects of one transmitter modulates the action of another but each retains an independence with respect to neuronal pathways, control of release and independent sites of action on the postsynaptic neurone.

With the recent awareness of the putative transmitter functions of endogenous polypeptides and the sophistication of modern neuroanatomical techniques for identifying and tracing polypeptide and amine-containing neurones, a plethora of new anatomical and pharmacological observations have been made, which have lead to a reappraisal of our classical notions of the mechanisms of neuro-transmission and the interactions between different neurotransmitters.

## SYNAPTIC ACTIONS OF CO-TRANSMITTERS

Of principal interest are the neuroanatomical observations showing that neurones may contain more than one neurotransmitter, but it will be my purpose to pro-pose some possible neuropharmacological and neurophysiological consequences and implications of the co-release of neurotransmitters.

There would seem to be little purpose in liberating more than one transmitter from the same nerve terminal unless one of two criteria were to be met. The argument would apply with equal force whether the transmitters exerted the same, different but synergistic or even opposite effects upon their target site, or even when the target sites themselves differed, for example, if one transmitter acted postsynaptically and the other acted presynaptically.

The two criteria to be met are: (1) either there should be some difference in the time-dependency of the release or action of the two transmitters: or (2) the relative rates of release of the two transmitters should change according to the functional activity of the terminal. An example of the first criterion could be that one neurotransmitter exerted an action which was more subject to desensi-tisation than the action of the other or that one was more rapidly inactivated or taken up than the other. The second criterion, possibly the most probable of the two, is that the two transmitters are released at rates which show different relationships to frequency of impulses in the presynaptic terminals.

As yet there is no evidence to show that co-release produces interactive effects which are time or frequency dependent. Such plasticity of synaptic efficacy by co-transmission could in part explain long-term chantes in functional activity at synapses.

By contrast, neuropharmacological and neurophysiological experiments have demonstrated that the polypeptides substance P and enkephalin, and perhaps even the monoamine 5-hydroxytryptamine, prime candidates for coexistence in and release from single neurones (see Hökfelt *et al.*, Chan-Palay and Gilbert *et al.*, this volume), have unusual features to their actions which could be autoregulatory in function and with clear implications for the mechanisms of co-transmission.

### Substance P and enkephalins as possible co-transmitters

On cat Renshaw cells the iontophoresis of substance P from multibarrel micro-pipettes selectively antagonises the excitatory effect of acetylcholine while leaving unchanged the excitation by amino acids (Belcher and Ryall, 1977; Ryall and Belcher, 1977; Krnjevic and Lekic, 1977; Davies and Dray, 1977). This indicates that substance P did not act by a non-specific inhibitory effect on the

Renshaw cell, such as is produced by inhibitory amino acids. Even more surprising was the observation that substance P did not antagonise the muscarinic component of excitation by acetyl-β-methylcholine (Belcher and Ryall, 1977; Ryall and Belcher, 1977), indicating a very selective effect on excitation mediated by way of the nicotinic cholinergic receptors.

It was therefore proposed that substance P modulates cholinergic transmission at the Renshaw cell by combining with the nicotinic receptor at an allosteric site or alternatively, that it modifies the coupling between receptor activation and conductance change in a specific but unknown fashion.

In keeping with these observations it was shown that substance P markedly reduced the early synaptically evoked discharge of Renshaw cells to submaximal stimulation of ventral roots, which is known to be antagonised by dihydro-β-erythroidine, a selective antagonist of acetylcholine at nicotinic receptors. However, substance P was not effective when much larger stimuli were used, presumably due to the intensity of activation in such conditions. This probably is the explanation for the failure of Krnjevic and Lekic (1977) to show an inhibition of responses evoked synaptically. On other spinal neurones and in the cerebral cortex excitation by acetylcholine, which is due to a muscarinic action, was either unaffected or only slightly reduced (Krnjevic and Lekic, 1977).

The action of substance P on nicotinic receptors is not confined to those on Renshaw cells. At the cholinergic synapse between giant fibres and Mauthner neurones in the hatchet fish (Steinacker and Highstein, 1976), substance P also has an anticholinergic effect in addition to presynaptic actions. Acetylcholine or nicotine, but not muscarinic agonists, release catecholamines from adrenal medullary neurones grown in tissue culture (Mizobe *et al.*, 1979). The release by nicotinic agonists but not that evoked by increased potassium concentrations was antagonised by substance P in concentrations of $10^{-7}$ to $10^{-5}$ M. Since extracellular calcium is necessary for the potassium-evoked release, inhibition of nicotinic stimulation by substance P was not due to interference with calcium transport. Neither was inhibition due to an action of substance P on the voltage-sensitive sodium channels, because the release of catecholamines by veratridine was unaffected (Dean and Livett, 1980).

The selective anti-acetylcholine effect of substance P is not confined to this polypeptide, because it has also been observed with Met-enkephalin on Renshaw cells (Davies and Dray, 1976) and with a number of substances P analogues, somatostatin and opiates on adrenal paraneurones (Dean *et al.*, 1981). However, the action of opiates was not stereospecific and was not reversed by selective opiate antagonists (Lemaire *et al.*, 1980). In bullfrog sympathetic ganglia it has recently been shown that 5-hydroxytryptamine antagonises acetylcholine-evoked depolarisation and nicotinic cholinergic transmission in an apparently competitive fashion (Akasu *et al.*, 1981), although concentrations of 5-hydroxytryptamine were in the range of $10^{-4}$ to $10^{-3}$ M and are unlikely to be of physiological interest.

There are no published observations on the action of substance P on nicotinic receptors at the neuromuscular junction. At a high concentration of $10^{-4}$ M, substance P reduced endplate and miniature endplate potential amplitudes at frog neuromuscular junctions (Steinacker, 1977) but it is not clear to what extent the depression was due to presynaptic depression of release or a post-synaptic block of receptors. The fact that the depression was reduced by high concentrations of calcium and that it was accompanied by reductions in minia-ture endplate potential frequency and quantal content of the endplate potential indicates that there was a large presynaptic component present. At concentra-tions of $10^{-5}$ to $10^{-6}$ M, after an initial transient depression, there was a pro-nounced increase in endplate potential amplitudes and in the quantal content of the endplate potential with only minor effects on miniature endplate potential frequency or amplitude. These observations suggest that substance P at moderate concentrations may have a presynaptic effect in increasing the number of quanta of acetylcholine released with each nerve impulse.

In preliminary experiments on chick neuromuscular junction (Ryall and Wallace, unpublished observations) substance P did not reproducibly antagonise contractures produced by carbamylcholine, although there was sometimes a small contraction caused by substance P itself. This is consistent with the observed facilitation of transmitter release in frog muscle (Steinacker, 1977) but suggests that nicotinic receptor activation in skeletal muscle is not antagonised by sub-stance P and that the polypeptide can differentiate not only between nicotinic and muscarinic receptors but also between different types of nicotinic receptors.

On cat Renshaw cells we also observed an initial excitatory effect of substance P which occurred less frequently than the inhibitory action on acetylcholine-evoked excitation and showed evidence of "desensitisation" with a time-course comparable to that of the acetylcholine antagonism (Belcher and Ryall, 1977; Ryall and Belcher, 1977). Furthermore, the excitation by substance P was antagonised by dihydro-β-erythroidine, clear evidence that substance P had a dual effect in first releasing acetylcholine from the cholinergic terminals and then antagonising its effect at postsynaptic nicotinic receptors.

Morphine administered iontophoretically also excited Renshaw cells and again this excitation was blocked by dihydro-β-erythroidine (Belcher and Ryall, 1977). Nistri (1976) has demonstrated by direct assay that morphine increased spontaneous release of acetylcholine from the spinal cord. Since morphine acts upon opiate receptors to which the endogenous ligands, the enkephalins, also bind, it seems likely that both substance P and the enkephalins have presynaptic facilitatory effects upon cholinergic transmission at spinal Renshaw cells, in addition to the antagonism at nicotinic receptors exerted by substance P and enkephalins. A facilitatory effect of enkephalins, rather than of morphine, has yet to be demonstrated.

On non-cholinoceptive spinal neurones and on cuneate neurones substance P causes a slow depolarization (Krnjevic and Morris, 1974; Henry *et al.*, 1975). This depolarisation is at least in part due to a reduction in membrane permeability to potassium ions (Krnjevic, 1977; Nowak and MacDonald, 1981). It may also be in part due to the release of non-cholinergic excitatory neurotransmitters since in tissue cultures substance P induced "bursting" behaviour which was blocked by tetrodotoxin (Nowak and MacDonald 1981).

A probable presynaptic facilitatory effect of enkephalins has also been described in hippocampal slices (Haas and Ryall, 1980). There was an increase in the amplitude of intracellularly recorded excitatory postsynaptic potentials and an increase in the number of synaptically-evoked action potentials, which was blocked by naloxone. However, there was little or no effect on resting membrane potential or conductance at this time and there was no change in the excitability of dendrites as judged by the inability of enkephalin to alter the excitatory effects of amino acids administered to dendritic or somatic regions of the pyramidal neurones. There was no change, or even a small increase in synaptica-ally-evoked inhibition, and it was concluded that the most probable action was a presynaptic facilitation of the release of excitatory neurotransmitters. Whether this mechanism also explains the exictatory effects of opiates on spinal non-nociceptive neurones (Belcher and Ryall, 1978) and elsewhere in the central nervous system remains to be established.

By contrast, inhibitory presynaptic effects of opiates on neurotransmitter release are well established. These include the well-known depression of acety-choline release from peripheral muscarinic synapses by opiates and the intriguing depression of substance P release by opiates in slices of trigeminal nucleus *in vitro* (Jessell and Iversen, 1977) and *in vivo* from the spinal cord in response to afferent nerve stimulation (Jessell *et al.*, 1979; Yaksh *et al.*, 1980).

Enkephalins and other opiates also block noxious inputs to a variety of spinal and supraspinal neurones. Often this depression is unaccompanied by a depression of the response evoked by a non-noxious input. Similarly, selective depression of noxious inputs to spinal interneurones is exhibited by 5-hydroxytryptamine (Belcher and Ryall, 1978). Such observations suggest that the depression is exerted presynaptically.

Substance P, enkephalins and 5-hydroxytryptamine are currently receiving considerable interest, as attested to by this symposium, as candidates for co-transmission. In this brief summary I have attempted to show that each of them has complex and unusual action composed of both presynaptic and postsynaptic excitation and depression.

The best established effects are those on cholinergic neurotransmission both in the central nervous system and in the peripheral nervous system. Substance P has now been shown by electrophysiological and pharmacological techniques to increase the presynaptic release of acetylcholine in the spinal cord and at the neuromuscular junction. However, postsynaptic depression, which is specific for exictation by way of nicotinic receptors for acetylcholine occurs simultaneously on Renshaw cells and is the only effect reported in adrenal medullary neurones in tissue culture. A similar postsynaptic depression seems to be absent at nicotinic receptors at skeletal neuromuscular junction indicating that substance P may distinguish between different classes of nicotinic receptors.

Morphine and enkephalins have both excitatory and inhibitory effects on central neurones and many of these are probably exerted presynaptically.


## CONCLUDING REMARKS

It therefore seems likely that if the polypeptides are co-released in physiological conditions then they will act either as modulators of the release of the primary transmitter by an autoregulatory facilitatory or inhibitory effect upon the terminals of the releasing or nearby neurones, or as very selective regulators of the postsynaptic action of the primary transmitters. In order to view these actions in physiological perspective, information is still required on the time-dependency of the release and action of the cotransmitters.


## REFERENCES

Akasu, T., Hirai, K. and Koketsu, K. (1981). 5-Hydroxytryptamine controls ACh-receptor sensitivity of bullfrog sympathetic ganglion cells. *Brain Res.*, 211, 217–220

Belcher, G. and Ryall, R. W. (1977). Substance P and Renshaw cells: a new concept of inhibitory synaptic interactions. *J. Physiol. Lond.*, 272, 105–119

Belcher, G. and Ryall, R. W. (1978). Differential excitatory and inhibitory effects of opiates on non-nociceptive and nociceptive neurones in the spinal cord of the cat. *Brain Res.*, 145, 303–314

Davies, J. and Dray, A. (1976). Effects of enkephalin and morphine on Renshaw cells in feline spinal cord. *Nature*, 262, 603–604

Davies, J. and Dray, A. (1977). Substance P and opiate receptors. *Nature*, 268, 351–352

Dean, D. M. and Livett, B. A. (1980). Study of mechanisms of peptide modulation of catecholamine release in bovine adrenal paraneurones. *Soc. Neurosci. Abstr.*, 6, 335

Dean, D. M., Boska, P., Day, R. and Livett, B. G. (1981). Peptide modulation of transmitter function. Symposium contribution to Transmission in the Autonomic Nervous System. *Proc. Austr. Neurosci. Soc.*, S7

Haas, H. L. and Ryall, R. W. (1980). Is excitation by enkephalins of hippocampal neurones in the rat due to presynaptic facilitation or to disinhibition? *J. Physiol. Lond.*, 308, 315–330

Henry, J. L., Krnjevic, K. and Morris, M. E. (1975). Substance P and spinal neurones. *Can. J. Physiol. Pharmac.*, 53, 423–432

Jessell, T. M. and Iversen, L. L. (1977). Opiate analgesics inhibit substance P release from rat trigeminal nucleus. *Nature Lond.*, 268, 549–551

Jessell, T. M., Mudge, A. W., Leeman, S. E. and Yaksh, T. L. (1979). Release of substance P and somatostatin *in vivo*, from primary afferent terminals in mammalian spinal cord. *Neuroscience, abstr.*, 5, 611

Krnjevic, K. (1977). Effects of substance P on central neurones in cat. In *Substance P* (ed. U. S. von Euler and B. Pernow), Raven Press, New York, pp. 217–230

Krnjevic, K. and Lekic, D. (1977). Substance P selectively blocks excitation of Renshaw cell by acetylcholine. *Can. J. Physiol. Pharmac.*, 55, 958–961

Krnjevic, K. and Morris, M. E. (1974). An excitatory action of substance P on cuneate neurones. *Can. J. Physiol. Pharmac.*, 52, 736–744

Lemaire, S., Lemaire, S., Dean, D. M. and Livett, B. G. (1980). Opiate receptors and adrenal medullary function. *Nature London*, 288, 303–304

Mizobe, F., Kosousek, V., Dean, D. M. and Livett, B. G. (1979). Pharmacological characterization of adrenal paraneurons: substance P and somatostatin as inhibitory modulators of the nicotinic response. *Brain Res.*, **178**, 555–566

Nistri, A. (1976). Morphine-induced changes in the spontaneous and electrically evoked acetylcholine release from the isolated spinal cord. *Brain Res.*, **110**, 403–406

Nowak, L. M. and MacDonald, R. L. (1981). Substance P decreases a potassium conductance of spinal cord neurons in cell culture. *Brain Res.*, **214**, 416–423

Ryall, R. W. and Belcher, G. (1977). Substance P selectively blocks nicotinic receptors on Renshaw cells: a possible synaptic inhibitory mechanism. *Brain Res.*, **137**, 376–380

Steinacker, A. (1977). Calcium-dependent presynaptic action of substance P at the frog neuromuscular junction.

Steinacker, A. and Highstein, S. M. (1976). Pre- and post-synaptic action of substance P at the Mauthner fiber – giant fiber synapse in the hatchet fish. *Brain Res.*, **114**, 128–133

Yaksh, T. L., Jessell, T. M., Gamse, R., Mudge, A. W. and Leeman, S. E. (1980). Intrathecal morphine inhibits substance P release from spinal cord *in vivo*. *Nature London*, **286**, 155–157

# 12

# Coexistence of adenosine 5'-triphosphate and acetylcholine in the electromotor synapse

H. Zimmermann (Fachbereich Biologie der Universität Oldenburg,
Postfach 2503, D-2900 Oldenburg, Federal Republic of Germany)

## INTRODUCTION

The neurotransmitter acetylcholine (ACh) is released from the presynaptic nerve terminal in the form of quantal packets. After diffusing through the synaptic cleft, it acts at the postsynaptic receptor. In the presynaptic nerve terminal ACh is stored inside synaptic vesicles which are thought to be the subcellular manifestation of quantal packaging. There is a "choline cycle" at the nerve terminal: ACh released is hydrolysed to form choline and acetate. An active transport system of high affinity supplies the nerve terminal with extracellular choline for renewed synthesis and release of ACh. Particularly for neuromuscular transmission these mechanisms would appear to be satisfactory for maintaining physiological levels of activation of the effector system.

However, during the past years new concepts have been introduced regarding the molecular aspects of peripheral cholinergic transmission both with regard to ACh and also to nucleotide function (see also Burnstock, chapter 6). Cholinergic nerve terminals like the postsynaptic membrane appear to contain ACh receptors and ACh may affect its own release via autoinhibition. In addition to ACh cholinergic nerve terminals may store adenine nucleotides, particularly ATP, at high concentrations inside synaptic vesicles. ATP can be released on stimulation. The physiological significance of this process is now becoming elucidated.

## VESICULAR STORAGE OF PURINES

### Molar ratios in synaptosomes and synaptic vesicle fractions

The only system in which molecular aspects of cholinergic function can be investigated in pure form is the electric organ. The electric organ of electric rays is derived from embryonic muscle tissue and its innervation corresponds to that of skeletal muscle. Following the pioneering studies of Sheridan *et al.* (1966) in Torpedo, methods for isolation of synaptosomes as well as synaptic vesicles of high purity were developed (see Zimmermann, 1982). Dowdall *et al.* (1974) found that synaptic vesicles isolated from the Torpedo electric organ besides ACh contain ATP at high concentrations. As can be seen from table 12.1 the

Table 12.1  Molar ratios of ACh and ATP in synaptosomes and synaptic vesicles from electric organ

|  | Species | ACh/ATP (molar ratio) | Reference |
|---|---|---|---|
| Synaptosomes | Torpedo marmorata | 3 | Meunier and Morel (1978) |
|  | Torpedo marmorata | 9 | Zimmermann *et al.* (1979) |
|  | Torpedo marmorata | 7 | Richardson and Whittaker (1981) |
| Synaptic vesicles | Torpedo marmorata | 5 | Dowdall *et al.* (1974) |
|  | Torpedo marmorata | 7 | Tashiro and Stadler (1978) |
|  | Narcine brasiliensis | 2.5 | Wagner *et al.* (1978) |

For comparison specific contents of ACh of 6.9 $\mu$mol mg protein$^{-1}$ have been reported for synaptic vesicles (Tashiro and Stadler, 1978) and 262 nmol mg protein$^{-1}$ for synaptosomes (Zimmermann *et al.*, 1979).

molar ratio of ACh/ATP in synaptic vesicles is around 5 with some degree of variation between investigators. If one vesicle contains about 200,000 molecules of ACh (Ohsawa *et al.*, 1979), its content in ATP molecules would be about 40,000.

It is interesting to note that the molar ratios in entire synaptosomes and in synaptic vesicles are about equal. This either means that the vast majority of nerve terminal ACh and ATP is stored in synaptic vesicles or that the substances occur in the same molar ratio inside and outside synaptic vesicles. The only other purely cholinergic tissue for which vesicular presence of ATP was reported is the electric organ of the electric eel with a molar ratio of ACh/ATP of 11 (Zimmermann and Denston, 1976). Since no more than 15 per cent of synaptic vesicles isolated from mammalian cortex are likely to be cholinergic, the presence of ATP in a brain vesicle fraction cannot be related to this particular transmitter. For comparison the molar ratio ACh/ATP recovered in a vesicle fraction isolated from guinea pig cerebral cortex was about 1, suggesting a relative higher contribution of ATP than in a pure cholinergic vesicle fraction (Nagy *et al.*, 1976).

## Is ATP contained in the same subcellular particles as ACh?

There is now good evidence that the ATP content of the vesicular fraction is not due to mitochondrial contamination and that the two compounds are indeed contained in the same particle. Under isoosmotic conditions both vesicular ACh and ATP are resistant to addition of hydrolyzing enzymes (Dowdall *et al.*, 1974). ACh and ATP not only co-sediment on sucrose density gradients as shown in figure 12.1 and are well separated from supernatant and membrane fractions.

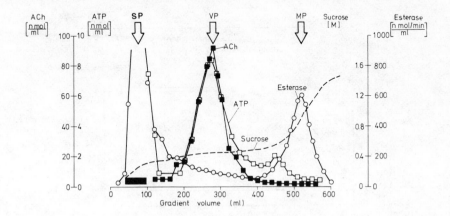

Figure 12.1  Separation of synaptic vesicles from Torpedo electric organ and co-sedimentation of ACh and ATP. Vesicles are extracted from frozen and crushed electric tissue and prepurified using differential centrifugation. Refractionated material is loaded (bar) on a shallow iso-osmotic NaCl/sucrose (sucrose) gradient and separated in a zonal rotor. Synaptic vesicles identified by their contents in ACh and ATP sediment as a sharp peak around 0.4 molar sucrose (VP) and become separated from a soluble supernatant fraction (SP) and a denser membrane fraction (MP) containing activity of cholinesterases (esterase). Material loaded corresponds to 33 g of fresh tissue.

They also co-sediment in gradient media containing membrane permable substances like glycerol and become eluted together from columns of porous glass beads (see Giompres *et al.*, 1981*a*). Furthermore, vesicular turnover of both ACh and ATP seems to occur at identical rate.

Repetitive stimulation of the nerve leading into electric tissue causes parallel depletion of vesicular ACh and ATP (figure 12.2*a*). The degree of depletion depends on frequency and time of stimulation. For example, application of 5000 impulses at 5 Hz reduces vesicular contents of both substances by 90 per cent. This is accompanied by an average loss of 50 per cent of synaptic vesicle counts as revealed by morphological examination of stimulated tissue. On the other hand low frequency stimulation at 0.1 Hz (1800 impulses) does not affect vesicle numbers but still reduces vesicular contents of both ACh and ATP by 50 per cent (Zimmermann, 1978). On subsequent recovery of tissue vesicular ACh and ATP become replenished *para passu* (figure 12.2*b*).

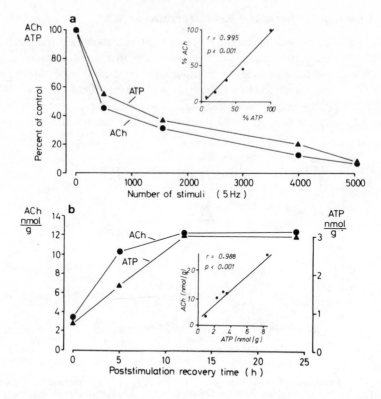

Figure 12.2  Correlated depletion of ACh and ATP from synaptic vesicles and correlated reloading during a subsequent period of rest. *a*, Continued stimulation *in vivo* of electric tissue at 5 Hz causes progressive depletion of both vesicular ACh and ATP. Values are means of three experiments. In each experiment one electric organ of the fish served as a control and the other one was stimulated. Inset: Correlation diagram of the same determinations (F-test). (From Zimmermann and Whittaker, 1974.) *b*, Parallel recovery of vesicular ACh and ATP after stimulation of electric tissue (1800 impulses, 0.1 Hz). Experiments were performed with perfused blocks of tissue in *in vitro* conditions. This is likely to explain the retardation in the recovery process after 12 h. All values are derived from one experiment in which four electric organs were used. Two independent tissue blocks were perfused for each time point and from each block 2-3 density gradient separations were performed. Values are means of the density gradient separations. Inset: In addition to the values presented in the graph the correlation diagram includes the value for vesicular control contents (unstimulated) of ACh and ATP (F-test) (From Giompres *et al*. 1981*b*.)

## Vesicular contents in other purine compounds

As can be seen from table 12.2 cholinergic vesicles also contain small amounts of ADP and AMP and even GTP. It is likely that the contents in these nucleotides reflect both the wide specificity of the vesicular "ATP" carrier described recently (Luqmani, 1981) and the cytoplasmic contents of the respective compounds.

Table 12.2 Contents in purines of cholinergic synaptic vesicles isolated from electric organ

| Species | ATP | ADP | AMP | IMP | Adenosine | GTP | GDP | GMP | Reference |
|---------|-----|-----|-----|-----|-----------|-----|-----|-----|-----------|
| Torpedo | 1* | 0.16 | 0.02 | N.D | N.D | N.D | N.D | N.D | Zimmermann (1978) |
| marmorata | 1** | 0.06 | 0.04 | 0.02 | 0.05 | N.D | N.D | N.D | Zimmermann (1978) |
| Narcine brasiliensis | 1* | 0.05 | 0.02 | N.D | N.D | 0.17 | 0.005 | 0.02 | Wagner *et al.* (1978) |

Values are relative to ATP contents. *Derived from measurements of total contents of vesicle fraction. **Derived from analysis of radiolabelled metabolites after extracellular application of [$^3$H]-adenosine. ND, Not determined.

## PRECURSORS OF VESICULAR ATP

### Uptake into synaptosomes

Experiments with synaptosomes isolated from the Torpedo electric organ show that both extracellular adenosine and adenine can be taken up into cholinergic nerve terminals. At concentrations of 0.3 $\mu$M both adenosine and adenine are taken up into isolated synaptosomes linearly at least up to 60 min (figure 12.3a). However, adenosine exceeds uptake of adenine by a factor of 10. In the same experiments and at similar extracellular concentrations isolated nerve endings showed no significant uptake of either inosine or hypoxanthine. In contrast to adenine and in analogy to the precursor of ACh, choline, adenosine is taken up into synaptosomes by way of a saturable uptake system of high affinity ($K_m$ = 2 $\mu$M, $V_{max}$ = 30 pmol min$^{-1}$ mg protein$^{-1}$ (figure 12.3b). This uptake is inhibited competitively by 2'-deoxyadenosine (Zimmermann *et al.*, 1979). Blockade of choline high affinity uptake with hemicholinium-3 does not affect adenosine uptake into nerve terminals (Zimmermann and Bokor, 1979).

The maximum uptake velocity of the preparation is of the same order as that observed for choline although both rates may be improved to a certain degree by modifications in the isolation procedure of synaptosomes (Richardson and Whittaker, 1981). Compared to the specific contents of the synaptosome fraction in ATP (see table 12.1) this would mean that isolated nerve endings could replenish about 1/1000 of their "adenosine" contents per minute. This does not appear to be very high but the situation is equivalent for choline recycling. Nerve endings *in situ* which have lost part of their ACh and ATP contents on stimulation take several hours to replenish their stores (figure 12.2).

### Intraterminal synthesis of ATP

Both adenosine and adenine can serve as precursors of ATP at cholinergic nerve terminals (figure 12.4). Adenosine becomes phosphorylated by adenosine kinase on its passage through the plasma membrane or immediately afterwards to form

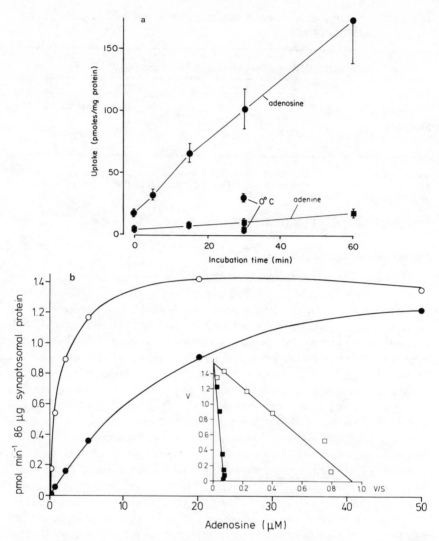

Figure 12.3 Uptake of extracellular precursors of vesicular ATP into synaptosomes isolated from electric organ. *a*, Time-dependent uptake was studied at room temperature with [$^3$H]-adenosine (0.31 $\mu$M) and [$^3$H]-adenine (0.36 $\mu$M). Uptake is linear up to 60 min. Uptake of adenosine ($\bullet$) exceeds that of adenine ($\blacksquare$) by a factor of 10. Additional values at the 30 min time point represent incubations at 0°C. Values are mean ± s.e. mean of six (adenosine) or five (adenine) determinations (from Zimmermann *et al.*, 1979). *b*, Concentration-dependent uptake of [$^3$H]-adenosine into synaptosomes and its inhibition by 2'-deoxyadenosine. Incubation was at room temperature for 30 min and terminated by filtration through Millipore filters. Values represent means of triplicate determinations for uptake in the presence of adenosine only (o, □) or means of duplicate determinations with 1 mM 2'-deoxyandenosine added to varying adenosine concentrations ($\bullet$, $\blacksquare$). Adenosine uptake is saturable. Inset: Eadie-Hofstee plot of the same determinations which show that 2'-deoxyadenosine is a competitive inhibitor of adenosine uptake ($K_m$ adenosine = 1.5 $\mu$M; $K_i$ 2'-deoxyadenosine = 91 $\mu$M). (From Zimmermann *et al.*, 1979.)

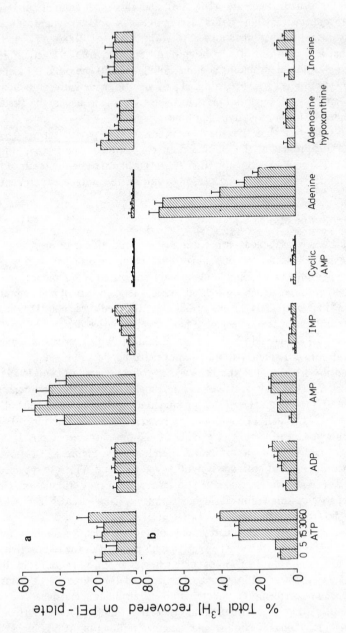

Figure 12.4  Metabolism of [³H]-adenosine *a* and [³H]-adenine *b*, after uptake into synaptosomes isolated from electric organ. [³H]-labelled products were analysed after incubation of synaptosomes for 0, 5, 15, 30 and 60 min at room temperature by two-dimensional thin layer chromatography on PEI cellulose plates. Values are mean ± s.e. mean of four (adenosine) or five (adenine) experiments. (From Zimmermann *et al.*, 1979.)

AMP. It does not accumulate inside nerve terminals. As shown by two-dimensional thinlayer chromatography on PEI cellulose plates, further metabolites formed inside the synaptosome are ADP, AMP and also small amounts of IMP and inosine. In contrast, adenine is first accumulated in isolated synaptosomes but eventually also becomes metabolised to form AMP, ADP and ATP. It is noteworthy that in conditions of rest insignificant amounts of 3', 5'-cyclic AMP are formed from either adenosine or adenine. Similar results are obtained if the two precursors are applied to perfused blocks of electric tissue with subsequent isolation and analysis of synaptosomes. Extracellular adenosine in the tissue becomes degraded to inosine and hypoxanthine.

These results suggest that the enzymes necessary for purine salvage (see Murray, 1971) are present at the cholinergic nerve terminal. The relative slow formation of ATP in our experiments (figure 12.4) is likely to be the result of a somewhat hypoxic state of the synaptosomes during the uptake experiment.

### Vesicular incorporation of ATP

Vesicular ATP becomes labelled on perfusion of isolated blocks of electric tissue with radiolabelled adenosine, in analogy to labelling of vesicular ACh with choline or acetate as precursor (Zimmermann and Denston, 1977b; Zimmermann, 1978). In experiments in which both choline and adenosine are applied simultaneously with different labels, labelled (newly synthesised) vesicular ACh and ATP comigrate on a sucrose gradient together with the native peak of ACh and ATP (see figure 12.1). Figure 12.5 shows an experiment which reveals vesicular heterogeneity after low frequency stimulation of perfused electric tissue.

As described in earlier studies and reviewed elsewhere (Zimmermann, 1979a; Zimmermann et al., 1981), synaptic vesicles are smaller in diameter and denser immediately after recycling. They have an increased uptake capacity for both newly synthesised ACh and ATP and may be separated (vesicle fraction, $VP_2$) by density gradient centrifugation or glass bead column chromatography from vesicles not yet involved in cycles of exo- and endocytosis. Figure 12.5a shows preferential incorporation of both newly synthesized ACh and ATP into recycled synaptic vesicles (denser vesicle peak, $VP_2$) after low frequency stimulation. On subsequent repetitive stimulation at higher frequency labelled ACh and ATP become lost again from vesicle fraction $VP_2$ (figure 12.5b).

Analysis by ion exchange chromatography of radiolabelled products in the synaptic vesicle fraction (or fractions) reveals that 85 per cent of the radioactivity derived from adenosine is in the form of ATP, whereas about 5 per cent is in the form of ADP. Only traces of AMP may be detected (see table 12.1). Thus, vesicular ATP becomes replenished directly from extracellular adenosine.

It is noteworthy that after stimulation vesicular refilling of ATP continues normally even if recycling of choline and vesicular refilling of ACh is blocked with hemicholinium-3. Thus, vesicles containing ATP with only traces of ACh may be produced (Zimmermann and Bokor, 1979; Giompres et al., 1981b).

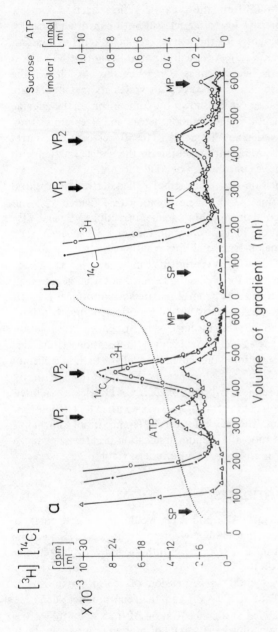

Figure 12.5 Parallel incorporation of [¹⁴C]-ACh and [³H]-ATP into synaptic vesicles derived from simultaneously applied [¹⁴C]-choline and [³H]-adenosine respectively. *a*, After 3 h of preperfusion with radiolabel 1080 impulses (0.1 Hz) were applied. In these conditions, [¹⁴C]-ACh and [³H]-ATP are preferentially incorporated into fraction $VP_2$ (Sucrose density gradient, zonal rotor). Vesicular fraction $VP_2$ appears in addition to vesicle fraction $VP_1$ (corresponding to vesicle fraction VP of figure 12.1) after tissue has been activated. *b*, After prestimulation (1080 impulses, 0.1 Hz) the tissue block was washed in the presence of the blocker of choline uptake hemicholinium-3 (100 μM) and the blocker of adenosine uptake, dipyridamole (5 μM). It was then re-stimulated at the higher frequency of 5 Hz (4500 impulses). There is a loss of total ATP as well as [¹⁴C]- and [³H]-label from vesicle fraction $VP_2$. The amount of parent fraction loaded on the gradient corresponded to 45 g (*a*) and 43.5 (*b*) of fresh tissue. SP, Supernatant fraction; MP, membrane peak; dotted line, sucrose gradient. (From Zimmermann, 1979*b*.)

## NERVE TERMINAL RELEASE OF ATP

As mentioned above (figure 12.2) repetitive nerve stimulation induces a *pari passu* loss of both ACh and ATP from the synaptic vesicle fraction. On low frequency stimulation a progressive loss of vesicles in both constituents can be observed, although vesicle counts in the nerve terminals remain constant (Zimmermann and Denston, 1977a;b). Although it seems likely that ATP is lost from vesicles by way of the same mechanism as ACh, it remains possible that the nucleotide becomes hydrolysed inside the vesicle in which its metabolites are retained. That this is not the case can be shown by comparison of the adenine nucleotide content in the synaptic vesicle fraction before and after stimulation. Even after depletion of the vesicular ATP content to 50 per cent of control values, ATP remains the most prominent nucleotide in the vesicle fraction with only minor changes in the relative contribution of ADP and AMP.

The same picture is obtained on analysis of radiolabelled derivatives of extra-cellularly applied [$^3$H]-adenosine. After vesicle isolation (see figures 12.1 and 12.5), [$^3$H]-ATP is the major component in both gradient fractions $VP_1$ and $VP_2$ before and after tissue stimulation. Relative contributions of [$^3$H]-labelled ADP, AMP, IMP, adenine, adenosine, inosine and hypoxanthine remain small (see table 12.2) (Zimmermann, 1978). These experiments can be regarded as indirect evidence for nucleotide release from the cholinergic electromotor nerve terminal.

Simultaneous release of ACh and ATP from stimulated synaptosomes isolated from the Torpedo electric organ has recently been demonstrated directly (Morel and Meunier, 1981). In this study synaptosomes were suspended in a solution containing (ATP-sensitive) luciferin-luciferase enzyme preparation. Using this method, released ATP can be monitored immediately as a light flash in a chemo-lumimeter. ATP release could be evoked either by $K^+$ depolrization or by application of the venom of the annelid *Glycera convoluta*. ATP release exhibited similar kinetics to ACh. The molar ratio of ACh/ATP was 45 after KCl depolriza-tion and 10 after venom action. The reason for this difference is not known but it is noteworthy that the molar ratio after venom application is in the same range as the molar ratio of ACh/ATP in isolated synaptic vesicles (table 12.1).

## FUNCTION OF ECTONUCLEOTIDASES

If both vesicular core components, ACh and ATP, would be released on axon depolarization one would expect that cholinergic nerve endings possess mechan-isms for rapid degradation, terminal re-uptake, resynthesis and vesicular refilling of adenine nucleotides as they do for ACh.

Our experiments further show that a suspension of sealed synaptosomes rapidly degrades external ATP to ADP, AMP and the final product adenosine (figure 12.6). If [$^3$H]-ATP is added at a concentration of 0.25 nmol ml$^{-1}$ to a synaptosome suspension corresponding to 20–40 $\mu$g of protein (containing about 1 nmol of endogenous ATP) already at sampling point 0 min more than 40 per

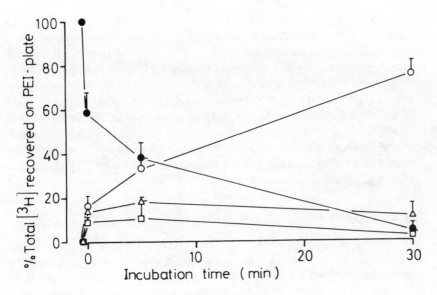

Figure 12.6 Activity of ectonucleotidases in a suspension of intact synaptosomes. After incubation of synaptosomes at room temperature with [³H]-ATP for 0, 15 and 30 min synaptosomes were sedimented at 44°C. The supernatant was analysed for [³H]-labelled products (ATP, ADP, AMP, IMP, cyclic AMP, adenosine, adenine, hypoxanthine and inosine) using two-dimensional thin layer chromatography on PEI cellulose plates. Besides a small contribution of inosine (8 per cent) after 30 min only significant contributions of the substances given in the graph were found. ●, ATP, ○, adenosine; △, ADP; □, AMP.

cent of the external ATP is found to be degraded. After 30 min at room temperature only 5 per cent of the extracellular radiolabel is left in the form of ATP. The major metabolite is adenosine. Only after 30 min could a significant amount of labelled inosine be detected. If synaptosomes are separated from the incubation medium by centrifugation they can be shown to have incorporated part of the radioactivity derived from external [³H]-ATP. Chromatographic analysis reveals the same purine pattern as after immediate application of [³H]-adenosine (see figure 12.4). On the basis of these results one would predict that ATP which appears in the interstitial fluid after release from nerve endings will be degraded extracellularly by nerve-terminal ectonucleotidases before reuptake in the form of adenosine. 5'-Nucleotidase activity was shown to reside at the outer surface of the nerve terminal membranes of electric tissue (Dowdall, 1978).

It is likely that ectonucleotidases for degradation of ATP to adenosine occur at the surface of a variety of cell types. Guinea-pig neocortical tissue degrades added ATP or AMP to adenosine (Pull and McIlwain, 1977). Pig aortic endothelial and smooth muscle cells in culture rapidly catabolize exogenous ATP, ADP or AMP.

Negative reports on release of ATP from cholinergic nerve terminals have to be discussed in this context. Due to the presence of ectonucleotidases sampling methods need to be immediate if native ATP is to be recovered in the perfusion or superfusion fluid. In contrast to Morel and Meunier (1981), when using electric organ synaptosomes incubated in suspension followed by subsequent centrifugation and pelleting of particles, Michaelson (1978) could not detect release of ATP. Similarly in the experiments of Kato *et al.*, (1974) at the perfused superior cervical ganglion of the cat, ATP released from nerve terminals would have needed to diffuse through the extracellular space and possibly pass capillary walls before collection. On this passage (which could not be mimicked by control perfusion of the ganglion with the nucleotide) released ATP would have become hydrolyzed.

## THE ADENOSINE CYCLE AT THE CHOLINERGIC SYNAPSE

Figure 12.7 presents a model for recycling of ACh and ATP at the electromotor cholinergic nerve terminal. It does contain some speculative features but these gain support from the evidence mentioned above. The choline cycle ensures the reformation of nerve terminal ACh after release whereby the extracellular hydrolysis products may be salvaged. Acetate diffuses back into the nerve terminal and can directly be reused for synthesis of acetyl-CoA (in contrast to brain tissue where

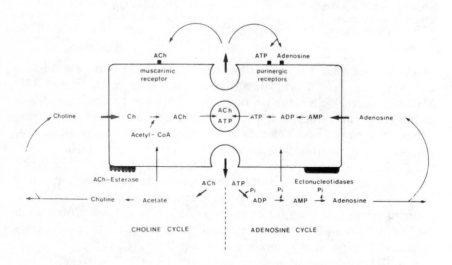

Figure 12.7  Model for recycling of acetylcholine and adenine nucleotides at the cholinergic electromotor nerve terminal. ACh and ATP are co-released on depolarisation of the axon terminal. Acetycholinesterase and ectonucleotidases ensure extracellular hydrolysis with choline and acetate and adenosine and phosphate as final products. Re-uptake into the nerve terminal of both choline and adenosine is by high affinity uptake mechanisms. Both ACh and ATP or adenosine may act on presynaptic receptors. In either case binding to the receptor results in depression of transmitter release. For further explanation, see text.

only pyruvate may serve as immediate precursor of the acetate moiety of ACh). Choline may be taken up into the nerve terminal by an active uptake system of high affinity ($K_m$ = 1 $\mu$m).

Similarly, the adenosine cycle ensures the reformation of nerve terminal ATP after release by salvage of extracellular hydrolysis product. ATP is completely hydrolysed by ectonucleotidases to adenosine which in turn may be taken up into the nerve terminal via n uptake system of high affinity ($K_m$ = 2 $\mu$M). It is likely to become phosphorylated to form AMP immediately on passage through the plasma membrane. The process of recycling of phosphate released from ATP has not yet been investigated. The nerve terminal possesses anabolic pathways to form ATP by way of AMP and ADP.

The mechanism of presynaptic release of ATP has not yet been explored to the same extent as that of ACh. As the plasma membrane is impermeable to ATP, special mechanisms have to ensure passage of ATP to the outside of the cell. The concomitant loss of ACh and ATP from synaptic vesicles on stimulation and the extracellular appearance of the two components (at least in certain experimental conditions) in the vesicular molar ratio would support the notion of co-exocytosis of both substances. On the other hand, ATP can be released from cells where it is not likely to be stored in vesicular form, for example, from isolated heart cells in response to hypoxia (Forrester and Williams, 1977). Furthermore, experiments with curarized preparations of Torpedo electric tissue suggest that the postsynaptic electroplaque cells also release ATP on activation and that this release exceeds the presynaptic contribution (Israël and Meunier, 1978). This suggests that mechanisms other than exocytosis can maintain cellular release of ATP. Regarding the scheme provided (figure 12.7) this also would imply that ATP released from the postsynaptic cell (not shown) can enter the presynaptic nucleoside cycle. Possibly the electroplaque cell also salvages nucleotides from extracellular (including presynaptic) sources.

## IS ATP A CO-TRANSMITTER?

There is now ample evidence that nerve activity is accompanied by release of purines. This includes peripheral tissues like adipose tissue, kidney, heart, vas deferens, stomach or taenia coli and also the central nervous system (see Fredholm and Hedquist, 1980). Purine release obviously is not restricted to cholinergic systems (see Burnstock, this volume). Furthermore, it is not always clear whether ATP or adenosine is the purine compound initially released and whether a pre- or postsynaptic contribution is dominating.

### The peripheral cholinergic neurone

Among cholinergic systems to date only for electric organs vesicular storage of ATP has been demonstrated. It remains to be established whether cholinergic vesicles from mammalian motor nerve terminals or sympathetic or parasympathetic neurones and also brain contain ATP.

The evidence collected at the cholinergic electromotor nerve terminal suggests that all the presynaptic criteria for transmitter function have been fulfilled for ATP. Sites of storage and enzymic mechanisms for synthesis and degradation have been identified and the substances may be collected in the extracellular medium on stimulation. On the other hand, no significant effect of either ATP or adenosine has so far been described at the cholinergic effector cell. However, ATP and/or adenosine have a pharmacological effect on cholinergic transmission: they inhibit transmitter release (for example, neuromuscular junction, Sawynok and Jahmadas, 1976; Torpedo electric organ, Israël and Meunier, 1978). The same result has been obtained for adrenergic systems where adenosine in addition may also have a postsynaptic effect (see Fredholm and Hedquist, 1980).

The effects of ATP and adenosine are antagonised by theophylline. Therefore, the presynaptic cholinergic element is likely to carry purinergic receptors (figure 12.7). These receptors could be activated by purines released from the nerve terminal resulting in autoinhibition and/or purines released from the postsynaptic effector cell resulting in retrograde inhibition. An inhibitory effect on its own release by way of presynaptic receptors has also been described for ACh (figure 12.7) (for example, guinea-pig myenteric plexus, Kilbinger and Wessler, 1980; Torpedo electric organ, Kloog *et al.*, 1980).

As it does not act trans-synaptically, it may be concluded that at least for the peripheral cholinergic motor synapse ATP (although it is coreleased with ACh) functions as a neuromodulator rather than a neurotransmitter. ACh may comprise both functions: transmission of the signal and modulation of its own release.

A possible role for vesicular ATP in the storage of ACh or in the process of vesicular exo- and endocytosis should not be excluded.

## Relation to the central nervous system

In the central nervous system adenosine has a number of significant effects: it depresses synaptic mechanisms as revealed by electrophysiological studies and it also enhances formation of cyclic AMP presumably by way of specific receptors (see Fredholm and Hedquist, 1980). Both high-affinity binding of [$^3$H]-adenosine to synaptosomal membranes from mammalian cortex ($K_m$ = 0.5–1.3 $\mu$M, Newman *et al.*, 1981) and high affinity uptake into brain synaptosomes ($K_m$ = 1 $\mu$M, Bender *et al.*, 1981; $K_m$ = 21 $\mu$M, Barberis *et al.*, 1981) have recently been described. It could be shown by the direct luciferase method that ATP is released from mammalian cerebral cortex synaptosomes following depolarization (White *et al.*, 1980; Potter and White, 1980). However, ATP release does not follow the same pharmacological properties as the neurotransmitter ACh ($Ca^{2+}$ dependence, sensitivity to botulinum toxin). Since brain synaptosomes present a mixture of transmitter types it cannot be established whether release of ATP was associated with any of the classical transmitters. ATP release may also be derived from possible brain endogeneous purinergic neurones (for discussion, see Burnstock, 1975; see also Burnstock, chapter 6). Furthermore, the contribution of contaminating glial particles is difficult to exclude. Using superfused pellets of hypothalamic synaptosomes with delayed purine analysis, Fredholm and Vernet (1979) have recovered mainly adenosine, inosine and hypoxanthine rather than nucleotides after membrane depolarisation.

To date, ATP has only been identified in storage vesicles of cholinergic and adrenergic peripheral neurones. It remains to be established whether there are transmitter-specific or rather general mechanisms of purine nucleotide or nucleoside function.

Finally, adenine nucleotides and adenosine can all act as vasodilators. ATP appears to be most potent (Wolfe and Berne, 1956). It is likely that nucleotide release on neuronal activity can result in an increase in blood supply in peripheral tissue and also in the brain, where blood flow is mainly controlled by functional activity of neurons (see Ingvar, 1976).

# REFERENCES

Barberis, C., Minn, A. and Gayet, J. (1981). Adenosine transport into guinea-pig synaptosomes. *J. Neurochem.*, **36**, 347-54

Bender, A. S., Wu, P. H. and Phillis, J. W. (1981). The rapid uptake and release of [3]H-adenosine by rat cerebral cortical slices. *J. Neurochem.*, **36**, 651-60

Burnstock, G. (1975). Purinergic transmission. In *Handbook of Psychopharmacology*, **5**, (ed. Iversen, L. L., Iversen, S. D. and Snyder, S. H.), Plenum Press, New York, pp. 131-94

Dowdall, M. J. (1978). Adenine nucleotides in cholinergic transmission: presynaptic aspects. *J. Physiol. Paris*, **74**, 497-501

Dowdall, M. J., Boyne, A. F. and Whittaker, V. P. (1974). Adenosine triphospahte, a constituent of cholinergic synaptic vesicles. *Biochem. J.*, **140**, 1-12

Forrester, T. and Williams, C. A. (1977). Release of adenosine triphosphate from adult heart cells in response to hypoxia. *J. Physiol. Lond.*, **268**, 371-90

Fredholm, B. B. and Vernet, L. (1979). Release of [3]H-nucleosides from [3]H-labelled hypothalamic synaptosomes. *Acta Physiol. Scand.* **106**, 97-107

Fredholm, B. B. and Hedquist, P. (1980). Modulation of neurotransmission by purine nucleotides and nucleosides. *Biochem. Pharmac.*, **29**, 1635-43

Giompres, P. E., Zimmermann, H. and Whittaker, V. P. (1981a) Purification of small dense vesicles from stimulated Torpedo electric tissue by glass bead column chromatography. *Neuroscience*, **6**, 765-74

Giompres, P. E., Zimmermann, H. and Whittaker, V. P. (1981b). Changes in the biochemical and biophysical parameters of cholinergic synaptic vesicles on transmitter release and during a subsequent period of rest. *Neuroscience*, **6**, 775-85

Ingvar, D. H. (1976). Functional landscapes of the dominant hemisphere. *Brain Res.*, **107**, 181-97

Israël, M. and Neunier, F. M. (1978). The release of ATP triggered by transmitter action and its possible physiological significance: retrograde transmission. *J. Physiol. Paris*, **74**, 485-490

Kato, A. C. Katz, H. S. and Collier, B. (1974). Absence of adenine nucleotide release from autonomic ganglion. *Nature, London*, **249**, 576-77

Kilbinger, H. and Wessler, I. (1980). Inhibition by acetylcholine of the stimulation-evoked release of [3]H-acetylcholine from the guinea-pig myenteric plexus. *Neuroscience*, **5**, 1331-40

Kloog, Y., Michaelson, D. M. and Sokolovsky, M. (1980). Characterization of the presynaptic muscarinic receptor in synaptosomes of Torpedo electric organ by means of equilibrium binding studies. *Brain Res.* **194**, 97-115

Lugmani, Y. A. (1981). Nucleotide uptake by isolated cholinergic synaptic vesicles: evidence for a carrier of adenosine 5'-triphosphate. *Neuroscience*, 6, 1011–22

Meunier, F. M. and Morel, N. (1978). Adenosine uptake by cholinergic synaptosomes from *Torpedo* electric organ. *J. Neurochem.*, 31, 845–851

Michaelson, D. M. (1978). Is presynaptic acetylcholine release accompanied by secretion of the synaptic vesicles contents? *FEBS Lett*. 89, 51–53

Morel, N. and Meunier, F. M. (1981). Simultaneous release of acetylcholine and ATP from stimulated cholinergic synaptosomes. *J. Neurochem.* 36, 1766–73

Murray, A. W. (1971). The biological significance of purine salvage. *A. Rev. Biochem.* 40, 811–26

Nagy, A., Baker, R. R., Morris, S. J. and Whittaker, V. P. (1976). The preparation and characterization of synaptic vesicles of high purity. *Brain Res.*, 109, 285–309

Nagy, A., Várady, G., Joó, F., Rakonczay, Z. and Pill, A. (1977). Separation of acetylcholine and catecholamine containing synaptic vesicles from brain cortex. *J. Neurochem.*, 29, 449–59

Newman, M. E., Patel, J. and McIlwain, H. (1981). The binding of $^3$H-adenosine to synaptosomal and other preparations from mammalian brain. *Biochem. J.*, 194, 611–20

Ohsawa, K., Dowe, G. H. C., Morris, S. J. and Whittaker, V. P. (1979). The lipid and protein content of cholinergic synaptic vesicles from the electric organ of Torpedo marmorata purified to constant composition: implications for vesicle structure. *Brain Res.*, 161, 447–57

Potter, P. and White, T. D. (1980). Release of adenosine 5'-triphosphate from synaptosomes from different regions of rat brain. *Neuroscience*, 5, 1331–56

Pull, I. and McIlwain, H. (1977). Adenine nucleotides and their metabolites liberated from and applied to isolated tissues of the mammalian brain. *Neurochem. Res.*, 2, 203–16

Richardson, P. J. and Whittaker, V. P. (1981). The Na$^+$ and K$^+$ content of isolated Torpedo synaptosomes and its effect on choline uptake. *J. Neurochem.* 36, 1536–42

Sawynok, J. and Jahmadas, K. H. (1976). Inhibition of acetylcholine release from cholinergic nerves by adenosine, adenine nucleotides and morphine: antagonism by theophylline. *J. Pharmac. exp. Therap.*, 197, 379–90

Sheridan, M. N., Whittaker, V. P. and Israël, M. (1966). The subcellular fractionation of the electric organ of Torpedo. *Z. Zellforsch*. 74, 291–307

Tashiro, T. and Stadler, H. (1978). Chemical compositions of cholinergic synaptic vesicles from *Torpedo marmonata* based on improved purification. *Eur. J. Biochem.*, 90, 479–487

Wagner, J. A., Carlson, S. S. and Kelly, R. B. (1978). Chemical and physical characterization of cholinergic synaptic vesicles. *Biochemistry*, 17, 1199–1206

White, T., Potter, P. and Wonnacot, S. (1980). Depolarization induced release of ATP from cortical synaptosomes is not associated with acetylcholine release. *J. Neurochem.*, 34, 1109–12

Wolfe, M. M. and Berne, R. M. (1956). Coronary vasodilator properties of purine and pyrimidine derivatives. *Circulat. Res.*, 4, 343–48

Zimmermann, H. (1978). Turnover of adenine nucleotides in cholinergic synaptic vesicles of the Torpedo electric organ. *Neuroscience*, 3., 827–36

Zimmermann, H. (1979a). Vesicle recycling and transmitter release. *Neuroscience*, 4, 1773–804

Zimmermann, H. (1979b). Vesicular heterogeneity and turnover of acetylcholine and ATP in cholinergic synaptic vesicles. *Progr. Brain Res.*, 49, 141–51

Zimmermann, H. (1982). Isolation of cholinergic nerve vesicles. In *Neurotransmitter vesicles*, (ed. R. Klein, H. Lagercrantz and H. Zimmermann)., Academic Press, London, pp. 241–269

Zimmermann, H. and Whittaker, V. P. (1974). Effect of electrical stimulation on the yield and composition of synaptic vesicles from the cholinergic synapses of the electric organ of Torpedo: a combined biochemical, electrophysiological and morphological study. *J. Neurochem.*, 22, 435–50

Zimmermann, H. and Denston, C. R. (1976). Adenosine triphosphate in cholinergic vesicles isolated from the electric organ of electrophorus electricus. *Brain Res.*, 111, 365–76

Zimmermann, H. and Denston, C. R. (1977a). Recycling of synaptic vesicles in the cholinergic synapses of the Torpedo electric organ during induced transmitter release. *Neuroscience*, 2, 695–714

Zimmermann, H. and Denston, C. R. (1977*b*). Separation of synaptic vesicles of different functional states from the cholinergic synapses of the Torpedo electric organ. *Neuroscience*, **2**, 715–30

Zimmermann, H. and Bokor, J. T. (1979). ATP recycles independently of ACh in cholinergic synaptic vesicles. *Neurosci. Lett.*, **13**, 319–24

Zimmermann, H., Dowdall, M. J. and Lane, D. A. (1979). Purine salvage at the cholinergic nerve endings of the Torpedo electric organ: the central role of adenosine. *Neuroscience*, **4**, 979–993

Zimmermann, H., Stadler, H. and Whittaker, V. P. (1981). Structure and function of cholinergic synaptic vesicles. In *Chemical Neurotransmission: 75 Years* (ed. L. Stjärne, P. Hedquist, H. Lagercrantz and Å. Wennmalm), Academic Press, London, pp. 91–104

# Index

*Index*

## DATE DUE

| | |
|---|---|
| | |
| | |
| | |
| | |
| | |
| | |
| | |
| | |
| | |
| | |
| | |
| | |
| | |

DEMCO, INC. 38-2971